# MAKE ROOM FOR BABY

# Also Available

*Psychotherapy with Infants and Young Children:*
*Repairing the Effects of Stress and Trauma on Early Attachment*
Alicia F. Lieberman and Patricia Van Horn

# Make Room for Baby

## Perinatal Child–Parent Psychotherapy to Repair Trauma and Promote Attachment

**Alicia F. Lieberman, Manuela A. Diaz, Gloria Castro,** and **Griselda Oliver Bucio**

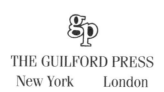

THE GUILFORD PRESS
New York     London

**Library of Congress Cataloging-in-Publication Data**

Names: Lieberman, Alicia F., author. | Diaz, Manuela A., author. |
     Castro, Gloria (Clinical psychologist), author. | Oliver Bucio,
     Griselda, author.
Title: Make room for baby : perinatal child–parent psychotherapy to
     repair trauma and promote attachment / Alicia F. Lieberman,
     Manuela A. Diaz, Gloria Castro, Griselda Oliver Bucio.
Description: New York : The Guilford Press, [2020] | Includes
     bibliographical references and index.
Identifiers: LCCN 2020019603 | ISBN 9781462543472 (hardcover)
Subjects: LCSH: Parent-child interaction therapy. | Parent-infant
     psychotherapy. | Perinatology—Psychological aspects. | Psychic
     trauma—Treatment.
Classification: LCC RJ505.P37 L538 2020 | DDC 618.92/8914—dc23
LC record available at *https://lccn.loc.gov/2020019603*

*To Patricia Van Horn,*
*whose gifts of wisdom and care continue*
*to enrich everything we do—her memory is an*
*inspiration and a blessing*

# About the Authors

**Alicia F. Lieberman, PhD,** is Irving B. Harris Endowed Chair in Infant Mental Health and Professor and Vice Chair for Faculty Development in the Department of Psychiatry at the University of California, San Francisco (UCSF). She is Director of the UCSF Child Trauma Research Program at Zuckerberg San Francisco General Hospital (ZSFGH) and Director of the Early Trauma Treatment Network. Dr. Lieberman is the senior developer of Child–Parent Psychotherapy (CPP). She is the author of *The Emotional Life of the Toddler,* for general readers, as well as professional books, articles, and chapters on childhood exposure to violence, mental health in infancy and early childhood, child–parent attachment, and cultural competence in intervention. Her cross-cultural background as a Jewish Latina informs her work with diverse children and families. Dr. Lieberman has received numerous awards, including, most recently, the René Spitz Award from the World Association for Infant Mental Health, the Hero Award from the San Francisco Department of Public Health, the Whole Child Award from the Simms/Mann Institute, the Blanche Ittleson Award from the Global Alliance for Behavioral Health and Social Justice, and the Paulina Kernberg Award from Weill Cornell Medicine.

**Manuela A. Diaz, PhD,** is a clinical psychologist in private practice in Berkeley, California, where she specializes in maternal and infant mental health and the application of mindfulness and neuroscience to the treatment of mood disorders and trauma. Dr. Diaz is an affiliated clinician at the UCSF Child Trauma Research Program at ZSFGH. Since the early 2000s, she has conducted clinical work and research in the area of perinatal mental health. She is a coauthor of the Mothers and Babies course, a maternal depression prevention program developed at UCSF, and a codeveloper of Perinatal Child–Parent Psychotherapy (P-CPP). Dr. Diaz has served as a trainer both nationally and internationally, in English and Spanish, and has published on reducing mental health disparities for racial and ethnic minority groups.

**Gloria Castro, PsyD,** a clinical psychologist and Certified Sexual Assault Counselor, is a bilingual psychotherapist at the UCSF Child Trauma Research Program at ZSFGH. In this role, she implements P-CPP throughout pregnancy, labor, delivery, and postpartum with women with histories of traumatic experiences. She also provides infant mental health services in the neonatal intensive care unit and the high-risk pediatric Kempe Clinic. Dr. Castro's interests include the impact of immigration on family systems, the intergenerational transmission of trauma, and the impact of trauma on children's development. She has consulted for, supervised, and trained mental health providers who work with immigrant families and their children, and has presented her work nationally and internationally.

**Griselda Oliver Bucio, LMFT,** is a psychotherapist in private practice in Walnut Creek, California. For over 14 years, she was a staff clinician and clinical supervisor at the UCSF Child Trauma Research Program at ZSFGH, where she also participated in clinical research. Ms. Oliver Bucio specializes in the treatment of young children exposed to trauma and of pregnant women exposed to domestic violence and other traumatic events. She has served as a CPP trainer and consultant since 2010, leading trainings and presentations nationally and internationally in both English and Spanish. Her major interests include infant mental health, the impact of early trauma within the dyadic relationship and pregnancy, disorders of attachment, the effects of paternal absence, the process of immigration in Latino families, and the dissemination of CPP and P-CPP.

# Acknowledgments

Pregnancy and the perinatal period evoke profound emotions, both as lived experiences in the moment and as remembered many years later. All four authors of this book are mothers whose children range in age from early childhood to midadulthood. Two of us (A. F. L. and G. C.) are also grandmothers. Each of us is profoundly grateful for this gift. Coming together as writers enabled us to give concrete expression to many years of personal reflection and clinical practice as Perinatal Child–Parent Psychotherapy (P-CPP) evolved, accruing new elements while retaining its primary goal of simultaneously healing the wounds of the past and preventing the repetition of those wounds with the future generation.

The cradle of P-CPP is the University of California at San Francisco's Child Trauma Research Program, which is now over 25 years old. Many cherished colleagues, supporters, and institutions make it possible for the program to continue to grow and thrive, generously giving us the resources to engage in this work. The Hebrew blessing "Shehecheyanu" gives specific cultural expression to the gratitude humans universally feel when pausing to acknowledge a moment of blessing in their lives. The publication of this new manual represents such a moment. The four authors are all immigrants to the United States, who grew up in different traditions in Paraguay, Peru, and Mexico while sharing cultural roots and most particularly Spanish as our beloved common language. We are united in saying "muchas gracias" to all those people—named or unnamed—who enabled us to arrive at this day.

The seeds of P-CPP go back to the 1970s, when Alicia Lieberman was supervised by Selma Fraiberg in the treatment of expectant parents whose joyful anticipation of their baby's birth was marred by the emotional weight of difficult childhood memories. Selma's mentoring had a transformational impact on a then young and inexperienced clinician and remains a source of deep gratitude and inspiration. Those early clinical experiences reemerged in 2004 in the aftermath of our randomized study of Child–Parent Psychotherapy (CPP) with preschoolers exposed to domestic violence. In leisurely conversations in the quiet of the office at the end of the day, Patricia Van Horn and Alicia Lieberman often talked about how much suffering might have been avoided if the parents of the traumatized young children in our study had been reached before or during their pregnancy. We soon translated wistfulness into proactive repair, crafting the application of CPP to pregnancy and offering treatment to women receiving prenatal care at the San Francisco General Hospital, where our program is located. In 2005 we established the *CTRP Pregnancy Project: Healthy Relationships, Healthy Motherhood* with the research and clinical support of Manuela A. Diaz and the clinical assistance of Maria Augusta Torres, both highly trained in implementing CPP with fidelity to ethnically and culturally diverse, high-risk populations.

A small team of outstanding caring clinicians were our partners in this effort. Manuela was the liaison between our program and the prenatal care clinic. She worked in close collaboration with Tahnee Gantt, who as the social worker in this clinic was invaluable in creating and maintaining a feedback loop of referral and primary care–mental health collaboration to maximize healthy outcomes for pregnant women and their babies. As P-CPP developed, Manuela added pregnancy-focused mindfulness- and body-based exercises, and Maria contributed infant massage to the menu of CPP intervention modalities. Griselda Oliver Bucio joined our team as a clinician skilled in understanding the symbolic meaning of pregnancy and the unborn infant for the mother and became an enthusiastic collaborator during the extended evolution of the treatment. Manuela, with Patricia's mentorship, documented this work in an early version of what would become the present treatment manual, with the valued research assistance of Mariana Cavallin.

When Gloria Castro joined our program in 2016, she brought the priceless contribution of many years of clinical service, of mental health consultation with primary care providers, and of teaching of residents in prenatal care, labor, delivery, and the NICU at our hospital. Her expertise rounded out and consolidated a versatile, but focused, intervention model that promotes multidisciplinary collaborations linking physicians, social workers, and mental health clinicians with the goal of providing outstanding care to each individual pregnant woman and her baby. We are particularly grateful to the medical providers who played a key role in giving us access and promoting integrated care—Anna Spielvogel at the high-risk OB/GYN clinic; Hayes Bakken and

Raul Gutierrez, pediatricians at the Children's Health Center; Gillian Otway, director of the Birth Center; and Shilu Ramchand, Nurse Manager at the NICU and Pediatrics—all of whom believed that the implementation of P-CPP would benefit hospital staff as well as the babies and the families they served.

From the beginning, we sought empirical confirmation that we were on the right track. Our early positive clinical results led us in 2005 to approach the Hedge Funds Care (HFC) Foundation for support in conducting a systematic evaluation of treatment outcomes. We are grateful to Bart Grossman in his role as HFC advisor for his advocacy and belief in the work. Subsequent funding from the Nathan Cummings Foundation expanded the HFC support, and we thank Adam Cummings for introducing us to the masterful body-based psychotherapist Al Pesso and for joining us in a weekend retreat with Al that enlarged our understanding of how the body speaks and how to promote healing after painful breaches of trust.

Systematic treatment outcome evaluation led in turn to several publications. We thank Arianna Gard, Melissa Hagan, and Iris Lavi for their research contributions showing the effectiveness of treatment to date.

Our work with pregnant women received new impetus in 2014, when our friend and partner William (Bill) Harris contributed his powerful intellect and commitment to young children and their families to the expansion and deepening of our approach. Bill had coined the term *angels in the nursery* back in 2004. This concept helped us realize that the exploration during therapy of benevolent memories of love and protection can be as transformational in the chiaroscuro of internal and external realities as grappling with the ghostlike reverberations in the present of early pain, conflict, and fear. He was a leading collaborator in a new study, BE SAFE, spearheaded with verve and vision by Angela Narayan with the inspired collaboration of Luisa Rivera and Rosemary Bernstein.

The BE SAFE study helped us understand how self-affirming and self-shattering experiences reemerge during pregnancy and the perinatal period and influence the formation of a new identity as a parent in a population of low-income, ethnically diverse pregnant women. We posted flyers inviting pregnant women receiving routine prenatal care at San Francisco General Hospital to tell us about their childhood, their present life, the circumstances of their pregnancy, and their hopes and fears for themselves and their baby. The participants answered our questions with raw honesty, thanks to the trust-promoting welcome of Tahnee Gantt and Esther Rodas at the prenatal clinics and the care and skill of the interviewers, including Ruby Jimenez, Kate Mallula, and Monica Rodriguez. Angela moved from her postdoctoral fellowship in our program to a faculty position at the University of Denver, where she is replicating and expanding this study with the participation of fathers as well as mothers—a much-needed contribution that includes the voices of expectant and new fathers in the dialogue. The data analysis is ongoing and continues to yield illuminating findings and numerous publications, with the much-valued participation of Ann Chu, Alagia Cirolia, Melissa Nau, Belen Rogowski, and Melanie Thomas at UCSF and Vicky Atzl, Jill Merrick, Laura River, Luisa River, and Madison Schmidt in Denver. We look forward to our continued productive collaboration.

The findings of the BE SAFE study called our attention to the high prevalence of conflictual, short-term intimate relationships resulting in unwanted pregnancies and absent fathers among a volunteer population of pregnant women who were not seeking mental health services. Women's candid responses during these interviews led us to expand the scope of the CPP motto "speaking the unspeakable." Their descriptions of their unborn babies' fathers taught us that the woman's attitudes toward her sexual partner have a profound influence on the mother–infant relationship and on who the baby will become. As a result, P-CPP incorporated the inclusion of fathers, whether as physical participants in treatment or as central emotional figures in the real and imagined family constellation. Women's descriptions of their reproductive health practices and whether the pregnancy was planned and wanted also emerged from the interviews as fundamental to understanding their decision making and future orientation. The treatment now includes nondirective reflection about family planning values and behavior as integral ingredients in promoting parental physical and mental health and preparing a safe space for the baby.

This manual benefited from the wisdom of cherished colleagues. Arietta Slade was both generous and generative in her substantive feedback and elegant editing suggestions. The National Child Traumatic Stress Network (NCTSN) of the Substance Abuse and Mental Health Services Administration has been our professional community since 2001, and we are immeasurably enriched by this collaboration. Our partners in the NCTSN Early Trauma Treatment Network—Julie Larrieu, Joy Osofsky, Carmen Norona, Paula Zeanah, and Charley Zeanah—help us expand the scope of our engagement with the systems of care serving traumatized young children and their families; Sheree Toth, Jody Manly, and Dante Cicchetti contribute to our knowledge with their groundbreaking research and innovative approaches to implementing CPP; Judy Cohen helped us clarify our conceptual frame and use behavior as one of the ports of entry into psychological growth; Lisa Amaya-Jackson brings her expertise in reconciling the often competing demands of evidence-based treatment with responsiveness to the clinical moment; Robert Pynoos has continually added to our understanding of trauma with his encyclopedic knowledge; and Bessel van der Kolk taught us the specifics of how the body keeps the score, an essential insight for understanding emotional experiences during pregnancy, the perinatal period, and the first years of life. In our own program, the fidelity measures spearheaded by Chandra Ghosh Ippen and the assessment protocols that Ann Chu helped create allow us to integrate clinical depth and operational clarity.

We are grateful for the long-standing support of foundations that are models of engaged philanthropy in supporting social justice. The Irving B. Harris Foundation continues the vision of its extraordinary founder in providing long-term support for innovation in infant mental health. Lisa Stone Pritzker and the LSP Family Fund enable us to maintain one of the defining missions we set for ourselves: training the next generation of clinicians committed to serving low-income and disenfranchised children and families. Ingrid Tauber and the Laszlo N. Tauber Family Foundation make it possible for us to pursue another defining mission of providing community-based services for hard-to-reach children and families in need. Daniel Lurie and the Tipping Point Community support our community mental health framework as they strive to create the conditions and offer the resources to make poverty preventable. The commitment to the shared goals of these supporters gives us roots that allow us to reach always higher.

We are grateful for our home team at the Child Trauma Research Program. To paraphrase the much-quoted African proverb, it takes a village to engage with trauma. We thank Laura Castro, Ann Chu, Nancy Compton, Chandra Ghosh Ippen, Miriam Hernandez Dimmler, Markita Mays, Vilma Reyes, and Barclay Stone for many years of loyal togetherness through the joys and tribulations of the work. We are appreciative of Tuesday Ray for upholding the day-to-day workings of the program and of Alagia Cirolia and Belen Rogowski for their energetic creativity in shepherding the many facets of our clinical training and research. Emily Cohodes, Aru Gonzalez, Laura Gildengorin, Maya Guendelman, Dione Johnson, and Leah Sodowick were their predecessors, and we continue to remember their outstanding contributions while they were with us. Over the years we have learned much from our students, and we thank them for their fresh thinking, incisive questions, and the vitality they infuse into our own work.

Each of the authors wants to give special thanks to our loved ones in our own words:

Alicia writes, "Michael and Lana, thank you for giving me the joy and wonder of becoming a grandmother. David, thank you for being with me in nurturing the next generations."

Manuela writes, "My deepest appreciation and gratitude go to *mi familia,* the rain in my forest."

Gloria writes, "Pablo and Andrea introduced me to the wonderful journey that is motherhood. *Amaya, mi nieta, tomémonos de la mano y caminemos juntas por la vida.*"

Griselda writes, "Brendan, Pablo, and Isabella Camille, thank you for your patience, trust, and for the gift of motherhood."

All of us are grateful to the mothers, fathers, and babies who entrust us with their most private feelings and teach us how to help.

Our final word of gratitude is always for Patricia. She nurtured the Child Trauma Research Program village for many years, and her legacy continues through our work. We dedicate this book to her as a token of how much she means to us.

# Contents

## Section II
# Perinatal Child–Parent Psychotherapy
### 45

## Section III
# Implementing P-CPP: Extended Clinical Cases
### 111

### Section IV

# Common Obstacles to Attuned Caregiving

*261*

## Section V
# Monitoring Fidelity:
# The "What" and "How" of P-CPP
### *319*

# Introduction

Perinatal Child–Parent Psychotherapy (P-CPP) is an application to pregnancy and the perinatal period of Child–Parent Psychotherapy (CPP), a relationship-based, trauma-informed treatment for children ages birth–5 years and their caregivers that has the goal of healing trauma and preventing the intergenerational transmission of psychopathology (Lieberman, Ghosh Ippen, & Van Horn, 2015; Lieberman & Van Horn, 2008). P-CPP starts during pregnancy, with the goal of guiding parents-to-be toward greater self-understanding and a more loving capacity to provide safe and nurturing care for their baby. Although pregnancy and the first months of the baby's life are normal developmental transitions, this time is also one of enormous physical and emotional vulnerability for parents and baby. P-CPP aims to provide mothers and fathers with the support they need when their adverse life circumstances and their emotional and interpersonal difficulties interfere with their ability to give their baby the love, care, and protection needed to promote healthy development. This P-CPP implementation manual addresses the unique challenges and opportunities of pregnancy and the perinatal period, which call for specialized clinical expertise and a specific training focus on the psychological, interpersonal, and concrete life issues that emerge during this extended adult developmental stage.

Even in optimal conditions, pregnancy and the postnatal period elicit a wide range of emotions as mothers and fathers encounter and prepare for the joys, challenges, and responsibilities of parenthood. Creating safe intimacy with a new baby calls for the parent to relive, consciously or unconsciously, what it was like to *be* a baby. For women, the bodily sensations of feeling the fetus growing in the womb and later holding, touching, smelling, listening to, and gazing at the newborn baby can evoke states of profound bliss that escape verbal articulation. For men, multilayered emotional processes unfold as they anticipate

*1*

becoming a father, while also relating to the changes in the intimate partner's body, moods, and behavior during pregnancy.

The earliest, preverbal experiences of helplessness and total dependence on others may re-emerge for expectant parents in unrecognizable forms. Pride in becoming pregnant, feelings of completeness, longing for complete fusion with the baby, and anticipatory joy in meeting the baby may alternate with self-doubt, anxiety, fear of entrapment, and anger in response to the physical challenges of the perinatal period or when the fetus/baby does not conform to the parent's fantasies of an idealized, contented, and well-behaved infant. The body changes and emotional processes set in motion by the pregnancy also transform the romantic relationship between the partners, with far-reaching implications for each partner's perception of themselves and each other in the new interpersonal context of parenthood.

Like all developmental transitions, pregnancy and the perinatal period open up new possibilities for emotional growth that can foster the mental health of the parents-to-be as individuals, their self-confidence as parents, and their baby's healthy development. Also like other developmental transitions, this period presents a heightened risk of psychological disorganization. The risk of emotional disequilibrium increases exponentially when expectant parents grew up in conditions that exposed them to unmanageable fear and/or when they are facing adverse or traumatic present circumstances with limited adaptive coping skills. The profound affective impact of pregnancy often creates a readiness for introspection, momentum toward change, and desire for help that make many expectant parents more receptive to services such as psychoeducation and psychological treatment. The anticipation of nurturing a new life gives many parents the impetus to come to grips with their past and to acquire the internal resources to build safety in the present and prepare for a more rewarding future.

Psychotherapy during pregnancy has the overarching goal of psychological reorganization and a higher level of emotional integration, including consolidation of a new maternal and paternal identity. The relationship with the clinician can be reparative in nature, with the clinician offering a nurturing, holding space to contain anxiety, work through intrapsychic and interpersonal conflicts, and receive developmental guidance and emotional support while grappling with the internal and reality-based challenges presented by pregnancy and upcoming parenthood. In this therapeutic process, the expectant mother and father (individually and/or together depending on clinical considerations) can gain insight into their positive and negative attitudes and unconscious attributions to the baby, allowing them to experience the baby as a separate person rather than a transference object for unresolved psychological conflicts (Fraiberg, 1980; Lieberman, 1983; Lieberman & Blos, 1980; Slade & Sadler, 2019). While becoming more attuned with the unborn baby, parents-to-be may also be more likely to change maladaptive behaviors to protect their own and their baby's health—for example, by improving nutritional habits, exercising, and/or discontinuing the use of harmful substances.

When treatment continues after the baby's birth, it can offer the parents opportunities to process the pregnancy and childbirth and to reflect on their emerging experiences as parents of this particular baby. A versatile therapeutic process promotes emotional growth while also building caregiving competencies that can translate into personal self-efficacy. Perinatal clinicians provide psychoeducation about babies' needs, helping the parents hone their caregiving skills through hands-on, individually tailored developmental guidance both in the moment and anticipating future developmental stages. The clinician can also provide parents with a safe interpersonal space to reflect on their emotional reactions, explore how their childhood experiences affect their adjustment to parenthood and their feelings for the baby, pursue the integration of positive and negative feelings, and modulate ambivalence in ways that summon love for the baby as a protective shield against anger and hate. Babies' urgent needs—as manifested, for example, in inconsolable crying or expectable biological dysregulations such as sleep disruptions in the first months of life—may act as triggers for the parents' reexperience of unresolved early conflicts or traumatic experiences. In the course of the treatment, the parents make use of the safe therapeutic space to identify and reflect on their emotional responses to the baby's signals, which become a concrete port of entry to help them examine how their own unmet emotional needs may continue to engulf the baby in negative perceptions and attitudes that interfere with attuned caregiving. For all these reasons, effective therapeutic intervention during and after pregnancy may help prevent the intergenerational transmission of psychopathology from parent to child.

This book provides guidelines that enable clinicians to implement P-CPP with fidelity to the conceptual frame and to the therapeutic modalities and strategies of the model. The book comprises five sections. Section I provides an overview of the theoretical contributions, scientific findings, and existing clinical interventions that frame pregnancy and the perinatal period as an extended developmental phase characterized by concrete biological and psychological manifestations that are profoundly affected by environmental circumstances and cultural meanings. Section II describes the P-CPP phases of treatment and therapeutic strategies and provides clinical examples that illustrate their application. Section III features four full-length case examples that follow a family from the beginning to the end of treatment, with each case illustrating a specific set of adverse circumstances that endanger the parents' loving commitment to their baby. Section IV consists of brief clinical vignettes that highlight therapeutic approaches to some common clinical presentations. Section V provides fidelity items to help clinicians monitor the extent to which they are following P-CPP guidelines for treatment, including their affective responses to the family and possible countertransference reactions that may negatively affect treatment outcome by interfering with the therapeutic alliance or their effectiveness as clinicians. All the clinical illustrations and case presentations in this book have been substantially changed in ways that preserve the confidentiality of the families, including changes in the description of the parents and composite clinical examples.

Although this book is structured as a P-CPP implementation manual, we do not prescribe a standardized, step-by-step approach to treatment. Our core clinical values are rooted in a psychodynamic understanding of emotional processes and therapeutic effectiveness that prioritizes the clinician's responsiveness to the themes and emotional tone of the clinical moment. Like CPP, this extension to pregnancy and the perinatal period is informed by the conviction that transformational treatment is co-created by the clinician and the recipient(s) of treatment. Each parent and each baby present a broad range of psychological strengths and vulnerabilities that contribute in unique and unpredictable ways to the relationship between them. Clinicians need to rely on their clinical judgment and their level of comfort with a range of therapeutic strategies to appraise the domain of intervention that might be most promising for promoting positive change at any given moment. The intersubjective space that unfolds between the treatment participants and the clinician is the essential container for effective clinical interventions but cannot be dictated or predicted in advance. Although P-CPP places great value on a clear clinical formulation that informs the treatment plan, the salient clinical issue and the nature of the intersubjective space in the moment help the clinician choose which of the relevant clinical formulation themes to pursue. The same versatility applies to the choice of a specific therapeutic technique in the moment. These techniques may include, for example, concrete assistance, developmental guidance/psychoeducation, insight-oriented interpretation, cognitive-behavioral interventions, and mindfulness or body-based interventions, which are flexibly deployed depending on the clinician's appraisal of which approach to intervention holds the greatest mutative potential at any given moment.

Along with their freedom to use their clinical judgment in choosing when and how to intervene, P-CPP clinicians have the sometimes daunting responsibility of learning the different bodies of knowledge that comprise the fields of developmental psychopathology and psychotherapy. These areas of knowledge include, but are not limited to, the domains listed below:

- Expectable developmental processes through the lifespan, with a specific focus on pregnancy, labor and delivery, and parenting during the first year of life as transformational adult developmental stages.
- Normative developmental milestones and caregiving practices in infancy and early childhood.
- Infant/early childhood and adult psychopathology, with a specific focus on manifestations of psychopathology during pregnancy and the perinatal period.
- Impact of trauma on development and mental health, including the neurobiology of posttraumatic stress disorder (PTSD) and depression and the trauma triggers emerging during pregnancy and the perinatal period.
- Cultural diversity in childrearing practices and sensitivity to racial, ethnic, religious, gender, and sexual orientation diversity as they manifest during pregnancy and the perinatal period.
- The theory and practice of psychotherapy, with special attention to attachment and psychodynamic theories.
- The systems relevant to pregnancy and perinatal care, including primary care for parent and child, reproductive health, substance abuse and domestic violence resources, and the legal system when maltreatment may be involved.

Each one of these domains calls for commitment to ongoing learning. To paraphrase Freud, becoming a skilled clinician involves a "terminable and interminable" personal process as each of us encounters the infinite variability of human experience and endeavors to respond to suffering in humane and effective ways. We hope that this book will be a useful tool in meeting this goal.

# Section I

# Pregnancy and the Perinatal Period

*Hope and Vicissitudes*

This section provides a conceptual framework and literature review documenting the biological, psychological, and interpersonal processes involved in pregnancy and the perinatal period and the influence of parental environmental and cultural circumstances. It includes succinct comments making explicit connections between the research findings described and their clinical implications for the treatment and prevention of trauma. For the purposes of this manual, we define the perinatal period as encompassing the entire pregnancy, childbirth, the postpartum period, and the baby's first year of life. This section also presents brief descriptions of existing clinical interventions during the perinatal period, which provide a context for the extended description of Perinatal Child–Parent Psychotherapy (P-CPP) in the rest of the book.

# Normative Processes in Pregnancy and the Perinatal Period

Pregnancy and the perinatal period comprise an extended developmental stage both for women and for men as they prepare to enter a new phase of their lives, either as first-time mothers and fathers or as the parents of a child who will expand the family and become a new sibling to their older children. There is extensive literature attending to the transformational experiences of pregnant women. Although less extensively studied, men's experience of their partner's pregnancy and preparation for fatherhood is receiving increasing attention as having enormous personal and social importance. The anticipatory psychological processes initiated during pregnancy set the stage for the new opportunities and challenges of the first year of life, when the here-and-now present baby is an active partner with immediate demands that contrast with the earlier role of the fetus as the relatively quiescent recipient of the expectant parents' wishes and fears.

## The Woman's Experience: Becoming a Mother

Pregnancy affects the woman's body, sense of self, and social conditions in ways that have profound implications for all aspects of her life, including her survival, health, and well-being. The physiological changes involved in gestation affect mood, states of mind, and basic bodily processes like appetite, digestion, and sleeping. Pregnant women navigate changes at these multiple levels simultaneously, so that physiological, psychological, social, and cultural factors interact to shape her physical well-being, transform her self-concept, and redefine significant aspects of her relationships and social roles. Her new state can, in turn, alter her aspirations and future life prospects, depending on her economic, social, and cultural circumstances (Benedek, 1970; Bibring, 1959; Buckwalter, Buckwalter, Bluestein, & Stanczyk, 2001; Narayan, Ghosh Ippen, Harris, & Lieberman, 2017; Slade & Sadler, 2019).

Similar to the developmental stages of adolescence and menopause, pregnancy and the perinatal period bring about a period of emotional disequilibrium that when all goes well resolves into a redefined identity, as the person adapts to the new circumstances by reorganizing existing schemas of the self in relation to others. In pregnancy and the year following the baby's birth, this process is crucial for the emotional health of both the mother and the child.

Pregnant women often report feelings of increased vulnerability and fear of losing control over their lives, partly in response to their realistic anticipatory anxiety about the physical ordeal of childbirth and uncertainty about their own and their baby's survival, and partly in reaction to transitions in their sense of identity and social roles (Darvill, Skirton, & Farrand, 2010; Stern, 1995). Pregnancy also triggers the reemergence of deeply embedded psychological processes that were first established during infancy and childhood and are revisited in this new maturational stage through the ongoing interplay between real-life events (including adversity, trauma, and loss) and psychic and interpersonal processes (Bradley, 2000; Slade & Sadler, 2019). When this process promotes emotional growth, the psychological reorganization that results from the resolution of intrapsychic and interpersonal conflicts culminates in the "development and acceptance of a coherent sense of self as person and parent" (Valentine, 1982, p. 244) that enables the woman to fulfill her mothering role while grounded in a firm sense of individual identity.

Achieving coherence in the new identity as a parent calls for the negotiation of a series of psychological milestones that received extensive attention in classic and more recent psychoanalytic writings (Benedek, 1970; Bibring, 1959; Bibring, Dwyer, Huntington, & Valenstein, 1961; Kofman & Imber, 2005; Slade & Sadler, 2019; Tilden, 1980; Valentine, 1982). In their book *The Birth of a Mother,* Daniel Stern and Nadia Bruschweiler-Stern (1998) describe this new identity in terms of a "maternal mindset" that may not always have center stage in the woman's inner life but becomes an integral part of her lifelong sense of self.

The formation of a maternal identity begins during pregnancy with the reemergence and reworking of early emotional experiences and unresolved conflicts from earlier developmental phases. Expectant women experience a renewed preoccupation with their own mothers and a reactivation of old conflicts, particularly when the mother-to-be perceives her mother as distant, absent, depriving, rejecting, and/or hostile, punitive, and abusive during her childhood.

This theoretical viewpoint has empirical support from research findings showing that the pregnant woman's perception of the mothering she received influences her attitudes about her own child (Benoit, Parker, & Zeanah, 1997; Main, Kaplan, & Cassidy, 1985; Slade & Cohen, 1996). For some women, pregnancy revives predominantly negative representations of their mothers that color their sense of self and interfere with the development of a stable and fulfilling maternal identity and positive perceptions of the unborn baby. For these women, psychotherapy during pregnancy offers an opportunity for resolution that if successfully addressed can lead to a stable reorganization of their identity as mothers by the time the baby is born (Slade et al., 2019).

Developing an emotional bond with the unborn baby occurs hand in hand with the effort to resolve intrapsychic conflicts (Leifer, 1977). Accepting and incorporating the fetus as part of the self are paramount undertakings during pregnancy, so much so that the growing emotional bond of the pregnant woman with her unborn child was compared to falling in love, because the baby becomes an intense focus of her inner life (Stern, 2005). Pregnant women express this prenatal affectional bond through heightened sensitivity to fetal/infant well-being, including caregiving behavior, such as eating well and abstaining from harmful substances, affectionate behaviors such as stroking their belly, and nesting behaviors such as preparing the home by making a physical space for the baby and buying baby clothes and equipment (Salisbury, Law, LaGasse, & Lester, 2003). The maternal–fetal bond is the necessary antecedent of the "primary maternal preoccupation," an inner state that Winnicott (1965) described as enabling the mother to give herself over to meeting her infant's physical and psychological needs in the months following the birth.

While accepting and incorporating the fetus into her body and sense of self, the pregnant woman must also recognize the separate individuality of the fetus and hold the baby in mind as independent of her wishes, fantasies, projections, and attributions. By acknowledging the fetus developing in her womb as intrinsically connected but separate, the mother-to-be is also maintaining her own connected but individual identity. The perception of the baby as a separate individual usually increases during the second trimester of pregnancy, when quickening takes place and the baby becomes more real because of fetal movement. When medical technology is available, the compelling images provided by ultrasonography have a profound impact on the sense of the baby as real (Birksted-Breen, 2000; Kofman & Imber, 2005). At this time, many pregnant women are able to describe with conviction and in vivid detail the characteristics they attribute to their fetus, and they often report dreams in which the baby appears with well-defined physical and psychological features. These observations suggest that the membrane between conscious and unconscious life becomes more permeable during pregnancy.

## Labor and Delivery:
### Sociological Realities and Psychic Experience

The physical experience of giving birth to the baby represents a decisive turning point that crystallizes the woman's identity as a mother, both to herself and to society. During the last part of labor, women know that they are performing a vital task. They know that two lives are at stake: her own life and her baby's life. There is a sense that what is happening is simultaneously because of her and in spite of her. Now there is no going back, for better or for worse.

Many women report a fear of death during labor. Stark statistics confirm the reality basis for this fear. The Pregnancy Mortality Surveillance System of the Centers for Disease Control and Prevention (CDC, 2019) shows a significant decline in public commitment to the health of pregnant women, as illustrated by statistics showing that the United States has the highest rate of maternal mortality among developed nations. Maternal mortality in the United States has more than doubled in less than 30 years, increasing steadily from 7.2 maternal deaths per 100,000 live births in 1987 to 17.2 deaths per 100,000 live births in 2015 despite great advances in medical technology and in sharp contrast to the steep worldwide decline in maternal mortality rates in the last decades. Maternal deaths in the United States are increasing across racial and ethnic groups, but African American women are dying in disproportionate numbers, with 40 deaths per 100,000 live births compared to 12.4 deaths per 100,000 live births for European American women. These inequalities highlight the inextricable connection between perinatal care and social justice and the importance of attending to the cultural and environmental circumstances in providing medical and mental health services for pregnant women.

The leading causes of maternal death involve severe bleeding, infection, high blood pressure (preeclampsia and eclampsia), delivery complications, and unsafe abortions (CDC, 2019). Half of these maternal deaths are preventable by improved prenatal, labor and delivery, and postnatal care (Petersen et al., 2019). These figures should be front and center in the consciousness of primary medical care and mental health providers working with pregnant women, who must be alert to all opportunities to improve the quality of service delivery at every stage of pregnancy, labor and delivery, and postnatal care.

While childbirth can and should become much safer with better public health policies, each individual woman in labor faces the duality of birth and death head on, often with the feeling that both are beyond her control. The last stages of labor and delivery stretch the woman beyond all her normal limits of purpose, concentration, pain tolerance, and endurance. One woman recalled, "*I was so frightened and in such pain that I found myself thinking . . . I'm getting out of here! But then I realized that I could not get out . . . that this was happening to me from the inside and not from the outside. I realized that I had to give in to what was happening to me.*" When the delivery results in a healthy mother and a healthy baby, the mother will feel relief and gratitude at having safely traversed the threshold between life and death—whether these feelings are consciously experienced and spoken or form the implicit emotional backdrop for the baby's entry into the world.

## Meeting the Baby

The physical act of delivering the baby is also a psychological transition, marking a profound change in the life of the woman. The baby has gone from being inside as an *intimate* experience to being outside of the mother, and the once "imagined baby" now becomes the "real baby." For many mothers, the baby's first cry and first gaze dramatically affirm the baby's personhood. One mother remembered that moment with a sense of revelation as she said, "*When I was pregnant I used to talk to my baby, and he would respond to me by moving. This was a very special way to communicate with each other. When he was born and the nurse held him up and he cried, I was surprised that he was real, a real baby. He was not inside me anymore, and he had his own voice, he was a real little person. . . . The first moment he looked into my eyes I had this beautiful experience . . . that we were two people together, but he was also a separate little baby, and I was his mother.*" This *moment of meeting* marks the beginning of a dialogue wherein the baby is first encountered as an interlocutor whose signals carry profound meaning in creating an emotional bond (Bruschweiler-Stern, 2009).

After the baby is born, the neonatologist performs a medical examination to check vital signs and indicators of health or medical concerns. The anticipation of the findings can be fraught with intense feelings as the mother is simultaneously recovering from the immense effort of giving birth and turning her attention to her baby's physical integrity. Once the exam is over, the neonatologist routinely places the baby on the mother's chest, and feeling her baby's weight and warmth on her body can be another powerful moment in the creation of what Stern (1995) referred to as the "motherhood mindset" or "constellation." When all goes well, this is an opportunity for bonding as the mother inspects her baby, looking, smelling, touching, and becoming viscerally connected with this new being she created. The feeling of connection becomes intensified when the newborn looks into the mother's eyes even for a brief moment. When the father is also present, a triadic relationship linking mother, father, and baby as a family unit begins to develop.

Meeting the baby is not always positive. The moment of meeting marks the beginning of a relationship that can start with a loving physical and emotional embrace, or with negative maternal attributions that may shape her caregiving and the baby's relational experience throughout development (Lieberman, 1999). Most women experience at least fleeting moments of aversion and even hatred of the baby that can become a source of secret worry and shame when mothers berate themselves for not living up to Madonna-like cultural archetypes of an unfailingly devoted mother. Many women also report disappointment or rejection when seeing their real baby for the first time. There are numerous reports of women who refused to look at their baby for many days because the baby did not conform to their expectations regarding sex, skin color, physical appearance, or health. Women also report momentary but recurrent fantasies of throwing the baby away and fears of smothering, dropping, or otherwise harming the baby, as well as fears of forgetting to pick up the baby from child care or other settings, or of leaving the baby in the car.

Concerns about the baby's well-being and survival also emerge at this time. Many mothers struggle with the real-life possibility of sudden infant death syndrome (SIDS). Anxiety over the risk of the baby dying while asleep may range from intermittent worry to an overriding concern that may lead to elaborate precautions in an effort to both protect the baby and alleviate the mother's fears.

CLINICAL IMPLICATIONS

The experiences of pregnancy, birth, and postpartum have important implications for treatment. Interventions focusing on the transition to motherhood need to include supportive normalization of maternal ambivalence as a universal human experience. This therapeutic attitude can serve as an antidote to the destructive cultural pressure to be a "perfect mother" that when internalized can lead to guilt, anger, and depletion, ultimately disrupting the mother–child relationship and jeopardizing the baby's overall development. Along with supportive normalization, interventions should also include ongoing clinical assessments to ascertain whether the mother's character structure and impulse control are sufficiently solid to contain negative feelings or if there is a risk that the mother will enact her negative feelings in ways that endanger the baby.

## The Medical Context of Childbirth and Delivery

The woman is not alone in giving birth to her baby. Every culture has developed practices designed to maximize maternal and infant survival during this life-and-death experience. Childbirth occurs in a medical context in technologically advanced societies, and the external world of doctors and nurses surrounding the family unit during labor and delivery can have a defining role in shaping this experience.

Perceiving the medical staff as competent and supportive or as incompetent, rushed, impersonal, or insensitive can have long-term consequences for the woman's self-confidence as a mother.

A casual comment by the medical staff can carry enormous emotional weight for the mother's perception of herself and her baby and set in motion lasting maternal attributions to the child. In one example, a lactation specialist tried to reassure a new mother who was having difficulty breastfeeding by blaming the baby, saying, "*You are doing a good job, but your baby is lazy!*" The mother felt protective anger at the lactation specialist on behalf of her baby, while also worrying that the specialist's expert knowledge gave her accurate insight into the baby's innate disposition. In other situations, the neonatologist may inform the parents about an infant medical condition in a factual manner that does account for the emotional impact of the information. For example, a doctor told a mother in a quick, matter-of-fact manner that the newborn had intracranial bleeding that might affect his development. In response, the mother chose to disregard this unsettling information. Once the doctor left the room, she told her baby, "*Everything is fine and we will go home soon. You do not have to listen to her.*" This example illustrates a loving mother's capacity to put herself in the baby's place as the object and recipient of this frightening information and to protectively reframe what the doctor said to reassure herself as much as the baby. At the same time, this mother's outright dismissal of the doctor increased the risk that she might not bring the baby for follow-up postnatal care because the doctor failed to establish a supportive context that gave the mother time to ask questions and gain an understanding of the baby's medical condition.

Cultural beliefs, values, and practices suffuse all aspects of pregnancy, including labor and delivery. The experience of giving birth may pose a particular challenge for immigrant women or those from marginalized minority groups because they often have less access to skilled, timely, and culturally respectful care and because they may feel alienated from the prevailing social expectations at a time of great physical and psychological vulnerability. This sense of uncertainty extends to the anticipation of what it will be like to raise a baby in an unfamiliar culture. In Jhumpa Lahiri's *The Namesake* (2004), a fictional account of an Indian woman's immigration experience in the United States, the writer portrays the inner experience of the pregnant protagonist as follows:

> Nothing feels normal. . . . It's not so much the pain, which she knows . . . she will survive. It's the consequence: motherhood in a foreign land. For it was one thing to be pregnant, to suffer the queasy mornings in bed,

the sleepless nights, the dull throbbing in her back, the countless visits to the bathroom.

Throughout the experience, in spite of her growing discomfort, she'd been astonished by her body's ability to make life, exactly as her mother and grandmother and all her great-grandmothers had done. That it was happening so far from home, unmonitored and unobserved by those she loved, had made it more miraculous still. But she is terrified to raise a child in a country where she is related to no one, where she knows so little, where life seems so tentative and spare. (pp. 5–6)

The reader can empathize with this young woman's anticipated experience of childbirth and childrearing in a country whose cultural assumptions and practices are unfamiliar. The specific manifestations of this uncertainty vary from woman to woman. For the protagonist of *The Namesake*, the main source of anxiety is the prospect of raising her child in a culture that feels alien and where she lacks deep and loving interpersonal connections. Other women respond with fear to what they perceive as the intrusive medicalization of childbirth. For example, a woman from a rural village in Pakistan was shocked when she found out that episiotomy is a routine procedure in the United States to prevent vaginal tears. She cried in disbelief, *"How can a doctor cut you in advance to make sure you don't tear? They are just trying to make their job easier!"* Different cultural values and practices can generate negative attributions to doctors and the medical system that detract from a woman's trust that she will be safe and well cared for during delivery.

CLINICAL IMPLICATIONS

The heightened sensitivity of parents to the input of medical providers during prenatal care, labor, and delivery is an important reason for adopting a culturally informed, linguistically appropriate, and multidisciplinary approach to the care of mothers, fathers, and babies during pregnancy and the postnatal period. Care providers need to cultivate an awareness of how cultural factors can shape the perceptions and expectations of the woman in labor and how the bedside manners of medical providers may affect their patients. The onsite presence of a culturally informed infant/early childhood mental health provider in the range of primary care settings serving pregnant women and newborns (OB/GYN, labor and delivery, NICU, pediatric clinic) is emerging as best practice for coordinated and culturally respectful medical, developmental, and mental health care. Perinatal intervenors can play a pivotal role in promoting a collaborative relationship between the expectant parents and the medical providers by serving as "cultural translators" that help to clarify medical procedures, explain parental wishes, and repair mutual misperceptions between parents and medical providers. These interventions enable them to become effective mediators of cross-cultural differences that, if left unaddressed, can lead to the family being misunderstood, pathologized, and/or ostracized.

## The Man's Experience: Becoming a Father

The journey to fatherhood begins the very moment a man hears the news that his partner is pregnant. The entire history of the couple's emotional and sexual relationship comes into play at this moment: How reciprocal is their perception of their relationship? Is there a shared commitment to be together? Was this a planned or unplanned pregnancy, and is the pregnancy now wanted or not by both partners, by one of them, or by neither? Is the first emotional response to the news of the pregnancy one of joy, worry, dread, anger, numbness, regression, or a mixture of positive and negative reactions? Does the man lean into the implications of the pregnancy by embracing fatherhood as the next stage in his life, or does he flee—physically or emotionally? Although men's bodies do not experience the intense physicality and medical risks of the pregnancy, the physiological, psychological, and social reverberations of becoming a father can change a man's sense of self and reorganize the trajectory of his life.

The socioeconomic context influences the couple's response to pregnancy and adjustment to parenthood. Financial instability can put a significant strain on the relationship, increasing the risk of dysfunction in the process of transitioning to parenthood. Are there enough financial resources to provide for stable housing, sufficient food, and other basic needs? Is the financial burden of adding a new member to the family shouldered by one of the partners only or shared in a mutually acceptable way by both of them? Do cultural values or immigration status play a role in the distribution of these financial responsibilities within the couple?

Rapid cultural changes in family structure and gender role allocation of the past decades set in motion new and sometimes contradictory societal perceptions and demands involving fatherhood. These external pressures influence the internal transformation that begins as men prepare for fatherhood. The changing nature of economic pressures, the rapid rise in the prevalence of full-time working mothers, and the psychological, sociological, and political changes brought about by feminism and by greater representation of cultural diversity in mainstream societal values are bringing about rapidly changing expectations of fathers by their intimate partners, by the father himself, and by the larger society.

Greater involvement of fathers in the day-to-day caregiving of their children has become an expectation among many but not all social groups. When the woman and social group expect the father to be an integral partner in childrearing, there may be large gaps between expected and actual involvement that create strain and resentment between the parents. There has also been an increase in the prevalence and social acceptability of single motherhood across different socioeconomic groups that renders the role of the father more ambiguous and perhaps more peripheral and open to disagreement among the mother, the father, and other parties involved. The African American community, for example, has adapted and redefined the experience of single motherhood into an extended family collaboration that may include grandparents and other family members as taking on caregiving roles (Jones, Zalot, Foster, Sterrett, & Chester, 2007).

All societies contain internal contradictions in values and practices that require painstaking efforts at resolution. Current definitions of masculinity are more likely to incorporate a demand for nurturance while also continuing to expect individual success and compliance with work pressures that interfere with time for the baby. Men confront a range of internal and external demands as they accommodate to the changes in their relationship with their intimate partner and take stock of their willingness and ability to care for their babies and provide for their families. These changes are happening just as women navigate shifting paradigms in the definition of femininity in societal and individual expectations of themselves. As individuals and as a couple, expectant men and women need to negotiate these changes and their effects on their relationship and their shared parenting of their baby.

The literature on becoming a father is less extensive than the literature on becoming a mother, but there is broad agreement that many men wish to become intimately involved with their infants. Benedek (1970) coined the term *genuine fatherliness* to describe what she regarded as an innate trait that enabled men to behave empathically and responsively toward their children. Nevertheless, there is also significant cultural uncertainty and perhaps ambivalence about the origins of this paternal desire. The motivations of motherhood are widely seen as biologically determined, whereas fatherhood is perceived as more dependent on cultural prescriptions to define its significance. However, greater social permission for gender fluidity and individual choice in gender roles are blurring the boundaries between biology and culture. New social mores consider maternal identity as biologically based, yet malleable to psychological and social influences. In this view, depending on her specific circumstances, the woman might either lovingly claim or self-protectively reject the baby through abortion, infanticide, or abandonment when the tradeoff between self-preservation and child care poses an unacceptably high cost to the woman and/or her older children (Hrdy, 1999). Reciprocally, the biological substrate of fatherhood is receiving increased research attention. Recent findings yield important new knowledge about significant physiological changes in fathers-to-be and fathers of newborns and about the associations between their physiological profiles and their interactive patterns with the baby.

## The Biology of Fatherhood

The biological processes that men experience in response to their partner's pregnancy are an important but often overlooked substrate of the transformation in their personal identities as they prepare to become fathers. Men's brains and bodies undergo biological changes during their partners' pregnancy and the perinatal period that may be an adaptation to their new role. Hormonal changes associated with social behavior in expectant fathers support the premise that men are biologically programmed to take care of their offspring and improve their survival and development. There are numerous examples. Men's prolactin levels increase during their partner's pregnancy, and fathers with higher prolactin levels are more responsive to infant cries and spend more time in play with their infants (Fleming, Corter, Stallings, & Steiner, 2002; Gordon, Zagoory-Sharon, Leckman, & Feldman, 2010; Storey, Walsh, Quinton, & Wynne-Edwards, 2000). A study of expectant parents found that they showed changes in both testosterone and estradiol, a hormone linked to bonding and caregiving in both humans and other mammals (Edelstein et al., 2014). The biological changes persist after the baby's birth, with brain growth and structural reorganizations occurring across the first 4 months postpartum (Kim et al., 2014). Fathers and mothers of 4- to 6-month-old infants had comparable levels of oxytocin in plasma, saliva, and urine, and this hormone was involved in parent–infant synchrony in both sexes, including the father's affect synchrony during social play with the infant (Feldman, Gordon, & Zagoory-Sharon, 2011; Gordon, Zagoory-Sharon, Leckman, & Feldman, 2010). Both human and animal fathers show decreases in testosterone, a change that might signify a shift from the motivation to mate toward a motivation to nurture and is associated with greater empathy and caregiving responses (Gordon et al., 2010; Saltzman & Ziegler, 2014).

Men often mirror in their own bodies the changes occurring in their wives' or intimate partners' bodies. Many men gain weight during and after pregnancy. Several longitudinal studies with large sample sizes showed that expectant fathers showed increased body mass index (BMI) and accelerated weight gain across the partner's pregnancy and the perinatal period when compared with childless men (Saxbe et al., 2018). Three possible clusters of factors may explain the association between fatherhood and weight gain: a hormonal cluster involving decreased testosterone; a behavioral cluster involving decreased sleep and decreased physical activity; and a psychological cluster involving stress resulting from the new pressures and responsibilities of becoming a father (Saxbe et al., 2018).

Men's somatic experiences and behavior may also mirror the woman's experiences. The fascinating cross-cultural phenomenon of *couvade* (also known as "male sympathetic pregnancy") involves somatic symptoms in the expectant father similar to those of his pregnant wife or intimate partner. They may include morning sickness, nausea, insomnia, food cravings, changes in appetite, indigestion or digestion changes such as diarrhea and constipation, stomachaches, back pain, breast growth, sore or hard nipples, and "labor" pains (Brennan, Marshall-Lucette, Ayers, & Ahmed, 2007; Gray & Anderson, 2010). Couvade symptoms usually begin in the first trimester of pregnancy, decrease in the second trimester, reappear in the third trimester, and may extend to the postpartum period. Studies report an incidence in the United States of 25–52%, of 61% in Thailand, and of 20% in Sweden (Brennan, Ayers, Ahmed, & Marshall-Lucette, 2007). Endocrine influences may provide a physiological substrate, but it is likely that psychological and cultural processes are also involved and lead to individual differences in the etiology, manifestations, and course of couvade. Theoretical explanations include the hypothesis that the man is simultaneously identifying with his pregnant partner and competing with the baby for the woman's attention. In this view, the transformational transition from being a couple to becoming a triad, marked in the woman by graphic bodily changes, leaves the man with a "disembodied experience" that triggers jealousy of the woman's procreative powers, conflicts about changing sexuality, and a rekindling of early conflicts that find somatic expression in the couvade symptoms (Klein, 1991).

Psychoanalysts trace the psychological roots of the impulse toward fatherhood to the pre-oedipal and oedipal stages, when 4- and 5-year-old boys can be quite articulate in expressing their wish to be pregnant, attribute their "big bellics" to carrying a baby, and speak about their wish to have a baby with their mothers. In the course of development, boys must come to grips with what is biologically and culturally impossible and cope with envy and competitiveness in response to the universal disappointment of discovering that they cannot have it all—they cannot have a penis and a baby at the same time, and they cannot marry mommy and have a baby with her. In the course of development, the quality of the boy's attachment to the mother and to the father has an important effect on his comfort with different aspects of relationships, including intimacy, nurturance, and self-assertion without fear of losing love.

As with any developmental transition, this process involves reevaluating existing self-perceptions and relational patterns, creating new ones, and gradually evolving toward a more integrated personal self in which achievements, aspirations, and disappointments coexist without excessive friction. When psychological obstacles or sociological conditions derail this process, the expectant father may experience a sense of marginalization, depersonalization, dislocation, denial, or anger. He may also degrade his pregnant partner, particularly when he feels that the pregnancy occurred without his conscious knowledge or consent. The changes to the woman's body may be perceived as "ugly" by both the man and the woman and exacerbate changes in sexual desire that may take different manifestations in the two partners, leading to strains in the intimate relationship. These internal and interpersonal conflicts may lead expectant fathers to distance themselves from their partner and/or unborn baby psychologically or physically, act out aggressively in the form of intimate partner violence (IPV), or revert to maladaptive patterns of coping, such as reckless behavior and illegal substance use.

When all goes well, fatherhood can give a man the opportunity to extend himself by passing on his positive experiences of growing up to the next generation. Fatherhood can also offer him a "second chance" to rework unresolved conflicts with his own father and mother and mature into a greater comfort with gender identity and with intimacy in ways that expand personal meaning and psychological safety. Becoming a father can dramatically stimulate a man's urge to nurture, which he might have suppressed earlier in life while pursuing traditional male goals. When men notice the beneficial effect of their caregiving and the baby's positive responses to them, they can undergo an internal transformation that enhances their self-esteem. This transformation may take the form of internalizing new caregiving practices, perhaps passed on from their own parents or learned from the baby's mother. It may also involve increased self-confidence about having something unique to give the baby that expands what the mother has to offer, for example, by engaging in more stimulating body-centered play (Pollack, 1995).

## Labor and Delivery

The vast cultural differences in how diverse ethnic, racial, religious, and national groups approach pregnancy, labor, and delivery apply also to the role of husbands and male partners during childbirth. In the United States, efforts to allow husbands and other supportive people into the delivery room comprised a major source of activism in the field of reproductive health in the 1970s, and most men are now present during the childbirth process (Steen, Downe, Bamfort, & Edozien, 2012). This cultural shift does not mean that their presence is always a welcome or positive experience for all involved. Like most cultural shifts, male partners' presence during childbirth evokes a range of individual responses that include anxiety as well as a wholehearted sense of belonging. Men interviewed about their impending participation in the birth process reported remarkably similar fears in two studies conducted almost 30 years apart (Shapiro, 1987; Steen et al., 2012). Their concerns included feeling unwelcome and out of place during prenatal visits, uncertainty about how they would respond during their partner's labor and delivery, discomfort with the OB/GYN establishment and hospital procedures, fleeting or persistent doubts about their paternity, fear of being replaced by the infant in their partner's affection, or—most terrifying—losing their spouse or child to death or ill health.

## Meeting the Baby

Many fathers fall in love with their babies at the time of the birth, a psychological state labeled "engrossment" in a study of first-time fathers whose babies were still in the neonatal unit (Bader, 1995). Engrossed fathers showed heightened visual and tactile awareness of the newborn's distinct characteristics, perception of the newborn as perfect, strong feelings of attraction that lead them to focus their attention on the newborn, extreme elation, and increased feelings of self-esteem. The study found that all fathers reported a significant degree of engrossment, although there were individual variations in the specificity of the response. Contact with the baby was the key factor in triggering engrossment. External factors were not relevant, including whether this was the first baby, the mother's or father's income, the length of the parents' marriage, or the age or weight of the newborn.

### IMPLICATIONS FOR CLINICAL PRACTICE AND SOCIAL POLICY

The extensive evidence of men's physical and emotional responses to pregnancy, childbirth, and the newborn supports the importance of comprehensive efforts to include fathers in the systems of care tending to pregnant women and newborns. In light of the variability of expectant fathers' responses to being present during childbirth, best clinical practice should involve careful consideration of both parents' wishes, strengths, and vulnerabilities when making decisions about who will be present to support the mother during labor and delivery. Medical practices that offer parents the flexibility to choose the best arrangement tailored to their specific needs should replace rigid expectations about the appropriateness of the father's presence or absence in the delivery room.

The importance of including fathers in the systems of care for pregnant women and newborns goes beyond considerations of their physical presence in the delivery room. This position stands in strong contrast to the consistent exclusion of fathers from most settings attending to maternal and child health. It is telling that the term *paternal and child health* is not in use as a routine complement to the term *maternal and child health* in medical settings. In a chapter calling for the consistent inclusion of fathers, Cowan, Cowan, Pruett, and Pruett (2018) list some of the elements that are too often missing from current parenting research and parenting interventions and call for interventions that include sustained attention to fathers' experiences and active efforts to include them in their babies' lives.

There is some progress toward fathers' inclusion. A federal multi-agency conference on Paternal Involvement in Pregnancy Outcomes expanded the existing fatherhood paradigm to include a new focus on men's preconception health that parallels the women's preconception health movement and the maternal and child health perspective (Kotelchuck & Lu, 2017). Fathers' participation in preconception health and health care is critical for healthy reproductive outcomes. This inclusive approach might help to counter the enduring and damaging politicization of access to reproductive health choices and services, in which external barriers often curtail women's freedom to make the decisions that are best for them and their families.

While the importance of policies that facilitate father inclusion in pregnancy and perinatal health services cannot be overstated, it is also important to keep in mind that the exclusion of an individual father may be necessary in specific situations of chronic paternal IPV, substance abuse, psychiatric problems, criminal lifestyle, and/or abandonment of the pregnant woman. In a study of second-trimester pregnant women interviewed at a public health hospital, 20% reported that they were no longer in an intimate relationship with the father of the baby, and more than 70% declined to invite the father of the baby to participate in the study (Narayan et al., 2017). These women had high prevalence of exposure to IPV prior to and during pregnancy, suggesting that many pregnant women might choose to exclude the father as a form of self-protection. In these situations, family-friendly public health policies must include coordinated multisystem approaches to create a collaborative safety net linking IPV intervention for victims and perpetrators of IPV to the mental health system, primary care providers, child welfare, and the judicial system. The safety of the woman and the baby must take priority in all these efforts, even at the cost of excluding the father in situations of risk.

## Life with Baby: Understanding the Dyad and the Triad in Their Social–Cultural Context

Each baby exists in a concentric circle of relationships with people who in turn have complex relationships with each other, and who together create an intricate tapestry of mutual influences that become part of the baby's sense of self. Efforts to understand how these influences shape the baby's development created a fertile field of diverse theoretical approaches and numerous empirical investigations about the transactional influences between the baby and its caregivers.

A key source of debate is the question: Is the affective bond between mothers and infants an exclusively important predictor of healthy emotional development? Attachment theory provided an evolutionary explanation for the emotional preeminence of the infant–mother relationship first proposed by Sigmund Freud and Donald Winnicott (Bowlby, 1969; Freud, 1926/1959; Winnicott, 1965). Attachment theory has roots in an ethological understanding of the infant–mother affective bond as a survival mechanism that evolved to counter the danger posed by predators in the Savannah environment where the human species originated (Bowlby, 1969). The premise that infants' seeking of proximity and contact with a preferred caregiver in situations of uncertainty and danger is a behavioral hallmark of attachment created a cross-cultural theoretical framework that enabled researchers to identify key behavioral manifestations of the infant–mother affective bond. These behavioral markers of maternal caregiving and infant attachment in turn allowed researchers to assess how these two domains predict other dimensions of the infant's functioning, both in the present and in the course of the child's long-term development. The impressive body of empirical research that documents the effects of early maternal care on multiple aspects of the child's present development and future functioning has made attachment theory the best-supported theory of child development to date (Ainsworth, Blehar,

Waters, & Wall, 1978; Main, Hesse, & Kaplan, 2005; Sroufe, Egeland, Carlson, & Collins, 2005).

Alternative theoretical paradigms emerged almost in tandem with this focus on the centrality of the mother–infant relationship. Soon after the publication of Bowlby's (1969) hugely influential first volume of his attachment trilogy, Michael Rutter (1972) published an equally influential treatise on maternal deprivation that identified other important mechanisms predicting child psychopathology, such as the impersonal care of young children raised in institutions, the absence of emotional bonds with mother substitutes, and chronic family discord. The importance of fathers as attachment figures was elucidated by early research from Michael Lamb (1976a, 1976b, 1978) and by the theoretical and clinical contributions of Kyle Pruett (2000), who coined the term *fatherneed* to describe the specific contributions that fathers make to child development. The role of environmental influences other than the parents became a focal point of study pioneered by Uri Bronfenbrenner (1979), who advocated for an ecological approach incorporating the transactional processes linking different levels of interpersonal, community, institutional, and societal contexts (micro-, meso-, exo-, and macrosystems) to predict child outcomes. The field of developmental psychopathology emerged in response to growing evidence for the heterogeneity of biological, interpersonal, social, and cultural factors that influence individual functioning. This field adopted a lifespan approach that integrates multiple disciplines and theoretical perspectives, investigates continuities and discontinuities between normative and atypical development, and understands that psychopathology emerges from the interplay between risk and protective factors whose influences are probabilistic rather than deterministic in predicting outcomes (Cicchetti & Sroufe, 2000). All these scholarly contributions lead to the inescapable conclusion that, while the affective bond between mother and infant is a cornerstone of development, it is important to include a broad examination of caregiver influences in the understanding of individual and group outcomes starting in infancy.

Mothers and fathers show different parenting styles when studied as a group, although there are major individual differences within each group. Compared to mothers, fathers tend to spend a greater proportion of their time with their young children in active play that often involves highly stimulating physical engagement and encouragement of exploration, while mothers engage more in caregiving exchanges (Grossmann, Grossmann, Kindler, & Zimmermann, 2008). Infants, in turn, develop different patterns of relating to each of their caregivers. Regardless of the style of the interaction—whether it is more physically stimulating or more oriented toward caregiving—infants establish secure or anxious attachments with either parent or with both parents, depending on the parent's quality of attunement, temperamental affinities, and interactional synchronicity with the child.

Relationships are not only dyadic. The baby–mother–father triad is "the primary triangle" because of its centrality in the infant's emotional life, as babies absorb the emotional climate that the parents create with each other around the child (Fivaz-Depeursinge & Corboz-Warnery, 1999). Babies position themselves from the beginning within the relationship that exists between their mother and their father. Infants are keen observers of how their parents relate to each other, and they need permission from each parent to establish a close interpersonal connection with the other. The ability of mothers and fathers to balance each of their own dyadic emotional engagement and interactional styles with the baby to give space for the other parent's personal relationship and style of interaction is a key factor in the baby's healthy development. *Partnership parenting* is a term coined by Kyle Pruett and Marsha Kline Pruett (2009) to promote a collaborative stance between mothers and fathers that acknowledges and respects their unique and separate contributions to their child's healthy development.

Parents and caregivers engage in moment-to-moment negotiations with each other on behalf of the infant, and these exchanges occur along multiple dimensions of caregiving that include problem solving, conflict resolution, caregiving role allocation, instrumental and emotional communication, emotional investment, behavioral regulation and coordination, and sibling harmony. The quality of collaboration along these caregiving dimensions has profound implications for the baby's well-being as well as for each adult's identity as a caregiver. Winnicott (1965) famously stated that "there is no such thing as a baby"— meaning that a baby only exists in the context of the mother's care. It is equally valid to state that "there is no such thing as a mother," "there is no such thing as a father," and "there is no such thing as a family" because the quality of family life that mothers and fathers can promote is either supported or undermined by their material and psychological circumstances and social supports.

## Clinical Implications

The fetus and the newborn develop within a complex matrix of transactional biological, interpersonal, social, and cultural influences that has at its core the interconnections among the relationships between the baby and each of its primary caregivers, how these caregivers join together to nurture the baby, and how society supports the caregivers in nurturing the child. The clinical importance of this relational matrix is recognized in *Diagnostic Classification of Mental Health and Developmental Disorders of Infancy and Early Childhood* (DC: 0–5; Zero to Three, 2016). Axis II in DC: 0–5 addresses the young child's relational context and includes two separate sections, which respectively examine the caregiver–child relationship from a dyadic perspective and the quality of the caregiving environment from the viewpoint of the stability, predictability, and emotional quality of the relationships among the adult caregivers on behalf of the child.

P-CPP has adopted this relational matrix. Section II describes P-CPP in terms of an evolving assessment and treatment plan that includes ongoing attention to the range of factors affecting the expectant parents' readiness to love and care for their child. After the baby's birth, therapeutic attention focuses on the relationship that each parent establishes with the baby, the quality of the relationship among caregivers, and the sources of protection and risk in the caregiving environment that form the backdrop for the day-to-day experience of the child.

# The Central Importance of Community: Protective and Risk Factors

The concept of risk and protective factors is central to an understanding of developmental influences and clinical formulations. Risk factors are variables that increase the likelihood of an adverse outcome. Protective factors, on the other hand, are variables or processes that mitigate risk and promote successful outcomes. Developmental psychopathology emphasizes the importance of understanding the multilevel nature of the contexts that contribute to the development of psychopathology, including the dynamic interplay of risk and protective factors. A basic principle of developmental psychopathology states that a single discrete risk factor can be associated with a variety of outcomes (a principle known as *multifinality*). For example, child abuse may lead to different kinds of adult psychopathology or to successful adaptation, depending on a variety of other factors, including the child's constitutional characteristics and the presence of protective adults and other positive influences that buffer the impact of the abuse. Another developmental psychopathology principle states that different risk factors can lead to the same outcome (a principle known as *equifinality*). For example, aggressive behavior in childhood can result from injury to the frontal lobes, coercive parenting, child abuse, and/or the interplay of several different factors such as a constitutional predisposition and parental rejection (Hinshaw, 2013). This nuanced understanding of the human experience has created a sea change in research and clinical practice, leading to more sophisticated research methods, clinical case formulation, and treatment models. Among expectant parents struggling with environmental stressors and emotional difficulties, pregnancy and the perinatal period comprise a maturational stage that may be particularly receptive to positive influences that restore a healthy developmental trajectory.

There is a powerful allure to thinking of pregnancy and infancy as a time of promise and loving anticipation. This can indeed be the case when family and society converge to create favorable conditions that support the parents and the child. Basic resources for physical health and well-being are essential, in the form of adequate nutrition and safe living conditions. In addition, stable and supportive relationships while growing up and in the present are of particular value in supporting and promoting the parent's quality of caregiving. These relationships may include caring connections with the baby's father, family members, friends, and members of shared social and cultural groups, such as communities of faith and family resource centers that can provide emotional and concrete support at times of stress and need (Narayan, Rivera, Bernstein, Harris, & Lieberman, 2018). Being able to derive comfort from childhood memories of feeling loved also serve as protective factors for maternal mental health (Narayan et al., 2017; Narayan, Ghosh Ippen, Harris, & Lieberman, 2019).

Pregnancy can also be an unwelcome occurrence, as evidenced by the frequency of abortion, infanticide, offspring abandonment, and offspring abuse both among humans and in the natural world (Hrdy, 1999). Motherhood and fatherhood are costly to the individual woman and man, and the parents' material, psychological, and social circumstances may force them to make choices that put other priorities above those of a new baby.

Women carry the unborn baby within their bodies, making fetuses susceptible to environmental conditions that affect the physical and emotional health of their mothers.

These risks include the numerous markers of poverty, including but not limited to food insufficiency, inadequate housing, neighborhoods with high levels of community violence and unhealthy conditions such as pollutants and lead, scarcity of financial resources, and lack of access to medical care. These risk factors often coexist and have a direct cumulative impact on the pregnant woman's physical health, raising her risk for psychiatric conditions such as anxiety, depression, and posttraumatic stress disorder (PTSD). Toxic social conditions also include racism, discrimination, and marginalization of minority racial and ethnic groups. Other risk factors include medical conditions, a history of psychopathology, substance abuse, past or current trauma exposure, such as childhood maltreatment and/or current IPV, unwanted pregnancy by the woman and/or her partner, and prior pregnancy loss (Kofman & Imber, 2005; Muzik, Cameron, Fezzey, & Rosenblum, 2009; Ostler, 2009; Slade & Sadler, 2019).

## Unwanted Pregnancy as a Risk Factor

Unplanned pregnancies are common. In 2011, 45% of the 6.1 million annual pregnancies in the United States were unintended. Of these, 27% of all pregnancies were "wanted later," and 18% of pregnancies were "unwanted." Women without a high school degree had the highest unintended pregnancy rate, and rates declined with each additional level of educational attainment (Finer & Zolna, 2016). The proportion of births that fathers report as unplanned is similar to that reported by mothers (Lindberg & Kost, 2014).

Specific individual responses to an unintended pregnancy may vary depending on many factors. However, unintended pregnancy is a predictor of negative maternal and fetal outcomes that include low birthweight, preterm birth, later initiation of prenatal care, maternal health risk behaviors, and maternal perinatal depression (Abajobir, Maravilla, Alati, & Najman, 2016; Gipson, Koenig, & Hindin, 2008; Hall, Benton, Copas, & Stephenson, 2017; Kost & Lindberg, 2015).

Important findings emerge when the investigator asks each partner separately whether she or he wants the pregnancy. Measures of wanting or not wanting the pregnancy at the couple level reveal important findings about the sequelae of agreement or disagreement between the partners. Couple-level pregnancy wantedness is defined as both partners wanting the pregnancy, and couple-level pregnancy discordance is defined as only one partner wanting the pregnancy. Couple discordance is associated with inadequate prenatal care, increased risk of preterm birth, adverse fetal health outcomes, rapid repeat pregnancies, and children's poorer social–emotional development (Cha, Chapman, Wan, Burton, & Masho, 2016; Hohmann-Marriott, 2009; Korenman, Kaestner, & Joyce, 2002; Saleem & Surkan, 2014). In a recent study with a sample of low-income, racially diverse pregnant women, women who reported that they wanted the pregnancy more than their partner had significantly higher prenatal and postnatal depression symptoms, prenatal PTSD symptoms, and prenatal and postnatal relationship conflict than women who reported that both partners agreed on their wanting or not wanting the pregnancy (Atzl, Narayan, Rivera, & Lieberman, 2019). This recent literature on the adverse sequelae of unwanted pregnancies adds to long-standing research findings showing that children from unwanted pregnancies are more likely than children from accepted pregnancies to experience negative outcomes even when followed 30 years later (Kubička et al., 1995).

## Clinical Implications

These findings highlight the negative social and psychological consequences of unwanted pregnancies, both at the individual and the couple level and both for the mother and the child. At a time when reproductive health choice is under siege, these findings are a stark reminder of the power of unwanted pregnancies to damage mental health and create or exacerbate conflict in the couple relationship. Clinical care, whether it involves medical or psychological treatment, should include routine engagement of women and men of reproductive age in a dialogue about their plans and wishes regarding pregnancy, family size, spacing of children, attitudes and values regarding conception and contraception, and the specific behavioral choices they are making with respect to conception and contraception. Given the central role of pregnancy in physical and mental health, questions about reproductive choices should be as routine as questions about smoking, drinking, substance use, and other medical screening questions. The goal is not to prescribe specific reproductive outcomes but to help bring attention to reproductive choices as an integral component of self-care, because mindful reproductive health practices go hand in hand with quality of parenting, physical health, and mental health for parents and babies.

## Interpersonal Trauma as a Risk Factor

Exposure to interpersonal trauma and other adversities during childhood is the norm rather than the exception among respondents from all socioeconomic levels and racial/ethnic backgrounds, as documented in the paradigmatic Adverse Childhood Experiences (ACE) study (Felitti et al., 1998) and epidemiological surveys (Finkelhor, Ormrod, Turner, & Hamby, 2005). There is also extensive evidence that chronic and cumulative exposure to childhood adversity and trauma predicts a plethora of medical and psychiatric conditions. A recent systematic review and meta-analysis replicated the findings of the original ACE study, showing that participants with four or more ACEs were at significantly increased risk for a range of poor outcomes, most significantly exposure to interpersonal violence and mental illness (Hughes et al., 2017).

Interpersonal trauma such as child abuse and witnessing or experiencing IPV affects the health of the mother and the fetus and has lasting effects after the baby is born. Risk factors routinely overlap, resulting in complex profiles of risk because the range of negative outcomes increases as risk factors increase. Women abused as children are more likely to engage in violent relationships as adults, and the combined effect of childhood maltreatment and current IPV increases the odds of PTSD during pregnancy when compared to the effects of either condition alone (Becker, Stuewig, & McCloskey, 2010; Finnbogadóttir, Dykes, & Wann-Hansson, 2014; Sanchez et al., 2017; Whitfield, Anda, Dube, & Felitti, 2003; Woods, 2005).

There is also strong comorbidity of postpartum depression and PTSD among mothers with histories of childhood trauma, as revealed by individual studies and a systematic review of more than 40 studies showing that women with a history of childhood maltreatment and/ or IPV are more likely to experience peripartum depression (Alvarez-Segura et al., 2014; Oh et al., 2018).

The co-occurrence of trauma and depression has significant clinical implications for parenting. In a study of first-time pregnant women in the Healthy Families America home visiting program, 30% had clinical depression and 70% reported at least one episode of violent trauma, with the combination of depression and trauma predicting less maternal sense of control and social support and an increased risk of child abuse (Stevens, Ammerman, Putnam, & Van Ginkel, 2002). Women with a history of childhood abuse and IPV also have more difficulty establishing an emotional connection with the fetus (Schwerdt-feger & Goff, 2007).

Substance abuse of alcohol and drugs often originates in childhood interpersonal trauma and becomes a powerful contributor to the intergenerational transmission of trauma because it affects the parents' capacity to provide safe and predictable caregiving (Suchman, Pajulo, & Mayes, 2013). The pernicious effects of substance abuse on the baby begin *in utero*. Fetal exposure to the direct impact of substances is often compounded by the transactional effects of maternal malnutrition, IPV, and other stressors associated with poor perinatal outcomes, such as premature birth; low birthweight; slowed growth; and long-term physical, emotional, behavioral, and cognitive problems (Behnke, Smith, & Committee on Substance Abuse, 2013; Hopping-Winn, 2012). Substance abuse is also frequently associated with other risk factors, such as parental mental illness, health problems, interpersonal violence, poverty, homelessness, criminal behavior, and unpredictable life circumstances that affect the capacity to provide safe and predictable care (Suchman et al., 2013). Parental substance abuse is associated with a range of maladaptive caregiving practices that include impulsive interactions, inconsistent discipline, and inattention (Boris, Renk, Lowell, & Kolomeyer, 2019). Substance abuse is often an intergenerational problem, with recent findings inducing a mean heritability rate of 40–70%, equal or higher than the rate for many chronic medical problems (Kendler, Myers, & Prescott, 2007).

It is widely acknowledged that parental substance abuse represents an important public health problem, with almost 10% of newborns exposed to alcohol and about 5.4% exposed to illicit drugs *in utero* (Substance Abuse and Mental Health Services Administration, 2014). The current epidemic of opioid use has given new urgency to this problem, with the rate of opioid use in pregnancy increasing 127% between 1999 and 2011 and higher rates of deaths, cesarean births, and preterm births among opioid-using mothers compared to controls

(Maeda, Bateman, Clancy, Creanga, & Leffert, 2014). In tandem, the last decade saw a threefold increase in the rate of neonates with neonatal abstinence syndrome, the cluster of neonatal symptoms associated with maternal opioid use (Patrick et al., 2012). The increase in opioid use coincided with an increase in involvement of the child protection system. In Minnesota, for example, the leading cause for foster care placement of young children is parental drug or alcohol abuse (30%), and the second leading cause is neglect (20%), which is often associated with parental substance abuse (Wright, Dallas, Moldenhauer, & Carlson, 2018).

The interplay of genetic, interpersonal, and environmental factors that coalesce in parental substance abuse creates a complex clinical picture that combines with the chronic lack of public investment in substance abuse prevention and treatment to place millions of children in inadequate caregiving environments and leaves expectant mothers and fathers in situations of despair. The voices of women and men who abuse substances are largely missing from the public perception of the problem, amid an often blaming and derogatory portrayal in the media. Compared to the magnitude of the problem, there is an indefensible lack of systematic investment in prenatal substance abuse treatment programs that meet the demand and in treatment outcome research to ascertain effective intervention strategies (Boris et al., 2019).

Increasing understanding of the neuroscience of addiction and parenting offers hope that effective strategies are emerging. Neuroimaging studies suggest that women with histories of chronic substance abuse may experience the normative practices of caregiving as less rewarding than controls (Kim et al., 2017; Landi et al., 2011). This insight led to the hypothesis that an attachment-informed, mentalization-based intervention with mothers in addiction treatment may improve the quality of parenting and the quality of child attachment, with the findings confirming these expectations (Suchman, DeCoste, Borelli, & McMahon, 2018). Building reflective capacity also informs the intervention strategies of Project NESST (Newborns Exposed to Substances: Support and Therapy), a multiservice program that pairs clinicians with paraprofessionals (Mentoring Moms) with lived experience in substance recovery, to help substance-abusing pregnant women use their pregnancy as an incentive to recovery (Spielman, Herriott, Paris, & Sommer, 2015). These promising approaches offer support for the idea that parents who abuse substances are receptive to the same foundational principles of effective psychotherapy: a dignity-affirming, caring therapeutic alliance in which their experiences are understood and affirmed and their personal goals for their child and for themselves inform all aspects of the intervention.

## The Intergenerational Transmission of Adversity

How are infants affected by maternal history of trauma? Biological and interpersonal processes are involved in the intergenerational transmission of risk. At the biological level, "fetal programming" is a phenomenon that links prenatal stress to alterations of fetal development and an increased risk of psychiatric conditions later in life (St-Pierre, Laurent, King, & Vaillancourt, 2016). Pregnant women's distress may influence fetal functioning through changes in placental gene DNA methylation (Monk et al., 2016). Maternal childhood maltreatment/trauma is associated with placental-fetal stress physiology and newborn brain structure (Moog et al., 2016, 2017).

A recent research review of both human and animal studies described parents' childhoods and epigenetics as the first exposure in the intergenerational transmission of disadvantage (Scorza et al., 2018). Maternal adversity before the baby's conception and maternal stress during pregnancy make separate and independent contributions to infants' respiratory sinus arrhythmia (RSA), a biological marker of infant self-regulation linked to physical and mental health outcomes across the lifespan. A recent publication entitled "Thinking Across Generations" documented these independent contributions with findings that high maternal ACE scores before conception were associated with lower infant RSA as measured in the still-face paradigm, while maternal prenatal stress was associated with the infant's failure to recover following the stressor of the still-face paradigm (Gray, Jones, Theall, Glackin, & Drury, 2017). These findings illustrate the extraordinary interconnection between maternal and infant biological systems during the course of pregnancy and the postpartum period.

## Intimate Partner Violence (IPV) and Perinatal Trauma

Partner violence often begins or escalates during pregnancy and more often than not continues after childbirth, with minority women at increased risk (Charles & Perreira, 2007; Martin, Mackie, Kupper, Buescher, & Moracco, 2001; Sharps, Laughon, & Giangrande, 2007). Estimates of IPV frequency during pregnancy vary widely across individual studies, but a recent meta-analysis of 92 studies revealed an average prevalence of 28.4% for emotional abuse, 13.8% for physical abuse, and 8% for sexual abuse (James, Brody, & Hamilton, 2013).

## Impact of IPV on the Pregnant Woman

IPV during pregnancy can have devastating consequences. Injuries to the woman can result in femicide and fetal death (Coker, Sanderson, & Dong, 2004; El Kady, Gilbert, Xing, & Smith, 2005; Martin, Macy, Sullivan, & Magee, 2007; Morland, Leskin, Block, Campbell, & Friedman, 2008; Silverman, Decker, Reed, & Raj, 2006; Yost, Bloom, McIntire, & Leveno, 2005). Medical risks are exponentially higher even when the violence is not lethal. When compared with pregnant women in nonviolent relationships, battered pregnant women face greater risk of medical complications, such as insufficient or excessive weight gain, urinary tract infections, kidney infections, anemia, preeclampsia, severe nausea and/or vomiting, dehydration, placental abruption, uterine rupture, and vaginal hemorrhage (El Kady et al., 2005; Johnson, Hellerstedt, & Pirie, 2002; Silverman et al., 2006). Brain injury is a possible undiagnosed outcome of IPV, as it emerged from a community-based study in which 81% of IPV-exposed women reported a head injury and 83% reported being choked, findings suggesting that blows to the head and oxygen deprivation may be involved in the etiology of the women's memory loss, difficulty understanding, trouble with vision and hearing, and other cognitive and affect-regulation problems (Nemeth, Mengo, Kulow, Brown, & Ramirez, 2019). Compounding these medical risks, IPV in pregnancy is associated with a greater risk of maternal behaviors that further compromise maternal and fetal health, such as smoking and use of alcohol and illicit substances (Huth-Bocks, Levendosky, & Bogat, 2002; Martin, Beaumont, & Kupper, 2003).

The climate of unwanted control and fear that exists in violent relationships can also influence women's ability to control their fertility and lead to unwanted pregnancies, which in turn raises the risk of unfavorable maternal and infant health outcomes (Goodwin, Gazmararian, Johnson, Gilbert, & Saltzman, 2000; Pallitto, Campbell, & O'Campo, 2005). IPV is also associated with delayed prenatal care and/or more missed appointments, compromising the quality of prenatal care and increasing the possibility of poor perinatal outcomes (Goodwin et al., 2000; Huth-Bocks et al., 2002; Jasinski, 2004). Depression and PTSD are psychiatric problems commonly identified during pregnancy and significantly correlated with IPV (Beydoun, Al-Sahab, Beydoun, & Tamim, 2010; Jones, Hughes, & Unterstaller, 2001; Seng, Low, Sperlich, Ronis, & Liberzon, 2009).

## Impact of IPV on Infant Well-Being

In addition to inflicting injury to the woman and contributing to high-risk pregnancies, violence during pregnancy endangers the well-being of the fetus and the child. IPV has been identified for decades as "the single major precursor to child abuse and neglect fatalities in the United States" (U.S. Advisory Board on Child Abuse and Neglect, 1995, p. 124), because infants and very young children are most vulnerable due to their susceptibility to injury from harsh parenting and/or abuse or from accidental injuries associated with neglect. National statistics document that a child's risk of maltreatment increases substantially from the moment a child is born into a violent home. Up to 70% of children who witnessed IPV are also victims of child abuse and/or neglect, and the incidence is highest in the first 4 years of life, with children under 1 year having the highest rate of victimization (Child Welfare Information Gateway, 2019; U.S. Department of Health and Human Services, Children's Bureau, 2019).

The risk to infants as the result of IPV starts at the biological level. A meta-analysis of 19 studies found that IPV was associated with low birthweight and preterm birth (Hill, Pallitto, McCleary-Sills, & Garcia-Moreno, 2016), which are among the leading causes of neonatal deaths and physical and mental disabilities in children (Asling-Monemi, Peña, Ellsberg, & Persson, 2003; Office of the Surgeon General, 2005; U.S. Advisory Board on Child Abuse and Neglect, 1995). Babies of IPV-exposed mothers also tend to have more health problems than babies whose mothers did not experience IPV, including more neonatal intensive care admissions, more frequent hospitalizations, and more outpatient visits other than well-baby check-ups (Huth-Bocks et al., 2002; Silverman et al., 2006; Yost et al., 2005).

The overlap between IPV and child abuse shows that the quality of parenting is also affected. Mothers involved in violent relationships are less nurturing; have more negative perceptions and more developmentally unrealistic demands of their children; and show more hostility, disengagement, and punitiveness (Huth-Bocks, Levendosky, Theran, & Bogat, 2004; Letourneau, Fedick, & Willms, 2007; Levendosky, Leahy, Bogat, Davidson, & von Eye, 2006; Lutenbacher, 2002). Men who batter are likely to display more anger and physical punitiveness and less positive engagement with their children than other fathers (Edleson & Williams, 2006).

These conditions have grave consequences for infants and young children, who are simultaneously helpless and terrified when witnessing violence and cannot turn to their parents for protection in the middle of a physical fight. Symptoms of affect dysregulation include excessive fussing and crying, difficulty soothing, feeding and sleeping problems, hypervigilance, and heightened fear responses, including symptoms of increased arousal and numbing that mirror the PTSD symptoms of their traumatized mothers (Bogat, DeJonghe, Levendosky, Davidson, & von Eye, 2006; Carpenter & Stacks, 2009; Schechter & Willheim, 2009).

## Long-Term Sequelae of Childhood Exposure to IPV

The repercussions of witnessing IPV in childhood last well beyond the early years. Women who grew up witnessing recurrent incidents of IPV against their mothers are at increased risk of becoming IPV victims, and men in the same circumstances are at greater risk of becoming IPV perpetrators. The risk of becoming either a victim or a perpetrator increases more than threefold when exposure to IPV overlaps with child maltreatment, as is often the case (Whitfield et al., 2003). Children who have increased episodes of witnessing IPV also have a greater likelihood of reported alcoholism, illicit drug use, IV drug use, and depression in adulthood (Dube, Anda, Felitti, Edwards, & Croft, 2002). These findings highlight the importance of considering early IPV exposure as a potential lifelong and intergenerational risk factor.

## Clinical Implications

The damaging impact of IPV on every family member involved makes it imperative to make it an unwavering focus of therapeutic intervention. Women exposed to IPV need to receive medical care that is responsive to the possible links between the specific types of violence they endured and their medical and psychiatric health problems. For example, domestic violence programs in Ohio are implementing a model called CARE (Connect, Acknowledge, Respond, and Evaluate) to encourage systematic attention to the diagnosis and treatment of possible traumatic brain injury (TBI) when warranted by symptoms and when there is a history of head injury and strangulation as forms of IPV (Nemeth et al., 2019).

There is empirical evidence that focusing on IPV in therapy with young children can have beneficial effects for the parent, the child, and their relationship. Child–Parent Psychotherapy (CPP), involving joint child–mother sessions with preschoolers and their mothers in the aftermath of father-perpetrated IPV, showed significant decreases in PTSD and other emotional problems in both the child and the mother immediately after the end of treatment and in a 6-month follow-up

(Lieberman, Ghosh Ippen, & Van Horn, 2006; Lieberman, Van Horn, & Ghosh Ippen, 2005). Another intervention, Fathers for Change, is an individual treatment for fathers with histories of IPV and substance abuse that includes optional co-parenting and child–father sessions and that showed postintervention reductions in the father's IPV, PTSD, depression, and anxiety symptoms and improved child symptoms as reported by the child's mothers (Stover & Carlson, 2017).

The effectiveness of interventions with IPV victims and perpetrators calls for their acknowledgment that violence took place and their motivation to change. Systematic screening for IPV should start with the initial clinical assessment, using a nonjudgmental approach that emphasizes conditions of safety for the baby and the parents. Victims and perpetrators may deny or hide IPV due to shame or fear of the consequences of the disclosure. The abstract term IPV is often alien for its victims and its perpetrators, who are more likely to recognize and relate to concrete experiences such as slapping, pushing, hitting, throwing objects, or other forms of physical violence. Clients are more likely to disclose painful, frightening, and dangerous experiences when clinicians use everyday words rather than technical words to inquire about sensitive topics.

Clinicians need to be alert to subtle manifestations of fear, anger, and danger in the intimate relationship between pregnant women and their partners, include regular individual sessions with each partner during the assessment phase, and remain ready to explore this topic supportively throughout the course of treatment.

# The Value of Psychotherapy Starting in Pregnancy

There is substantial empirical evidence demonstrating the success of interventions that begin in pregnancy and continue after the baby's birth. These interventions share the goal of promoting maternal and infant health and well-being but differ in theoretical orientation, intervention focus and modalities, inclusion of father, format (for example, home visiting versus office based), professional discipline of the intervention provider, number of providers, and length of the intervention. The *Nurse–Family Partnership* (Olds et al., 2007) is a 2-year home visiting psychoeducational intervention provided by nurses to first-time mothers living in poverty that starts during pregnancy and focuses on promoting healthy maternal behaviors, enhancing maternal sensitivity, teaching effective parenting skills, and improving the maternal life course through family planning, stable work, and educational attainment. This program improves a large number of both maternal and child outcomes (Kitzman et al., 2010), but research shows limited effects in reducing the incidence of child abuse and neglect when there is IPV in the home (Eckenrode et al., 2000). *Minding the Baby* (Sadler et al., 2013; Slade et al., 2018, 2019) is an intensive home visiting intervention that focuses on increasing the mother's reflective capacities during pregnancy and through the first 2 years of the child's life through integrated nursing and mental health services provided by a pediatric nurse and a master's-level social worker. Findings show improvements in maternal reflective functioning, higher rates of infant secure attachment, lower rates of disorganized attachment, and lower levels of child protection involvement (Sadler et al., 2013; Slade et al., 2019); at graduation, program toddlers were less likely to be obese (Ordway et al., 2018). At follow-up, preschoolers showed fewer externalizing behaviors (Ordway et al., 2018); school-age children were also less likely to manifest behavioral problems, and their parents were more likely to parent in a supportive and reflective way (Londono Tobon et al., 2018). *Mom Power* is a time-limited intervention that integrates concepts from attachment theory and trauma theory for pregnant women with histories of trauma who are at a high psychiatric risk (Rosenblum et al., 2017). It consists of a 10-week group model led by two group facilitators and includes three individual sessions that allow for an individually tailored approach. Groups comprise six to eight mothers, who are invited to bring their children under age 6 to the sessions. The groups begin with a shared meal, followed by separate Mom Power groups and child groups and then by a reunion. A randomized controlled trial found improvements in mental health symptoms, reflective capacity, parenting stress, and maternal representations (Rosenblum et al., 2017).

Interventions that include fathers are also available. The *Supporting Father Involvement (SFI)* intervention project, sponsored by the California Office of Child Abuse Prevention to reduce child abuse and maltreatment risk factors, involved low-income couples from a range of ethnic and racial backgrounds who were collaborating in the care of their young child, whether or not they were married or living together (Cowan, Cowan, Pruett, & Pruett, 2019). Fathers were recruited directly by the staff from family resource centers, schools, and child welfare services who highlighted the father's importance to the well-being of his child and his partner. The 16-session curriculum focused on domains empirically connected to the reduction of child abuse. These domains include parents' individual well-being such as depression and anxiety; co-parenting and parenting discipline, parenting styles, and stress; the couple relationship, including conflict, communication, and problem-solving style; intergenerational influences; and the balance between life stress and social support from family, friends, and organizations. Findings showed significant reductions in couple conflict, which was in turn related to decreases in both parents' anxious and harsh parenting and their children's internalizing and externalizing behavioral problems (Cowan et al., 2019). *Figuring It Out for the Child (FIOC)* is a time-limited intervention conducted with unmarried African American parents expecting their first child together and offered during the second and third trimesters of pregnancy (McHale, Salman-Engin, & Coovert, 2015). It is an adaptation of Focused Coparenting Consultation (FCC) for pregnancy, initially developed for parents living together and later expanded to include divorced parents and unmarried parents living apart. The guiding premise is that even parents who experience acrimony in their personal relationship with each other can collaborate effectively as co-parents when they are committed to setting aside their mutual animosities and creating a protective family structure that serves the child's best interests. The intervention is based on family therapy and brief psychotherapy conceptual frameworks and promotes mindfulness, empathy, and conscious awareness by guiding parents through structured exercises that help them make intergenerational connections to their own experiences of being co-parented as children, highlight similarities and differences in parenting perspectives, and practice problem solving and conflict resolution. Unmarried parents expecting their first child who completed the intervention together showed reductions in negative behavior and improved co-parenting communication and problem solving as observed during mother–father conflict discussions (McHale et al., 2015).

## Attending to the Experience of Trauma in Clinical Interventions

The consensus that trauma is both prevalent and harmful to physical and mental health has spurred the recognition that best medical and mental health practice should include routine screening for childhood adversity and exposure to violence both in the past and in the present (Burke Harris, 2018). This is not a new insight. As early as 2006, Steven Sharfstein announced the formation of an American Psychiatric Association task force to address the effects of violence on children with the statement that "interpersonal violence, especially violence experienced by children, is the largest single preventable cause of mental illness. What cigarette smoking is to the rest of medicine, early childhood violence is to psychiatry" (Sharfstein, 2006).

In spite of this knowledge, trauma screening continues to be inconsistent at best in medical and mental health practice. The reasons include service providers' reluctance to ask, insufficient training about *how* to ask, uncertainty about what to do with the information that may emerge in response to asking, scarcity of trauma-informed services to refer people who disclose trauma exposure, and a lack of training in trauma-informed therapeutic approaches among mental health providers. These obstacles are stark reminders that trauma screening is a necessary but not sufficient first step in addressing the lasting sequelae of trauma on a person's physical and emotional health. Once screening identifies trauma exposure, it is also necessary to provide trauma-informed assessment and treatment. The next section provides an overview of the specific features of trauma-informed mental health interventions.

## What Is Unique about Trauma-Informed Treatment?

Trauma treatment cannot be "treatment as usual" because the threat that trauma poses to survival and personal integrity becomes a powerful organizer of personal meaning and pervades all aspects of personality and daily functioning. Trauma evokes intense feelings of terror, horror, helplessness, rage, and the wish for revenge. It transforms previous expectations of safety and danger to such an extent that following a traumatic event the person may misperceive safe situations as threatening while dangerous situations may be mistaken as safe. These distorted perceptions may make the person respond to neutral situations as if they represented personal threats, engaging in behaviors that appear to be impulsive, aggressive, or self-endangering, but can be understood as misguided efforts at self-protection when assessed from the perspective of traumatic expectations.

The biologically rooted survival behaviors of "fight, flight, and freeze" are internalized in the form of coping mechanisms involving aggression, emotional withdrawal, and dissociation in response to situations that are reminders of the trauma. Traumatic reminders—also known as "traumatic triggers"—operate mostly outside consciousness and influence behavior in ways that seem incomprehensible to the individual and others unless they understand how the behavior originated in the traumatic experience.

The biological imprint of traumatic responses is manifest in changes in the physiology of stress and fear among traumatized adults, including structural and functional brain changes and neuroendocrine alterations in cortisol and norepinephrine levels that hamper the effectiveness of the stress response system (Olff, Langeland, & Gersons, 2005; Yehuda & LeDoux, 2007). Focusing only on behavioral change can be ineffective or insufficient in managing traumatic responses because these body-based automatic reflexes operate independently of the individual's conscious efforts. The failure to bring about behavioral change may in turn perpetuate the feelings of impotence, guilt, shame, rage, and self-blame that so often torment survivors of acute and chronic trauma before they find coping strategies that support their recovery (Pynoos, Steinberg, & Piacentini, 1999; van der Kolk, 2014).

Trauma-informed treatment involves a systematic approach to understanding whether the presenting symptoms may be an expression of trauma exposure. The *Diagnostic and Statistical Manual of Mental Disorders* (5th ed.; DSM-5) defines a traumatic event as exposure to actual or threatened death, serious injury, or sexual violence by direct experience, witnessing the event, learning that it occurred to a close family member or close friend in a violent or accidental manner, and/or repeated or extreme exposure to aversive details of the traumatic events (American Psychiatric Association, 2013).

Trauma-informed assessment and treatment involves a systematic identification of the possible links between traumatic events and presenting symptoms, because these links enable the clinician to target for intervention the specific traumatic reminders that trigger maladaptive perceptions, feelings, thoughts, and behavior. There can be profound therapeutic value in the ostensibly simple therapeutic intervention of helping clients explore the potential relationships between what happened to them and the symptoms that brought them to treatment. One of the most insidious effects of trauma exposure is cognitive and emotional disorganization, which happens because the person is flooded by the bombardment of overpowering sensory stimuli that occur in the traumatic moment (terror from seeing, hearing, smelling, tasting, moving, and touching). Self-protective efforts to cope with these overwhelming experiences involve automatic freezing, fleeing, or fighting, and these instinctive responses are cut off from the logical thought processes that in everyday life give meaning to experiences. The crippling shame and guilt that often accompany unresolved trauma can be relieved when people understand that their present suffering might stem from the enduring emotional impact of events that created past suffering. Helping the person recognize the impact of trauma on self-perception and behavior is a prerequisite for the recovery process.

There are significant commonalities among the diversity of approaches to the treatment of trauma, all of which involve helping the person recognize the impact of trauma on different aspects of functioning and creating strategies to promote physical and relational safety and affect regulation. The common features of treatment modalities target symptoms of traumatic response and are briefly listed below (Marmar, Foy, Kagan, & Pynoos, 1993):

1. Return to normal development, adaptive coping, and engagement with present activities and future goals.
2. Increased capacity to respond realistically to threat without minimizing danger or over-reacting to it.
3. Maintaining regular levels of affective arousal by identifying and addressing hyperarousal, numbing, and other forms of emotional dysregulation.
4. Reestablishing trust in bodily sensations by cultivating safe body-based experiences of pleasure.
5. Restoration of reciprocity in intimate relationships by promoting safe conflict resolution and problem-solving strategies.
6. Normalization of the traumatic response by framing trauma responses as understandable responses to imminent and unpredictable danger.
7. Increasing the capacity to differentiate between reliving and remembering by identifying traumatic triggers and responses to them.
8. Placing the traumatic experience in perspective by acknowledging its impact without becoming the defining feature of the person's life and personal identity.

Section II describes P-CPP as a trauma-informed treatment and preventive intervention that is guided by these goals and mechanisms, and that starts in pregnancy and continues into the baby's first year. The impact of interpersonal violence on the well-being of pregnant women and their offspring makes it imperative to ask pregnant women referred for treatment about their trauma exposure both during childhood and in the present. We argue that prenatal care should include routine screening for physical, sexual, and emotional maltreatment and other trauma both currently and during childhood, and treatment must include a specific trauma lens when the client reports exposure to traumatic events. This clinical stance aligns with the position of the National Child Traumatic Stress Network (NCTSN; *www.nctsn.org*) about the importance of identifying trauma exposure and providing trauma-informed treatment across the age range.

# Section II

# Perinatal Child–Parent Psychotherapy

P-CPP is a relationship-based, trauma-informed treatment and preventive intervention that begins during pregnancy and continues after the baby's birth. Treatment during pregnancy may include the woman and her partner, either individually and/or together depending on clinical considerations. The baby is consistently included as an integral participant of treatment, using a dyadic or triadic format after the baby's birth, depending on whether one or both parents participate in treatment. The length of treatment takes clinical considerations into account. The clinician conducts a comprehensive evaluation of the parent(s) and infant when the baby is 6 months old, and the treatment comes to a close at that time if the parents are providing safe, protective, and loving care and if the baby is developing as expected. When clinical concerns remain at the 6-month assessment, the clinician ascertains the clinically appropriate next steps and provides this feedback to the parent(s) to plan for an appropriate course of action. Options may include continued P-CPP, individual psychotherapy for one or both parents, couple therapy, developmentally focused interventions if the baby is lagging behind in areas of development, and/or other clinically appropriate intervention modalities.

Research findings with mothers who received P-CPP starting in pregnancy and ending when the baby was 6 months old showed significant improvement in depression, PTSD, and parenting attitudes (Lieberman, Diaz, & Van Horn, 2011), with the greatest improvement for those mothers who had the lowest maternal–fetal attachment at intake (Lavi, Gard, Hagan, Van Horn, & Lieberman, 2015). These are promising findings that point to the effectiveness of P-CPP in the treatment of trauma during the perinatal period.

# Therapeutic Context: Basic Principles of Child–Parent Psychotherapy (CPP)

As we have noted, P-CPP is an application to pregnancy and the perinatal period of CPP, a relationship-based, trauma-informed, manualized treatment intervention for trauma-exposed young children in the birth–5 years age range and their primary caregivers (Lieberman & Van Horn, 2005, 2008; Lieberman et al., 2015). Rooted in Selma Fraiberg's (1980) psychoanalytic "ghosts in the nursery" model of the intergenerational transmission of psychopathology, the primary CPP innovation consists of a simultaneous focus on the child's and the parents' dual experience of real-life traumatic events and the impact of their experiences on the child's quality of attachment and the parent's capacity to protect and nurture. Key contextual factors are the child's and parents' developmental stage, the family's cultural background, the interplay of risk and protective social factors that may include the enduring impact of historical trauma, and childrearing attitudes and practices.

CPP shares the therapeutic goals and mechanisms of other trauma-informed treatment approaches described in "What Is Unique about Trauma-Informed Treatment?" in Section I (Marmar et al., 1993), but uses the parent–child relationship as the preferred vehicle for implementation, because the attachment relationship is the most powerful mutative factor in young children's development. CPP includes six conceptual premises that frame the mental health of infants and young children in the context of their relationships with their parents and other primary caregivers (Lieberman et al., 2015):

- *Premise 1.* The attachment system is the main organizer of children's responses to danger and safety in the first years of life.
- *Premise 2.* Emotional and behavioral problems in infancy and early childhood are more likely to improve when the child's attachment figures are proactively engaged in the treatment.
- *Premise 3.* The cultural and socioeconomic ecology of the family must inform all clinical formulations and treatment plans.
- *Premise 4.* Interpersonal violence is a traumatic stressor that harms those who witness it as well as those who experience it, with the result that witnessing IPV, community violence, civil disorder, and war is pathogenic for children and their parents.

- *Premise 5.* The empathic quality of the therapeutic relationship is a fundamental mutative factor in treatment.
- *Premise 6.* Effective treatment must include identifying traumatic experiences and a supportive approach to "speaking the unspeakable" as core mechanisms to correct negative attributions and pathogenic beliefs, promote safety, and instill hope.

This section provides a brief synopsis of CPP as relevant context for the theoretical orientation and clinical principles of P-CPP, because throughout pregnancy, the P-CPP clinician must keep in mind how the expectant parents' clinical presentation might affect their capacity to provide safe caregiving that prevents trauma exposure and promotes the baby's capacity to love and learn. After the baby's birth, the clinician shifts the primary focus of therapeutic attention to the mother's and father's quality of parenting and uses what the parents reveal as a guide to addressing the obstacles that interfere with protective and emotionally invested caregiving.

CPP's therapeutic modalities are versatile and tailored to the specific clinical case formulation and clinically salient themes. The basic treatment format includes joint sessions with the child and the primary caregiver, but both parents, siblings, and/or other key family members may join either consistently or intermittently depending on the family circumstances and clinical needs. The CPP manual describes these basic therapeutic modalities, which include psychodynamic interpretation, unstructured developmental guidance, somatic processing, and cognitive-behavioral strategies in the context of emotional support and developmental and cultural considerations (Lieberman et al., 2015). The application of these therapeutic modalities in P-CPP is described in later sections.

CPP has shown efficacy in five randomized studies conducted with multicultural samples of varied socioeconomic status and risk factors, which consistently demonstrated significant improvements in biomarkers of stress, quality of attachment, perception of self and others, clinical symptoms, and cognitive functioning (Lieberman et al., 2015; Toth, Michl-Petzing, Guild, & Lieberman, 2018).

# The Theory and Practice of P-CPP

As a CPP extension into pregnancy and the postnatal period, P-CPP is trauma-informed, grounded in psychoanalysis and attachment theory, and guided in its clinical application by developmental and cultural considerations that include attention to historical trauma as a possible factor in the etiology of the presenting problems (Lieberman, Diaz, & Van Horn, 2009; Narayan, Oliver Bucio, Rivera, & Lieberman, 2016). P-CPP conceptualizes becoming a parent as a key phase of adult development and aims to promote psychic reorganization by addressing the traumatic triggers and psychological conflicts that emerge during the unfolding stages of pregnancy and thereafter. The goals of treatment are to ensure safety, foster affect regulation, and prepare the expectant woman and man to become protective and loving parents. The clinical focus is initially on the experience of pregnancy, influenced by the real-life experiences of the parents and each parent's fantasies, fears, attributions, and hopes for the unborn child. After the baby's birth, the therapeutic focus turns to the experience of what happened during labor and delivery, perception of the newborn baby, and the harmonies and dissonances of the rhythms co-created between mother, father, and baby.

## The Origins of Perinatal Child–Parent Psychotherapy (P-CPP): Perinatal IPV in the Context of Adversity and Trauma

P-CPP originated in findings from a randomized CPP study with preschoolers exposed to IPV against their mothers, who in a high percentage of cases disclosed that their partner's violence started during their pregnancy (Lieberman et al., 2005). This finding launched a secondary prevention effort to recruit and provide treatment to pregnant women who disclosed IPV in the course of receiving prenatal care (Lavi et al., 2015; Lieberman et al., 2011).

Data from the first 41 pregnant women referred for treatment showed that other traumatic stressors in addition to IPV were also common in the women's early life and in the present, including childhood physical, sexual, and emotional abuse; victimization by crime; witnessing community violence; accidental injury; and traumatic separation and/or loss of one or more attachment figures. All the women in this clinical sample were low income and publicly insured, and only 24% were working. About half of the women (40%) were expecting their first child. More than half of the women (52%) experienced pregnancy complications during the current pregnancy, with vaginal bleeding and hypertension as the most frequent problems. The majority also reported clinical symptoms of depression (73%) and PTSD (60%). About half of the women (48%) reported living with the baby's father. Only 26% reported using birth control, and 69% reported that the pregnancy was unplanned, representing an additional stress in already difficult socioeconomic circumstances. An unexpected finding was the self-report that 30% of the women engaged in physical violence against their partners by slapping, shoving, or throwing objects at them. The use of knives, guns, or other lethal objects was infrequent, but a few women reported that their violent actions led to their partners' severe injury and hospitalization. This finding underscores the importance of assessing and treating maternal and mutual violence in addition to the violence perpetrated by the male partner when working with battered women and their young children.

Another study involving 101 low-income pregnant women replicated the finding of a high prevalence of multiple adversities and trauma preceding and during pregnancy (Narayan et al., 2017). This was a nonclinical sample, and the only criteria for inclusion were that the woman was pregnant, 18 years or older, and spoke English or Spanish. Participants responded to flyers posted in the women's clinic and the pediatric clinic of a public health hospital. Although this sample of women were not seeking mental health services, almost half of the participants reported clinical levels of depression, one third reported clinical levels of PTSD, and more than half reported a lifetime exposure to IPV, both as victims and as perpetrators. More than half also reported growing up with at least four adverse childhood experiences (ACEs) and at least two forms of childhood maltreatment, a finding associated with negative health outcomes in previous research (Dube et al., 2002). Their experiences of pregnancy were often difficult, with 62% reporting that the current pregnancy was unplanned, 44% reporting at least one unwanted pregnancy in their lifetime, 14% reporting IPV from their partners, and 20% reporting IPV against their partners in the current pregnancy. These findings lead us to conclude that prenatal clinics should expand the definition of what constitutes a clinical population of pregnant women to identify and address risk factors and to offer services that include reproductive health and perinatal mental health.

## An Integrated Model of Care: Embedding P-CPP in Prenatal Medical Care

While developing the P-CPP model, we found that the women's experience of trauma influenced their choices for primary care, both for themselves and for their babies. They tended to start prenatal care late in the second trimester or in the third trimester of pregnancy, and many of them used the emergency room rather than regular pediatric appointments for their infants' health care, resulting in less appropriate pediatric care and posing a burden for the increasingly stressed public health system. When asked about their reasons for choosing the emergency room, the mothers said that clinic-based care was for serious medical problems only, and they worried that regular contact with the medical system increased their chances of doctors or nurses reporting them to child protective services or to immigration authorities.

The mothers' worries were understandable in the context of concerted federal efforts at present to deport undocumented immigrants and the lack of cultural understanding, unconscious bias, and institutionalized racism that often permeate systems of care. In the hurried pace of medical clinics, with long waits and overburdened primary care providers, there is often little time for meaningful doctor–patient communication and exploration of different perspectives. Cultural factors, including unfamiliarity with the U.S. health care system among immigrants, can lead to misunderstandings between mothers and pediatric providers. Lack of knowledge and belief in conspiracy theories are also factors. For example, some mothers worried that vaccinations could cause AIDS or that bringing a healthy baby to the pediatric clinic could make the baby sick from exposure to pathogens. Many mothers believed that their pediatric providers discriminated against them by not offering the expected treatment, for example, by not prescribing antibiotics to treat a baby's flu symptoms. The health providers at times voiced negative perceptions of the mothers. Even medical providers who were committed to under-served populations sometimes expressed the opinion that the mothers were neglectful when they did not comply with medical recommendations, especially if language or other cultural barriers made it difficult to understand the reasons for the mothers' behavior.

Maternal descriptions of their attitudes toward medical care highlighted the importance of understanding the cultural background for their choices. This understanding enables P-CPP clinicians to serve as cultural mediators between parents and pediatric care providers.

Active engagement with primary care providers to foster better communication between doctors and nurses and their patients is an integral component of P-CPP. Clinicians take the time to understand the specifics of mutual misconceptions between parents and primary care providers and to help frame them in a cultural context that avoids blaming either side.

## Pillars of a Therapeutic Attitude

All psychotherapies share a commitment to human values of emotional support, empathic understanding, and relief of suffering. This attitude is necessary but not sufficient to promote positive change. Clinicians need to cultivate specific therapeutic skills to convert their emotional commitment into effective mental health practice. CPP and P-CPP adopted the following easy-to-remember mottos to guide intervention.

- *Notice feelings in the moment.* This pillar involves attunement to present emotional experience as a port of entry to understanding. It also involves tracking body movement and posture as other ports of entry to identifying the manifestations of traumatic reminders and other strong emotions in the body.
- *Speak the unspeakable: Dare to use concrete words to describe the trauma.* Guilt and shame can silence a person's voice. Hearing the clinician model how to articulate unspeakable experiences, overwhelming feelings, and bodily reactions using a calm and supportive stance can normalize the experience and restore a sense of belonging rather than alienation from self and others.
- *Find connections between experiences.* Following the person's free associative flow of thoughts and feelings can guide the clinician to an understanding of unconscious motives, fears, and wishes and make them amenable to reflection and the creation of new meaning.
- *Remember the suffering under the rage.* Anger is often a form of self-protection against unmanageable fear. Offering protection, safety, and understanding helps to modulate rage, promotes self-understanding, and relieves shame and guilt.
- *Seek out the benevolence in the conflict.* Bitter disagreements often stem from a clash between competing but equally legitimate values and priorities. Bowlby (1969) described security of attachment after infancy as a "goal-corrected partnership" in which both partners endeavor to negotiate mutually acceptable solutions when conflicts arise. Building reciprocal emotional relationships involves a conscious effort to

understand and legitimize the other's perspective even when it is not feasible to agree with it.

• *Offer kindness.* This component of the therapeutic attitude involves remaining empathically curious and nonjudgmental. Kindness and compassion generate healing by relieving the self-recrimination, shame, and guilt that are universal components of traumatic stress.

• *Encourage hope.* Trusting that things can get better provides the emotional energy and commitment to action to make it happen. The effectiveness of treatment relies on trust in the possibility of improving the present and the future. Clinicians need to foster this trust by noticing and highlighting examples of the treatment participants' strengths and harnessing these examples to the goals of treatment.

### Addressing Defenses: Negative Parental Attributions and Projective Identification

Children and parents influence each other through verbal and nonverbal interactions involving cycles of synchronicity, disruption, and repair that often occur outside consciousness (Beebe, Lachmann, & Jaffe, 1997; Emde, 1990; Stern, 1995). These interactive patterns are internalized through repetition into mental representations that become internal working models of the self in relation to others, shaping attitudes and behaviors that regulate emotional closeness as a hallmark of danger or protection (Bowlby, 1980).

Parental attributions to the child are one manifestation of these mental representations, defined as fixed beliefs about the child's existential core that the parent holds as if these perceptions were objective and accurate appraisals of the child's essence. Babies have immense meaning for their parents. They can become in the parents' minds the carriers of what is best in themselves and the hope for the fulfillment of what has remained unrealized in their own lives. This emotional investment gives rise to positive attributions that engender joy and reciprocity in the parent–child relationship. Babies can also become the recipients of the parents' most painfully hidden impulses and fears when the child embodies repressed or disowned parts of the parents' sense of self. These negative attributions can be more or less rigid or amenable to correction in response to disconfirming data; they can also be relatively contained or permeate the parent's entire perception of the child. Negative attributions often begin during pregnancy and may change or become entrenched when the imagined baby becomes a real human being after the birth.

Early negative attributions can have a powerful impact on parental behavior from the first moments after the baby's birth. The traits attributed to the infant help determine how the parent perceives the baby's signals and responds contingently or misinterprets or ignores these cues. Daniel Stern (1985) coined the term *selective attunement* to describe how mothers shape their babies' subjective experiences by responding to some kinds of cues but not to others and by projecting their own fantasies, desires, fears, and prohibitions into the baby's emerging sense of what feelings and behaviors are allowed and what is not allowed. Christopher Bollas (1987) used the compelling image of the mother as a "transformational object" whose actions shape the baby's sense of self. The same is true of fathers, who also engage in selective attunement and also form and transform the baby's sense of self.

Projective identification is a powerful defense that gives rise to negative parental attributions. Melanie Klein (1946/1980) is the originator of this important clinical construct, which received multiple elaborations in subsequent years (e.g., Bion, 1959; Ogden, 1982; Seligman, 1999; Silverman & Lieberman, 1999). P-CPP considers that projective identification is a core mechanism in the intergenerational transmission of trauma. Parents can feel intolerable unconscious memories in response to their infants' states of helplessness, dysregulation, or rage. The baby's inconsolable crying or angry rejection of the parent's caregiving efforts when these ministrations do not meet the baby's unarticulated but urgently felt need can trigger the parent's body-based memories of having been ignored, punished, or rejected. The parent may then respond in the punitive, frightening ways she experienced as a child. This identification with the aggressor protects the parent from reexperiencing her childhood terror but does so at the cost of inducing in her child the fear and anxiety that she is unable to tolerate in herself.

It is important to remember that the *events* of abuse, neglect, abandonment, loss, violence, or other trauma may be clearly remembered; what is absent from consciousness is the *affective experience* associated with those violations. P-CPP monitors parental negative attributions and their behavioral expression as a defense against the affective experience and engages the parent in tracing the origins of these expressions, giving words to previously unspeakable experiences as the key to interrupting the transmission of past trauma onto the present baby. Selma Fraiberg wrote, "Our hypothesis is that access to childhood pain becomes a powerful deterrent against repetition in parenting, while repression and isolation of painful affect provide the psychological requirements for identification with the betrayers and the aggressors" (1980, p. 195). P-CPP endeavors to guide the parents in gaining access to their childhood pain as the pathway to healing for the parent and protection for the baby.

# P-CPP Therapeutic Modalities

Trauma-informed treatment is based on the premise that the negative impact of traumatic experiences are alleviated when the client can integrate body-based sensations, feelings, and thinking into a set of coherent trauma narratives and protective narratives that promote realistic meaning making; foster appropriate self-protection; and relieve pathogenic self-blame, shame, and guilt. P-CPP applies and extends the CPP intervention modalities to promote the parent's physical and emotional health, bonding with the fetus, and protective attunement to the baby's signals; to promote eliminating or decreasing negative parental attributions and maladaptive caregiving practices; and to promote fostering a constructive parenting partnership between the baby's mother and father. The following sections describe each of the therapeutic modalities deployed toward these objectives.

It is important to note that not every P-CPP clinician uses all these modalities. Like all clinicians, P-CPP clinicians may prefer and be particularly skilled at a subset of these modalities. Beyond the individual differences among clinicians, different clinical needs call for different strategies or combinations of strategies depending on what seems to be the best fit with the wishes and personal style of the parents. The common denominator linking all the modalities are the shared objectives of addressing parental emotional problems and promoting the mother–infant, father–infant, and mother–father–infant protective and nurturing relationships both during pregnancy and after the baby's birth.

## *Emotion Regulation*

Emotion regulation consists of "the processes by which individuals influence which emotions they have, when they have them, and how they experience and express these emotions" (Gross, 1998, p. 275). The ability to manage emotions entails the capacity to identify, express, and modulate emotional experience. Many therapeutic interventions include an emotion regulation component in response to evidence that deficits in this area play a central role in the etiology and symptomatology of various mental health problems (Gratz & Tull, 2010). These interventions are associated with improvements in physical health and psychological functioning and decreases in symptoms of stress, depression, anxiety, PTSD, and other conditions (Baer, 2003; Gratz & Gunderson, 2006; Grossman, Niemann, Schmidt, & Walach, 2004; Hofmann, Sawyer, Witt, & Oh, 2010; Kimbrough, Magyari, Langenberg, Chesney, & Berman, 2009).

Cultures have evolved a variety of practices that have an implicit affect regulation outcome while addressing different values and needs. Exercise, sports, dance, and music are prime examples. Religious or spiritual rituals and practices help calm the body as well as the spirit. Some specific examples include the observance of Shabbat and prayers that mark specific times of the day to sanctify time in Judaism; praying the rosary in Catholicism; ritual ablutions for purification before daily prayer in Islam; small acts of charity that punctuate daily activities, such as the offering of flowers or foods to the gods and offerings of a little water in memory of the ancestors in Hinduism; and silent meditation in Buddhism. Many parents report that prayer is a source of great comfort and helps them maintain emotional balance or restore serenity at times of fear or distress. P-CPP supports parents in their personal practice of activities that help them cultivate spiritual meaning and maintain emotion regulation.

The emotion regulation modality adopted in P-CPP incorporates body-based practices to help the parents become aware of negative affective and bodily sensations that interfere with emotion regulation, cognitive coherence, and goal-oriented behavior.

*Tracking/tracing of feelings and bodily sensations* is a method used to observe the parent's verbal and nonverbal behavior, including facial expression, vocal tone, movements, and body posture as they occur in the moment. When dysregulation in these areas interferes with therapeutic goals, the clinician may guide the parent's attention to the bodily sensations and encourage reflection on the emerging feelings and associations, a process that may lead to the retrieval of painful or traumatic memories that can promote insight and bring about experiential relief.

During the postpartum period, *tracking/tracing* in the session aims to uncover the origins in the parent's past of present feelings and behaviors toward the baby, including attributing to the baby adult characteristics (such as being manipulative, aggressive, or greedy) that lead to ignoring the baby's needs or responding in ways that exacerbate those needs. For example, the clinician tracks the mother's or father's affect and its manifestations in body postures and movements as they interact with the baby, and when these interactions are aversive the clinician may direct the parents' attention to their bodies and ask them to describe how they are feeling in the moment, both emotionally and physically. The clinician then uses the new understandings emerging from this conversation to engage the parent in creating and practicing more lovingly reciprocal ways of relating with the baby. These new forms of interaction become self-sustaining, because the baby's positive response reinforces the parents' pleasure in their own competence and in their growing intimacy with the baby. Through this practice, the clinician brings the parents' attention to the present and helps them differentiate between remembering their painful past experiences and reliving/reenacting them in the moment through emotional and somatic dysregulation with the baby.

This approach also relies on using observations of the parent's behavior to provide psychoeducation about the mind–body relationship, offering specific examples of how it helps to explain the mother's somatic and emotional difficulties in the perinatal period. During pregnancy, the woman learns that her body is the first to respond to stress through physiological changes that manifest as symptoms of pain, fatigue, muscle tension, headaches, sadness, and other painful feelings and sensations. When somatic symptoms are a prevalent manifestation of emotional distress, the clinician may ask the woman to mentally scan her body for areas of tension and discomfort, an exercise that teaches her to "actively listen" to what her body is communicating to her through physical signs and symptoms. As the woman becomes more aware of how her body signals stress, she is better able to recognize these signs when they occur and resort to specific strategies to regulate her emotional state.

*Diaphragmatic breathing,* also called deep abdominal breathing or belly breathing, is a basic relaxation technique that involves the expansion of the abdomen and that can be taught to encourage self-regulation both during the session and in daily life. Before first teaching the exercise, the clinician may use handouts and other visual aids to provide psychoeducation about the features and benefits of diaphragmatic breathing. The clinician then models the exercise and encourages the woman to practice it in the session and at home. Other relaxation techniques involve graduated relaxation, progressive or passive muscle relaxation, and visualization/imagery. Grounding and the creation of visualized safe spaces are particularly helpful to address reexperiencing symptoms. P-CPP clinicians also make referrals when appropriate to programs that offer pregnancy yoga, exercise, meditation, and massage.

*Touch* represents an integral part of the human experience with critically important functions for early development, particularly in the physiological and social–emotional realms. Described as the first act of communication between a mother and her baby, the act of touch represents the earliest and most essential nonverbal means of communication, eliciting not only reciprocal behavioral exchanges between mother and baby, but also influencing the affective quality of these exchanges. Through touch, the infant forms enduring emotional bonds with significant figures that lay the foundation for healthy growth and development. Touch comforts and soothes the infant in times of distress. The lack of adequate social and sensory stimulation that includes touch has detrimental consequences for the physical, cognitive, and social–emotional functioning of young children (Carlson & Earls, 1997; Chugani, Behen, Muzik, Juhász, & Chugani, 2001).

P-CPP implements interventions that encourage touch starting in pregnancy. Traumatic experiences violate the body's sense of integrity, and trauma-related symptoms are frequently manifested or experienced in the body, with the result that the body itself may become "something to be feared and avoided, defensively shutting down sensations and closing off the possibility of intimacy and pleasure with another" (Lieberman & Van Horn, 2005, p. 16). The goal of touch-based interventions is to help the parents reestablish trust in bodily sensations so that they can experience physical intimacy with others, mainly their baby, by realizing that "one can safely touch and be touched and that the pleasure of safe touching is something to be cherished" (Lieberman & Van Horn, 2005, p. 17). The clinician helps the parent achieve this by encouraging free expression of affection through touch. During pregnancy, the clinician acknowledges and provides positive reinforcement when the woman engages in positive tactile communication with her unborn baby (e.g., when she caresses her belly to calm the active fetus). In the postpartum period, the clinician may encourage the parent to hold and rock the baby and carry the baby in ways that are conducive to positive interactions. P-CPP clinicians are also encouraged to be receptive to the mother's physical expression of trust toward the clinician within the boundaries of the therapeutic relationship.

*Infant massage,* perhaps the oldest touch therapy known to humans, may be incorporated in P-CPP due to its many therapeutic benefits. Infant massage involves gentle tactile and kinesthetic stimulation in the form of stroking and rubbing each part of the infant's body, usually applying slight pressure (Bennett, Underdown, & Barlow, 2013; Field, 2014). Frequently called "nurturing touch," infant massage promotes weight gain, less crying, lower salivary cortisol levels, and more alert states in at-risk infants, including preterm infants, infants of depressed mothers, cocaine- and HIV-exposed infants, and infants with different medical conditions (Bennett et al., 2013; Field, Diego, & Hernandez-Reif, 2010; Field, Hernandez-Reif, Diego, Schanberg, & Kuhn, 2005). Infant massage may help the mothers as well. There is research evidence that teaching mothers to massage their infants is effective in improving mood in depressed mothers, increasing maternal warmth, and showing increased attentiveness and more positive affect in the mother–infant interaction (Feijo et al., 2006; Onozawa, Glover, Adams, Modi, & Kumar, 2001).

These findings have clinical implications for treating traumatized mothers who are often depressed and who may struggle in their mothering roles. Infant massage can be particularly useful as a concrete intervention for mothers who find physical contact aversive as the result of coercive sexual experiences and physical abuse. Massaging the baby can offer a developmentally acceptable framework that helps mothers feel safe touching their babies with the protective guidance of the clinician. The infants' increased relaxation and pleasure in response are powerful sources of positive reinforcement for the mother. Infant massage can also become a strategy to soothe the baby that promotes a greater sense of maternal self-efficacy.

P-CPP may incorporate infant massage as an adjunct treatment for traumatized mothers and their infants. P-CPP clinicians may become certified infant massage therapists and offer this modality to mothers who have difficulty holding or touching their babies or whose babies have trouble achieving homeostasis and experience sleep problems, fussiness, and difficulty soothing. Clinicians may also make a referral to a certified infant massage therapist when clinically appropriate. Mothers usually require two-to-three sessions to learn a massage routine for their infants, which they can then practice at home with their babies. During these sessions, the mothers receive instruction and training in how to gently massage different parts of the infant's body. The lessons involve following a particular sequence and massaging the infant at a time when the baby will be most receptive (i.e., active alert or quiet alert behavioral states). The mothers are also encouraged to observe and respond to their infants' cues throughout their interactions and to become aware of how they can positively influence the baby's sensory experiences.

Clinicians should make a careful assessment of the mother's and infant's needs before suggesting infant massage as a possible adjunct modality. Babies vary widely in their needs for tactile experiences and in their response to tactile stimulation (Barnett, 1972). Some infants may dislike tactile stimulation; they may be extremely sensitive to different aspects of touching or may have sensory integration difficulties. Massage may not be appropriate for these infants, and clinicians seeking a way to promote maternal contact should explore other activities that encourage positive mother–infant interaction.

### Unstructured Reflective Developmental Guidance

P-CPP tailors developmental and caregiving information to specific clinical needs to enhance the physical and mental health of the parents and the baby. Many expectant parents have a rudimentary or inaccurate knowledge of pregnancy-related body changes, fetal development, health care considerations, and caregiving during pregnancy and after the baby's birth. Reflective developmental guidance aims to foster in the parents a "theory of mind" attitude wherein interest and empathy for their own and their baby's needs, inner life, and emotional experiences become their prevailing approach in attempting to understand themselves and the baby.

Many mothers report a fear of labor and delivery. First-time mothers are likely to report "fear of the unknown," because experiences surrounding labor and delivery are all novel to them. This attitude is also frequently the case among immigrant mothers, who are often unfamiliar with childbirth medical practices in the United States. The P-CPP clinician elicits the mothers' description of what is happening to their bodies; provides reflective developmental information about the meaning of these changes; and explains medical practices during prenatal care, labor, delivery, and the postpartum period, as well as the reasons for specific medical practices. They also encourage mothers to attend prenatal classes and support groups led by childbirth educators to supplement their knowledge and to obtain additional support, which may be particularly relevant for immigrant mothers who often have inadequate networks of support.

After the baby's birth, the clinician engages the parents in conversations about what the baby's behavior might mean, expanding on the parents' responses to provide developmental information about the baby's capacities. Joint parent–baby sessions provide opportunities to help parents notice the baby's ability to remember; to communicate with crying and other behaviors; to recognize people using sight, hearing, smell, and touch; to feel emotions that include pleasure, joy, fear, distress and pain; and to manifest emerging interpersonal preferences that become attachments in the course of development. The clinician also elicits conversations about feeding, sleeping, bathing, crying, and caregiving routines to offer reflective developmental information as needed.

The process of discovering the infant through loving observation promotes parents' sense of wonder about their baby's capacities to communicate and respond from the first moments after birth. Many P-CPP clinicians incorporate the Newborn Behavioral Observations (NBO) or the Neonatal Behavioral Assessment Scale (NBAS) as adjunct tools to show parents in graphic detail that their babies are born with a repertoire of skills to adapt to their environment, to communicate how they feel, and to adapt to stress (Nugent, Keefer, Minear, Johnson, & Blanchard, 2007). Infant observation, whether spontaneous or involving the use of structured instruments, helps parents to recognize their babies as unique individuals and starts a dialogue about the baby's temperament and the areas of "goodness of fit" and mismatches between infant and parent temperaments. These interventions help normalize infant behavior and have the potential to defuse negative parental attributions.

### Insight-Oriented Interpretation

Insight-oriented interpretations enable the parent to explore the possible links between life events, memories, and feelings that might give meaning to symptoms and to maladaptive reactions. Insight-oriented interpretations also involve exploring traumatic reminders to understand the underlying triggers for dysregulated emotional reactions and incoherent thoughts patterns.

Negative parental attributions are a focal point of therapeutic attention. The clinician monitors the parent's free associations as she or he moves back and forth between different topics both in the past and in the present, seeking the unconscious associations that may guide the parent's speech and behavior. Specific attention is devoted to the possible origins of the parents' negative attributions to the fetus/baby in their unresolved feelings about conflicts, adversities, and traumatic experiences with the purpose of elucidating how these "ghosts in the nursery" may interfere with their emotional claim on the baby (Fraiberg, 1980). Using tactful interpretation can help parents become aware of the unconscious repetition of their past in their present, reframe distorted perceptions of the fetus/baby, clarify the origins of pathogenic beliefs, correct these beliefs in the context of reality testing, and help create a more coherent and self-forgiving sense of self. This psychological reorganization at the individual level extends to the parent's relationship with the baby.

The concept of *angels in the nursery* (Lieberman, Padron, Van Horn, & Harris, 2005) evokes early memories of moments when the parent felt loved, accepted, and protected by a parent or other adult. Just as P-CPP clinicians ask parents about moments of fear, anger, and pain while growing up, clinicians also ask parents to remember benevolent memories from the time when they were children. When parents cannot recover benevolent memories (either because they had few loving experiences or because these are lost to retrieval as a function of trauma), the clinician helps them realize that the baby can represent a new and more fulfilling beginning for memory making. Memories are created constantly, and good moments with the baby in the present can create the kind of memories the parents wish they had while growing up. This aspect of the therapeutic work aims to redirect the parents' psychological energy from despair to hope, helping them to imagine scenes of loving reciprocity with the as-yet-unborn baby and then to enact these scenes after the baby is born.

## Reproductive Health and Family Planning

Unintended and often unwanted pregnancies are common sequelae of childhood trauma, because women may learn that they have no control over their bodies. Sex can be a primary motivation among people of childrearing age, and for that reason family planning values and practices are naturally relevant topics of clinical inquiry during the perinatal period. Sexuality, fertility, family size, birth control, and reproductive choices are often emotionally charged issues that remain unspoken when expectant parents do not know how to address them owing to a lack of information and feelings of powerlessness and shame. There is much potential for emotional growth when the clinician brings these topics up respectfully and tactfully.

Family planning is an extremely complex issue. Psychodynamic processes; real life circumstances; and social, cultural, religious, and political factors contribute consciously and unconsciously to the parents' perceptions of what is right or appropriate and what is immoral or forbidden. The P-CPP clinician explores with the mother-to-be the circumstances of the current pregnancy as a port of entry to learn about her attitudes about her own fertility and childrearing. This is a rich opportunity to help resolve internal conflicts and build a greater sense of personal agency and responsible freedom of choice.

Ultimately, clinicians do not have the moral right to make direct recommendations about family planning issues. It is their professional responsibility, however, to help clients examine their sexual and reproductive behavior when it can have harmful consequences for themselves or their children. This therapeutic endeavor needs to occur in ways that are kind, respectful, and nonjudgmental, but also straightforward and clear-eyed when there is a clinical need for intervention. Treatment providers need to cultivate the courage to examine and address unrealistic fantasies, ambivalence, and unsafe practices. Failure to do so represents an omission of best practice when the parents' histories include unwanted pregnancies; repeated therapeutic abortions; closely spaced young children who are taxing parental resources; and/or children who have been abused, neglected, relinquished, or removed from their care. These events represent risk factors for the unborn baby because parents' attitudes toward their own fertility are good predictors of their attitudes toward childrearing. Family planning is a major clinical issue for many parents, and skilled intervention can have beneficial effects that compensate for the challenge of addressing it.

## Emotional Support and Empathic Communication

All effective therapies require a foundation of trust that evolves from the clinician's emotional availability. Supportive interventions take the form of conveying, through words and actions, sincere caring for the parent and child, a realistic hope that the treatment goals can be achieved, empathic resonance with life circumstances and emotional reactions, noticing and pointing out progress, satisfaction and joy at milestones and achievements, encouraging self-expression, and supporting reality testing (Luborsky, 1984).

## Crisis Intervention and Concrete Assistance with Problems of Living

Real-life circumstances matter, and living conditions help to shape the emotional world of parents and children. Many expectant parents referred for treatment live in precarious financial and social circumstances that drain their proactive energy and contribute to feelings of dejection, helplessness, worry, and despair. Poverty, inadequate housing, lack of a steady income, and the threat of deportation among undocumented immigrants are frequent sources of crippling concern. Clinicians should define their role as attending to the basic needs of parents and infants in addition to their emotional needs, and they should intervene as needed by helping to make safety plans, promoting a resolution of concrete problems, making referrals for needed services, explaining how systems work, and helping to secure material resources.

These interventions are important for promoting safety, health, and well-being, but they are not ends in themselves in the implementation of P-CPP. The clinician needs to remain conscious of her ongoing role as a clinician who uses concrete assistance as a tool to promote inner change and not as a stand-alone intervention. The rationale and methods for concrete assistance occur in partnership *with* the parent, rather than as something that the clinician does *for* the parent. The clinician helps the parents reflect on what they need and how to secure it, and then helps the parents monitor what happened and engage in problem solving. These interventions promote the parent's growth as an increasingly knowledgeable, self-reliant, and competent adult. This is an important developmental process promoted by this intervention modality.

# Implementing P-CPP

P-CPP involves the same treatment phases as CPP (Lieberman et al., 2015). Treatment begins with the referral process because *how* the referral source explains the rationale for recommending treatment to the prospective client affects the perception of treatment and motivation to accept the referral. Following the referral, P-CPP involves the following treatment phases: (1) foundational phase: assessment and engagement, (2) core treatment phase, and (3) recapitulation and termination. The *foundational phase* takes place at best sometime in the first two trimesters of pregnancy to give time to develop a solid therapeutic relationship and start implementing the treatment frame. The *core treatment phase* includes labor and delivery, meeting the baby, and joint sessions with the parent(s) and the baby. The *recapitulation and termination phase* builds on the accomplishments of the core treatment phase to revisit the therapeutic trajectory, reflect on the progress made and the challenges that remain, plan for coping strategies in response to these challenges, and promote sustainability of therapeutic gains.

## The Referral Process

Our model of primary care-mental health collaboration links trauma-trained infant mental health providers, obstetrical providers, and pediatrics. A P-CPP clinician (G. C.) spends time onsite at the OB/GYN clinic, labor and delivery, and NICU to provide mental health consultation to nurses, physicians, and social workers, offer onsite psychoeducation and mental health services to pregnant women, and make referrals for P-CPP when she identifies the need for clinical treatment. Referrals for P-CPP are also made by social workers in the OB/GYN department, who ask pregnant women coming for prenatal care about their emotional state, life circumstances, and exposure to environmental adversities. When a woman reports clinical symptoms or traumatic stressors, the social worker gives a brief description of P-CPP and asks whether she would accept a referral. If the woman agrees, the P-CPP clinician either makes a telephone call or meets her at the following prenatal care appointment to offer weekly counseling through pregnancy and delivery and until the baby is at least 6 months old. After the baby's birth, the pediatric care provider is also included in the service team. All the providers are located at the county general hospital, a colocation that facilitates collaboration.

Although the integration of primary care and mental health is a core value, we regard it as a value-added component rather than an indispensable part of P-CPP. Clinicians can practice P-CPP successfully in a variety of settings, including home visiting programs, community-based clinics, and private practice. Attention to the medical needs of the mother and baby remains an important aspect of best practice regardless of the treatment setting.

## Starting Treatment: P-CPP Foundational Phase

All effective treatments begin with a process of creating a collaborative working relationship that engages the client's motivation and hope for greater well-being. "Getting to know each other" is the first step in this process. Many P-CPP clinicians use this phrase during the first session to describe the first few meetings as a time to think together about what the woman wants and needs, the clinician's ideas about how to best meet those wants and needs, and joint decision making about the next steps, which may involve continued meeting for treatment or other alternatives. For the client and clinician, getting to know each other involves the clinician's ability to provide a clear explanation of the treatment framework, what the clinician will do in her therapeutic role, expectations about the client's participation, and a sense of hope and possibility. For the client, the process involves at least a modicum of trust that the clinician can understand who she is or who they are if she is working with a couple, and guide her or them toward positive change.

P-CPP begins with an extended assessment phase that may last between three and five weekly 60- or 90-minute sessions and is designed to establish the foundations of treatment by developing a clinical formulation, as well as establishing a treatment format (individual and/or with the woman's partner), and treatment plan. In this process, the clinician must balance the importance of obtaining relevant clinical information with the need to respect the woman's timing in self-disclosure. Assessment always goes hand-in-hand with trial interventions to probe for psychological strengths and vulnerabilities, defensive structure, and the most-promising intervention strategies. Therapeutic interventions during this foundational phase have the goal of building the therapeutic relationship while also giving the clinician an understanding of the psychological characteristics of the pregnant woman in the context of her current circumstances and of her experiences both in childhood and as an adult, including her perceptions of the pregnancy and the unborn child. This phase is also the time to broach the feasibility of engaging the woman's partner.

The foundational phase culminates in a feedback session that takes place when the clinician believes that she or he has a clear enough understanding of the issues included in the list of foundational-phase topics to arrive at a preliminary clinical formulation. This emerging clinical understanding becomes the basis for offering feedback and engaging in a joint formulation of the treatment plan.

## Foundational-Phase Topics

• Presentation of P-CPP as an opportunity to prepare for the baby's arrival by reflecting on how the woman is feeling about herself and the people important to her, including the baby and the baby's father.

• Informed consent for treatment and discussion of legal constraints on confidentiality.

• Duration of treatment and an estimated date for the end of treatment, with an explanation that they can be revised as treatment progresses in response to the woman's needs and other considerations, which may involve, for example, agency regulations regarding treatment length and funding sources.

• Circumstances of the pregnancy and whether the woman and her partner have similar or different views about the pregnancy, including whether or not it was planned and wanted by either the woman, her partner, or both; how the woman and her partner each responded to learning about the pregnancy; and how each of them feels about the pregnancy now.

• Relationship with the intimate partner or father of the baby, his personal characteristics as perceived by the mother, IPV risk assessment if clinically appropriate, and consideration of his possible involvement in treatment.

• Specific information about the woman's life history and current circumstances, including her relationship with attachment figures, positive experiences, adversities and traumatic events (including violence in intimate relationships), and a description of current support networks. Structured assessment instruments are clinically useful to elicit systematic information about trauma exposure and life circumstances as a way of creating acceptance for "speaking the unspeakable" and normalizing traumatic events that routinely engender shame and guilt as a painful but frequent aspect of human experience.

• Specific information about the mother's symptoms, with a particular focus on symptoms of depression and posttraumatic stress. A suicide risk assessment should be included if the woman has a history of clinical depression and suicide attempts. Areas to be addressed include perception, attitudes, and feelings about the fetus and hopes and fears for the baby, including positive and negative attributions that reflect the woman's internal world in relation to the fetus and baby-to-be.

• Psychological strengths and vulnerabilities, including a capacity for self-reflection, insightfulness, and affect regulation; defense structure; coping strategies; and openness to trial clinical interpretations.

• The meaning that the woman gives to her real-life circumstances and psychological experiences, including a sense of self as an individual and as a mother; the role of the baby's father; and pathogenic beliefs about herself, the baby and others that may interfere with psychological growth and the capacity to love.

• Cultural background, including historical trauma and culturally rooted values and attitudes about pregnancy and childrearing practices and acculturation level.

## Tailoring the Foundational Phase to the Stages of Pregnancy

Women who experienced physical or sexual violence, whether as children or adults, may become emotionally disorganized when the physical sensations that accompany pregnancy become trauma reminders, as may be the case with—for example—fetal movements or with the repeated medical examinations that are part of routine prenatal care.

Different issues may emerge depending on the stage of pregnancy. When the referral occurs during the *first trimester,* the woman may still be grappling with the circumstances of the pregnancy, her own emotional response, her partner's reactions, her family's responses, whether she wants to keep the pregnancy, and the emerging realization of how the new baby will change her life. In the *second trimester,* positive and negative attributions to the fetus usually become more distinct in response to the growing reality of the baby. Women may attribute malevolent intentions to the fetus, equating the unborn baby to the trauma perpetrators in their present or their past. At the same time, women form a more specific attachment to the fetus as it becomes more real through its physical growth and increasing movement. Positive, negative, or contradictory feelings and perceptions may coexist outside awareness when the woman's defense mechanisms involve avoidance, splitting, isolation of affect, dissociation, or depersonalization. Other women may feel consciously conflicted between love, fear, anger, and even hate. When the referral takes place in the *third semester* and close to labor and delivery, fears about childbirth or conflicts about becoming a mother may predominate in the clinical presentation. Women may have conscious or unconscious self-perceptions of being physically damaged persons, fear that that they will be harmed by labor and delivery, or worry that their damaged bodies may harm the fetus. They may also fear that they will repeat their childhood abuse by maltreating their babies.

The fluidity of emotional life means that any and all of the themes that predominate at the different stages of pregnancy may recur or disappear at subsequent stages. The clinician needs to be mindful of these themes while exploring the key topics of the foundational phase. Foundational-phase intervention strategies are geared to the specific clinical issues that emerge, while also helping the woman learn self-regulation strategies to regain a sense of calm when dysregulated; engage in problem solving about concrete life decisions; and anticipate the themes that will emerge as treatment progresses, including preparing for labor and delivery and for life with the baby.

## Feedback Session: Presenting the Clinical Formulation Triangle

An overriding consideration during the foundational phase is to ensure that the clinician gathers information and offers initial interpretations in a collaborative manner that helps the woman gain a growing understanding of the links between what happened to her, the feelings and symptoms that she is experiencing in the present, and the strategies she developed to cope with her circumstances. Throughout the foundational phase, the clinician engages in therapeutic strategies that begin to contextualize and normalize the traumatic response, differentiate between reliving and remembering, promote self-understanding and emotional regulation, and address distorted perceptions of the fetus as understandable but inaccurate generalizations of the woman's traumatic responses that will be explored during treatment. The feedback session is an opportunity to bring together all the pieces that emerged in previous sessions into a coherent narrative that will provide the rationale for the invitation to treatment.

The clinician begins the feedback session by asking the woman about her experience of the previous few sessions and what she learned about herself. The woman's response becomes the matrix for presenting the clinician's perspective, affirming and elaborating on points of agreement, raising the need to explore pathogenic beliefs, and presenting possible connections between real-life experiences and the woman's psychological state.

The clinical formulation is described in shorthand as "the formulation triangle" (see Figure 1) because it links external reality, internal reality, and the treatment goals of creating safety, fostering protective attachments, and promoting well-being for the parent(s) and the baby.

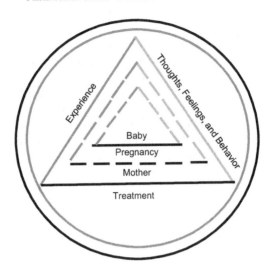

**FIGURE 1.** P-CPP clinical formulation triangle. Based on Lieberman, Ghosh Ippen, & Van Horn (2015, p. 85).

The clinician needs to think of this formulation as the elaboration of nested triangles involving the following components:

1. Links between the woman's real-life experiences, her psychological makeup, and treatment goals.
2. Links between the woman's psychological makeup, her attributions and feelings about the fetus, and treatment goals.
3. Links between the woman's attributions and feelings about the fetus, her emotional readiness to be a mother, and treatment goals.

### Clinical Illustration of the Foundational Phase with a Single Mother: Susan

The foundational phase with a single mother named Susan illustrates how the clinician used the emerging clinical material to promote increasing maternal self-awareness and improve self-care during the foundational phase. Susan was 12 weeks pregnant when the OB/GYN medical social worker referred her after she reported a recent separation from her abusive partner and moderate levels of depressive symptomatology. Susan was a 29-year-old European American woman with two older children, who at the time of the referral was living in an IPV shelter with her children. The social worker described Susan as difficult to engage and noncompliant with treatment for her recently diagnosed gestational diabetes, as shown in her not monitoring her blood glucose levels, failing to keep prenatal care appointments, and missing several sessions with the nutritionist. The social worker reported that the medical providers viewed Susan as "negligent" for not following medical orders and placing her fetus at risk, and commented that she was pleasantly surprised when Susan agreed to the referral to our clinic to help with her feelings of depression.

## GETTING TO KNOW EACH OTHER

In the first meeting with the P-CPP clinician (M. A. D.), Susan disclosed that her pregnancy was unplanned and initially unwanted, that she had considered abortion but did not follow through with the referral due to her Christian religious beliefs, and that she was now struggling with anger and fear about how she would raise three children with her meager income as a waitress. The clinician validated her concerns and said that she and Susan could meet for a few sessions to get to know each other, think together about Susan's needs as a person and as a mother, and make a plan about the best strategies to meet her and her children's needs.

In the course of the initial two sessions, Susan reported growing up in an area of the city ravaged by poverty where community violence was a daily occurrence. She and her two older sisters were raised by their single mother, whom she described as "*someone who was very cold, unaffectionate, and always working.*" She recounted that her mother was away for weeks at a time and left Susan under the care of her two teenage sisters, who often left her alone at home from a very young age. When she was 7 years old alone at home, Susan burned herself with boiling water while trying to make soup; the burn left a large visible scar on her left arm that she showed to the clinician with a mixture of anger and shame. The clinician looked closely at the scar and said how sad and wrong it was that Susan did not receive the care that she needed as a little girl and had hurt herself in a way that left lasting marks in trying to take care of herself.

When the clinician asked Susan about her father, she became tearful and expressed intense sorrow when disclosing that she last saw her father when she was 6 years old. She had a vivid memory of how her mother "*kicked him out of the house*" following a fight in which her mother blamed his addiction to alcohol for their precarious economic situation. Susan added sadly that to this day she did not know what had happened to her father, who in her words "*vanished*" from her life after this incident. The question of what happened to her father remained a major source of grief for Susan, who described his whereabouts as *"a mystery that haunts me to this very day."* When Susan became an adult, she traveled to her father's hometown on the East Coast looking for him, but was unable to find him. She added that no one, including her own mother and her paternal relatives, would tell her the circumstances behind her father's disappearance. She did not know if he was dead or alive, and all those who knew him said they did not know either.

When the clinician asked whether she had memories of specific childhood moments when she felt loved, understood, or safe (during the angels in the nursery interview), Susan responded that she only had those feelings about her father. Her face lit up as she described feeling *"true happiness"* in knowing that *"he cared so much"* about her when playing hide-and-seek in the park or being consoled by him after waking up from a bad dream or simply getting treats from him. After vividly describing these loving memories, Susan became overwhelmed with sadness by the fact that she *"never had a chance to grow up with him."*

The ongoing influence of her father's loss was evident in Susan's relationships with men. She related a history of failed relationships permeated by violence, and followed by abandonment. All her three children had different fathers. When the clinician asked what Susan thought were the main problems with her past relationships, she stated, *"As soon as things got serious between us, everything, as always, went sour."* She said angrily that her children's fathers *"refused to become responsible"* when they found out she was pregnant by them. She stated, *"These men simply got what they wanted, sex, and then disappeared from my life and the lives of my children."* She depicted her relationship with the father of her 13-year-old son as the most violent of the three, recounting several incidents in which he threatened her with knives and severely beat her. She required medical attention twice due to broken ribs and a scalp laceration. By her account, her most recent relationship with the father of the fetus *"was better than the two previous ones"* because the violence was *"mild."* Matter-of-factly, she described several incidents in which her inebriated ex-partner pushed, shoved, slapped, and pulled her by her hair. She noted that, like her previous partners, he too had *"a bad temper and a drinking problem."* The last violent incident happened 2 months before the referral, when he accused Susan of being unfaithful with one of her coworkers. The neighbors called the police after hearing Susan's screams while he was trying to strangle her. He fled when he heard the police cars, but was later captured and charged with assault and battery. Since that event, Susan said, he had vanished and nobody knew his whereabouts. Susan expressed openly her ambivalent feelings toward her partner, saying that she still had loving feelings for him but was also very mad at him for what he did. She added that she felt like she had failed her children, because once again a father figure had abandoned them.

## LINKING PAST AND PRESENT: ADDRESSING GHOSTS IN THE NURSERY

Susan's lingering pain and self-blame for her father's early abandonment were relived in the present, and the clinician used this opportunity to ask her how she understood her relationships with the partners who hurt and abandoned her. Susan responded that she did not know. She only knew that she got involved in intimate relationships very quickly with men who presented themselves as loving, but quickly became abusive after becoming sexually involved and then abandoned her when she became pregnant. The clinician pursued this line of thinking, asking, *"Do you think maybe you are so hurt for losing your father that you keep looking for someone who will make you feel safe and loved like he did?"* Susan nodded, and began crying. This marked the beginning of her mourning process for the loss of her father. The clinician added softly, *"And when they leave you, I wonder if it's as if your father were leaving all over again, and you blame yourself."* Susan nodded in agreement, and responded that her mother always blamed her for things that went wrong, including her burning herself when she was 7 years old. The clinician said, *"Little children take what their mothers say very seriously. You believed your mother, and you are still carrying that burden of guilt since you were a little girl."*

Susan responded to this comment by disclosing that she had a history of depression with her two previous pregnancies. She described the depressive episode during her second pregnancy as the most debilitating, saying that she spent her days crying and unable to find any pleasure in life. After she delivered, she wanted to sleep all day and *"did not want anything to do with the baby."* She said she felt *"blessed to have the support of the baby's godmother"* who helped her during this difficult time. When the clinician asked whether anyone else had helped, Susan responded that her medical providers referred her to a psychiatrist who prescribed medications and made a referral for individual therapy at a community agency. However, she did not follow through with the referral.

Anticipating the possibility that Susan might not follow through with the current treatment, the clinician asked her about her reasons for not accepting the referral at the time. Susan responded that she was *"not crazy,"* and did not want to take medication. The clinician addressed Susan's fear directly, saying, *"I have been talking with you about your life, and I agree that you are not crazy. The things that happened to you would make anybody angry and depressed. That is not being crazy. I*

*could help you with those feelings so that you don't continue blaming yourself
for the things that hurt you that were not your fault. Are you interested in
continuing to meet with me to think together about what you need to feel better?"* Susan responded, *"Yes. I don't want to be so depressed after this baby
is born that I can't take care of him like with my younger son."* This was the
first direct mention that Susan made of the fetus she was carrying and
her wish to take care of him. The clinician understood this comment
as an indication of Susan's readiness to explore the links between her
life experiences and her current emotional state.

ADDRESSING TRAUMATIC REMINDERS TO PROMOTE SELF-CARE

During the initial two sessions, the clinician kept in mind the concerns
expressed by the referring social worker about Susan's lack of compliance with medical recommendations, but could not find a promising port of entry to address those concerns. She decided to start the
third session by asking how the doctor's appointment had gone the
day before. Susan became angry instantly, saying, *"Can you believe that
I had to wait for 4 hours to be seen by my doctor? I waited and waited . . . I
got so tired of waiting for her!"* The clinician validated Susan's feelings of
frustration about receiving her prenatal care at a busy clinic known for
long patient waits. Susan responded angrily that her doctor had yelled
at her because she came to her appointment without her weekly dietary
log and because her levels of glucose were still very high. She said that
she had tracked her meals and snacks during the last week but she had
forgotten her log at home. The doctor told Susan that she would most
likely start insulin therapy (i.e., insulin shots) because diet modifica-
tion had not been sufficient to control her glucose levels. Susan's eyes
welled up with tears as she mumbled, *"I hate needles! I just hate them . . .
I cannot stand needles. The sight of needles makes me sick!"* The clinician
said with a tone of concern, *"It sounds like your whole body reacts to the
sight of needles. Needles can be frightening for some people . . . Did something
ever happen to you with needles?"* Susan began sobbing as she placed
her hands over her face. The clinician handed Susan a tissue, which
she accepted, and remained silently present as Susan continued to sob.
Once Susan calmed down, she began narrating how her oldest sister
used needles to discipline her. Whenever Susan misbehaved, her sister
threatened to poke her with a needle and had actually done it twice.
She remembered feeling terrified when her sister lifted up a needle
toward her as a threat. The clinician validated the legitimacy of Susan's
fear and asked whether anyone knew about her sister's cruel method of
discipline. Susan said that she told her father when her sister poked her
with a needle for the first time, and he punished the sister for hurting

Susan. Tearfully, she added, *"After he left, my sister continued doing this to me because the only person who could protect me was now gone, had disappeared, had left me. My father was gone forever."*

This disclosure helped the clinician gain a better understanding of a complex psychological picture. Susan was unconsciously equating her doctor's statement that she would need to start insulin therapy with her sister's threats to discipline her with a needle. The doctor had become a transference object for the sister, responding punitively to Susan's failure to bring her glucose levels down and to show that she was logging her meals and snacks. This equation was linked in Susan's mind with the loss of her father as a protector. The clinician realized that she would need to become the protector in the moment to provide Susan with a reparative experience for her entwined fears of body damage and abandonment.

## THE CLINICIAN AS PROVIDER OF A PROTECTIVE CORRECTIVE EXPERIENCE

In response to Susan, the clinician created an emotional space where she could express her feelings of grief about the loss of her father, including her anger at him for abandoning her. The clinician then restated the link she made in the previous session between Susan's grief for the loss of her father and the despair of the breakups with her children's fathers. Susan responded that this was the first time she talked about her father and about the void that he left in her life, adding that she never realized how much his loss had continued to affect her.

The clinician used this exchange to provide psychoeducation about the sequelae of trauma exposure, giving Susan examples of how the body, through physiological changes, remembers and reacts to traumatic memories and sensory stimulation as a form of self-protection. She then asked Susan to tell her doctor about her fear of needles and its relation to her punishments with needles as a young child. Susan was hesitant, saying that the doctor would not believe this explanation. The clinician offered to speak with the doctor, and Susan responded, gratefully, *"Are you really willing to do that? Yes, please! I don't really like her. . . ."* The experience of protective help was *new* and welcome to her.

The doctor's first response to the clinician's request to speak about Susan's medical care was to express frustration about Susan's unwillingness to cooperate with the treatment and the danger to the fetus. The clinician validated the doctor's frustration and talked about Susan's fear of needles stemming from a childhood trauma. The doctor was receptive and suggested a meeting with Susan and the clinician to discuss implementing a more effective treatment plan. During this meeting, Susan agreed to follow an appropriate meal plan devised by the nutritionist to control her blood glucose. They also discussed a plan of progressive desensitization to help Susan overcome her fear of needles so that she would be able to self-administer the insulin shot if it was ever required. Through these supportive interactions, the doctor also built greater rapport with Susan, and Susan's feelings toward the doctor began shifting. In later sessions, she told the clinician, "*I guess the doctor is not too bad . . . she's an OK doctor.*"

### FEEDBACK SESSION: FORMULATION TRIANGLE AND INVITATION TO TREATMENT

The clinician used the first four meetings of the foundational phase to help Susan learn about the enduring effects of her early traumatic experiences of abuse and abandonment and create a concrete system of support for her self-care with her medical condition. It was now time to consolidate the new understanding and start building a safe physical and emotional environment for labor and delivery and for welcoming the baby.

The clinician started the feedback session by asking Susan how she had experienced their meetings to date. Susan said that she was grateful to learn that she was not crazy and had a right to feel angry and sad for the way she was treated as a little girl. The clinician agreed, saying that losing her protective father and not knowing what had happened to him was a great burden that made it hard to know how to have safe relationships with men. The clinician added that Susan was still dealing with the hurt of losing her partner and was putting all her energy in trying to care for herself and her older children. She then asked, "*I am wondering if maybe you feel at times that there is little energy left to prepare yourself for the coming baby so that you can try to prevent the depression you told me about with your earlier pregnancies.*" Susan listened carefully, nodding and elaborating as the clinician spoke. The clinician said, "*You know, Susan, it doesn't need to stay that way. You are really using what you are learning about yourself to take care of yourself. Would you like to continue meeting with me to talk about what you want for yourself and for your new baby as he joins the family?*" With Susan's agreement, the foundational phase was completed, and the core phase of treatment began.

### REFLECTIONS ON THE FOUNDATIONAL PHASE WITH SUSAN

The foundational phase involves not only information gathering, but also treatment as well. In this sense, assessment and treatment always go together, because new information invariably emerges in the course of treatment and influences the clinician's always-evolving clinical formulation and treatment plan. The 10 key topics of the foundational phase (see pp. 65–66) provide a rich opportunity to engage in trial interpretations and assess the client's response, which in turn helps the clinician to tailor the future intervention strategies that are most likely to be effective.

Clinicians learning a new treatment model sometimes worry that asking about traumatic experiences or intervening "too fast" may jeopardize the process of building a therapeutic relationship. This is a valid concern when clinicians are insufficiently attuned to the client's verbal and nonverbal communications and priorities, perhaps because they are too intent on following a treatment protocol. The case of Susan illustrates the usefulness of integrating clinically informed assessment with initial intervention strategies from the beginning. It is through the process of offering themselves as supportive, interested, useful, and competent partners while gathering information that clinicians most effectively start to create a transformational therapeutic relationship that starts during the assessment process.

### *Promoting Co-Parenting: When the Intimate Partner/Baby's Father Joins the Foundational Phase*

P-CPP shares the clinical dilemma that all perinatal treatment models must grapple with: Whether, when, and how to include the baby's father in the treatment. The father is seminally important as an attachment figure, and even his absence constitutes a presence in the psychological landscape of mother and baby. As a key member of the "essential triad," the absent father exists in fantasy rather than as a real life partner in the emotional life of the mother and child. Women have intense feelings about the man who impregnated them, whether these feelings are conscious or suppressed, and the fetus/baby may become a negative transference object for those feelings. Whether or not the baby's father joins the treatment, the pregnant woman's experience of him and of his imagined connection with the fetus/baby needs to become an integral part of the issues discussed during treatment, both during the foundational phase and as the treatment unfolds.

P-CPP makes the question of including the father an integral component of the foundational phase. The answer to this question depends primarily on the woman's wishes, but the clinician helps her explore the rationale for her wishes and engages in an open and ongoing dialogue about the ambivalent feelings she might have about the role that she imagines for the father in her own and in the baby's life. Assessing the balance between reality-based factors and wish-based factors is an important part of this therapeutic endeavor. When IPV, criminal behavior, or other threats to safety are part of the picture, the clinician guides the woman in exploring the psychological meaning of these issues for her and helps her to take steps for self-protection and protection of the fetus/baby.

The increased risk of IPV during pregnancy is a powerful but undervalued indicator of the stress that impending fatherhood may pose for a man. While a woman's pregnancy sets in motion prenatal and perinatal care for the mother-to-be, there are no formal services to educate men about the emotional challenges that they are likely to experience during their partner's pregnancy and to help them plan for their new responsibilities. Men's consistent inclusion in services offered to pregnant women remains a rarity.

The general omission of fathers as active participants in their partner's pregnancy can become actual ostracism on the part of the medical establishment when men have perpetrated IPV, and there is much debate about the desirability of including them in treatment (Groves, Van Horn, & Lieberman, 2007). To address the questions of whether, when, and how to involve fathers in treatment, we developed a set of assessment procedures to evaluate the safety and clinical appropriateness of engaging the father. The first consideration continues to be whether the mother wants her partner to be involved. Many mothers in violent relationships use treatment as a private opportunity to explore whether they want to remain in the relationship and how they want the relationship to change now that there is a baby at stake. It is important to honor the mother's motivations and enable her to use the treatment as a tool to plan for a safer future for herself and her baby. The second consideration is safety for the mother, the baby, and the clinician. Many women describe their baby's fathers as unpredictably violent; others report stalking after the relationship ends. Court orders restricting the father's access to the mother and/or the child may be in place, but restraining orders are notoriously ineffective in preventing violence. Each situation needs careful evaluation in the decision to extend fathers an invitation to treatment.

If the mother wants the father to be involved in treatment, the clinician makes clear that before treatment can be offered the father needs to participate in an initial assessment to ascertain his capacity for self-reflection and remorse, potential for violence and lethality, and commitment to parenting prior to offering treatment. We adopted six criteria that must be met before offering to start the foundational phase with a violent father (Groves et al., 2007), as outlined below.

1. The mother wants the father to participate in the treatment.
2. The father acknowledges that he engages in violent behavior that is dangerous to his partner's and his baby's well-being.
3. The father expresses the wish to change and makes a commitment to refrain from violence during treatment.
4. The father agrees to participate in a concurrent anger management program or treatment for perpetrators of IPV. If alcohol or substance abuse are involved, he agrees to attend an alcohol or substance abuse program. He agrees to give signed permission for regular communication between the P-CPP clinician and the anger management program or substance abuse program providers to monitor his compliance.
5. The father signs releases of information that enable the clinician to obtain information about him and stay in communication with all relevant resources, including his probation officer, attorney, child welfare worker, anger management and/or mental health provider, and the courts.
6. The father agrees that the foundational phase of treatment will involve an assessment of his commitment to treatment and ability to abide by the agreements he made to refrain from violence, to attend concurrent intervention programs, and to maintain safety. The clinician informs the father that the agreement to offer treatment will be revisited during the feedback session that is the culmination of the foundational phase.

The format of treatment when the father is involved can be adapted in response to clinical needs, but the focus remains on the safety and well-being of the mother and the baby. The clinician asks that the couple together develop a proposed format for the father's participation. The most frequent format involves a joint session with the couple to talk about their respective perceptions and wishes. This joint session also provides the forum for an agreement about the confidentiality of personal information each of them will share with the clinician. The clinician makes a clear statement about the limits of confidentiality, adding that while each partner has the right for specific clinical information to remain confidential, the clinician will encourage communication about issues that interfere with their ability to create a partnership on behalf of the baby. The initial joint session sets the stage for a combination of individual and joint sessions that follow. The format of these sessions covers the 10 key topics of the foundational phase (see pp. 65–66), while simultaneously supporting the development of a partnership around the shared role of parents. At the same time, parents are learning about their partner's individual experiences and psychological makeup.

In some situations, the father attends every session. In other situations, he attends at regular intervals, but there are also separate sessions with the mother or, after the baby's birth, with the mother and the child. Safety remains a primary focus, and the P-CPP clinician deploys the therapeutic modalities described earlier to help the father grow in his capacity to become a safe partner and a competent parent.

## Clinical Illustration of the Foundational Phase with a High-Conflict Couple: Ana and Martin

The clinical work with Ana and her husband, Martin, illustrates the foundational phase with a pregnant woman and her partner involved in a high-conflict relationship. The father's participation enhanced the progress of treatment by keeping the unborn baby clearly present as an anchor to motivate and sustain positive change. The foundational phase spanned seven sessions, which included two initial individual sessions with Ana, a third session with Ana and Martin, a fourth individual session with Ana, a fifth individual session with Martin, another joint session with both parents, and a feedback and treatment planning session.

### REFERRAL PROCESS

Ana, a 31-year-old recent immigrant from Colombia, a war-torn country in South America, was 22 weeks pregnant with her second child when she was referred for treatment by the Women's Health Center medical social worker due to marital conflict and a history of depressive episodes. The social worker reported that in a recent prenatal visit Ana began to cry when asked whether she was satisfied with the level of involvement of the baby's father in her pregnancy. She denied physical violence, but disclosed that she was having frequent verbal arguments with her husband, whom she described as controlling and verbally abusive. The clinic's psychiatrist prescribed antidepressants for her anhedonia and difficulty concentrating, but Ana refused to take the medication after she learned about possible teratogenic effects. Ana was having moderate pregnancy complications and was being monitored for light vaginal bleeding, mild edema (abnormal buildup of fluid in the ankles, feet, and legs), and recurring urinary tract infections. She reported that her pregnancy had been unplanned, but that both she and her husband, Martin, now wanted the baby. The first session with the P-CPP clinician (M. A. D.) took place at the hospital following a prenatal checkup visit.

## GETTING TO KNOW ANA

During the first session, Ana discussed her concerns about receiving mental health services because she feared that people would think she was "crazy" because she was seeing a psychologist. This is a common concern among people from a variety of backgrounds and most particularly among those from countries or communities where mental health services are scarce and primarily available to the severely mentally ill, such as people with psychotic disorders. The clinician elicited Ana's perceptions of mental illness, provided psychoeducation about the stigma associated with mental health services in many Latin American countries, and explained that psychotherapy could be an integral component of her prenatal care focused on her emotional well-being. The clinician also used the session to gather sociodemographic information and to administer structured questionnaires to assess for IPV, depressive symptoms, quality of bonding to the fetus, and parenting attitudes and beliefs. Ana responded to the questionnaires in a matter-of-fact manner, with interest but without showing much emotion.

Ana stated that the baby's father was aware of the referral and that he had encouraged her to call so that "she could get help with her issues." The risk assessment revealed that Ana was involved in a high-conflict relationship with Martin but was not at imminent risk of becoming a victim of physical violence. When the clinician raised the possibility of including Martin in the treatment, Ana responded that she liked the idea but was unsure about Martin's willingness to participate. She added that he was waiting for her outside the clinic and that he usually accompanied her to all her appointments.

During the following session, the clinician explained that she wanted to learn about Ana's life experiences, because difficult events while growing up and in adulthood have a deep effect on how people feel about themselves and their loved ones. She administered a semi-structured interviewed about stressful life events and assessed current posttraumatic stress symptoms. Ana had experienced significant adversity and trauma exposure beginning in childhood. The most salient events included routine spankings with a belt by her mother and a severe burn that had left a large scar on the back of her right hand by her father, who had burned her with an iron when she was 4 years old to teach her that *an iron is not a toy to play with.*

During the following session, Ana devoted most of the time to talking about the history of her relationship with Martin, which began in their home country when she was 18 and he was 30 years old. He had been a member of his country's Special Forces at a time of civil war and terror attacks, but received a discharge due to a life-threatening injury after 5 years of service. He met Ana after his discharge at the factory where they both worked. Ana became pregnant very soon after they met and was very happy with the pregnancy. Martin, however, was not. When he learned of the pregnancy, he moved back to his hometown and visited Ana only three times during the ensuing months. He was present during the birth of their first baby girl and stayed with them for 2 weeks, before disappearing from their lives 2 months later after telling her that he would be leaving for a business trip for a few months.

During the ensuing 2 years, Ana attempted repeatedly but without success to locate Martin, and eventually gave up with the assumption that he had abandoned her and the baby. Ten years later, Ana heard from a neighbor that Martin was now living in his hometown with his mother and went there looking for him, but his mother told her that he was now living in the United States. His mother refused to give her information about his whereabouts, but she obtained his telephone number from one of his uncles, who believed her story that she had a daughter with Martin. Ana recounted how difficult it was to make that first telephone call because of the strong resentment she had harbored toward him throughout these years. She explained, "*I was very happy to finally find him, but I was also very angry at him for having vanished from my life.*" Ana narrated the first telephone conversation with Martin, when he told her that he had tried to contact her repeatedly but unsuccessfully after leaving their country, apologized for his absence, and promised her that he would make up for all the years that he had been gone. After 4 months of regular phone contact, Martin asked Ana to come to the United States and marry him. Ana accepted Martin's marriage proposal and agreed to leave their 11-year-old daughter with her grandmother only for a few months until she and Martin had the resources to bring her to this country.

When Ana arrived in the United States, she lived with Martin in an apartment they shared with his sister and her family. Ana reported that Martin's sister became jealous and made derogatory comments about Ana's physical appearance and behavior because Martin was spending more time with Ana than with his sister's family. Six months after her arrival, Ana became pregnant and had a miscarriage 5 weeks into her pregnancy. She blamed the stress from her sister-in-law's treatment of her for the miscarriage. Ana and Martin moved out a month after Ana miscarried and went to live with a friend, where they were still living at the time of the present referral. Ana reported that she did not have any contact with Martin's family and was very pleased about that, but he resented the rift that Ana's arrival had created in his relationship with his sister and her family.

When the clinician asked Ana how Martin expressed his resentment, Ana described for the first time several episodes of physical violence in addition to episodes of emotional and verbal aggression. On two occasions before the current pregnancy, Martin had pushed her against the wall and grabbed her roughly by the arms, leaving her with black-and-blue marks. She also described three additional "playful incidents" that occurred during this pregnancy, in which Martin had pinched her hard in the arms and left visible bruises. When the clinician asked Ana how she felt about these "playful incidents," Ana said she was very angry that he played with her in such a rough manner. She reported that he no longer "played" like that after she told him that her midwife had questioned her about the bruises during one of her prenatal visits. As the clinician continued to explore the relationship between Ana and Martin, Ana disclosed that she had never told him how angry she continued to be about his previous absence from her and her older daughter's life and about her ongoing separation from that daughter. She added, with remarkable insight, that the fights helped her express some of the anger she had been holding for so many years.

Ana's relationship with Martin was clearly the salient focus of her emotional life at the moment, and her candid acknowledgment of anger became a port of entry that suggested once again that she consider inviting Martin to join in preparing to become parents together. Ana agreed. To her surprise, Martin responded positively, saying that their fights were creating a lot of stress and made him worry about what would happen when the baby was born.

## MEETING MARTIN

Ana and Martin arrived promptly to the following session, with Martin following behind Ana looking serious and uncomfortable. The clinician welcomed him, trying to put him at ease by commenting lightly on the times they had waved at each other when he dropped Ana off at the clinic, and then asked whether he and Ana had talked about these meetings. Ana answered, saying she had told him that she was in psychotherapy to help her be in a good state of mind, and she wanted Martin to come so that they would learn not to fight so much and could care for the baby together. The clinician asked Martin what he thought about what Ana said, and he responded that he was nervous about becoming a father and was coming to this session only because Ana asked him. The clinician said she appreciated his coming and his wish to support Ana, and asked whether he had ever seen a clinician in the past. Martin smirked and said sarcastically that he always thought one needed to be crazy to see one. The clinician thanked Martin for his honesty and acknowledged that in many countries that was indeed the custom.

This exchange showed that Martin had a similar perception of psychotherapy as Ana had expressed during her first visit, but it also implied that Ana might be "crazy" for coming. The clinician chose to use supportive psychoeducation to offer a different perspective. She explained that pregnancy is a time when the mood of the couple and how they get along can affect the health and well-being of the mother and the fetus. Martin's facial expression changed from defensive sarcasm to cautious interest, and the clinician went on to elaborate on her work with pregnant women and their families. Specifically, she told Martin, "*I am a clinician who works with pregnant women who experienced difficult, traumatic things in their lives. In this program, we meet with the pregnant woman, and ideally also with the baby's father, during pregnancy and after the baby is born. We hope to help parents give their babies the best possible start, both physically and emotionally. Parents tell me about the difficult things that happened to them or between them that may affect how they feel and how they take care of their children. We think together about what they want for themselves and their child and how to create the family environment that they hope for.*"

Ana, who had remained quiet until now, said to Martin, "*Remember, I told you that I was coming to see my clinician because we were having problems . . . our arguments were affecting me.*" Martin remained quiet, and the clinician said, "*I understand that there has been a lot of stress between you during these past few months.*" Martin nodded his head slightly in agreement, but continued to stay silent. The clinician then added, "*The goal of our program is to help parents with their difficult moods so children are not exposed to difficult situations like yelling and fights, because this can be very frightening for young children, including babies.*" Martin then broke his silence, and said, "*Things have been difficult between us, but we are now getting along better.*" Ana responded, "*Maybe you think that but I don't. You insult me and call me stupid. You don't eat my food because you say it is not clean. You say that you don't see your family because of me. I don't even know why I came to this country and left my daughter behind.*" Martin looked very embarrassed, and said, "*I don't know what you are talking about!*" Ana responded, "*Yes, you do. Everything I am saying is true, and you just don't want the clinician to know.*"

Sensing the danger of polarization if Martin perceived her as taking sides, the clinician said, "*Ana and I have been meeting together, but you are just getting to know me. You don't yet know how much of your private life you want me to know. Do you think the two of you can find a way of making our conversation useful for both of you?"* Martin responded with contained anger, *"She is always angry. She trapped me getting pregnant with our first daughter 2 months after we met. I did not plan this baby either. Ana thinks that she can get pregnant, and then she can get me to do whatever she wants."* Ana burst into tears, and between sobs and in an angry tone of voice said, *"You sure like the sex, but you don't like the consequences . . . You are an irresponsible man!"*

This exchange gave the clinician a concise and stark picture of the parents' conflict. She sought to offer hope by normalizing their plight, explaining that pregnancies are very often unplanned and that men and women often respond differently to the news. She added that their talking about their different experiences was difficult but courageous, and offered the opportunity to think together about what each of them wanted of the other for the sake of their baby. There was a slight softening in the mood in both parents following this remark. The clinician commented that it was time to end the session, and asked if they wanted to meet together again the following week. Martin said that he had to work and could only continue coming if the day of the session was changed to his day off. The clinician said she would rearrange her schedule, and asked Martin if he would be open to an individual session so they could talk about his personal life in preparing for the baby, just as Ana had talked about hers. The clinician took some risk in making this offer because of how Ana might react, but clinical necessity guided her choice. Martin hesitated, and Ana said, *"That makes sense, Martin. I needed the time alone to learn to trust her."* They agreed that Martin would have an individual session 2 weeks later when the clinician could see Martin on his day off from work.

### EMERGING PATTERNS OF ABUSE AND ABANDONMENT

The fourth session was with Ana alone, and the clinician knew the themes of the joint session with Martin would need to be addressed. Ana greeted the clinician with a big smile, saying she was very happy because she had spoken on the telephone with her mother and daughter earlier that day. Her voice then broke, and her eyes welled up with tears as she said that this was the first time she had been apart from them. With an affectionate look, Ana said, *"I miss them so much. You know, I'm very blessed to have a mother who is strong, willful, and caring."* This statement contrasted with Ana's previous description of her mother's regular hard spankings with a belt, and the clinician answered, *"It sounds like you admire many qualities of your mother. Tell me a little more about her."* Ana responded, *"My mother is the rock of my life"* and went on to repeat her mother's words of encouragement when she found herself overwhelmed by raising her daughter on her own. Ana added, "*When I get sad about being so far away from my daughter, it helps me to know that my mother is with her; that she is there when my daughter gets sad. I know my mother is taking good care of her the way she took care of me when I was a child.*" Ana then went on to describe how her mother was a "true role model" for her and her siblings. She said, "*After my father left, my mother had to work very hard to raise her five children. She made sure that we had everything we needed. She worked long hours at the local market selling goods, and she never once complained when she came home to cook and help us with our homework.*" Ana also added that her mother was "*strict when she had to be*" but that she never abused them. She also attributed her own individual and maternal characteristics (e.g., caring, responsible, hardworking, and nurturing) to her mother's teachings—"*the way she raised me.*" As she spoke, Ana started to lovingly rub her belly, smiling and commenting that the baby seemed to be listening and agreeing with her.

The clinician realized that Ana needed this idealized identification with her mother as an ego ideal to give her guidance and hope at a time of fear and anger in her relationship with her husband. She validated the meaning of Ana's early experiences with her mother, and they talked for a while about the kind of relationship she wanted with her own children. She then moved on to bring the masculine element into the session, asking Ana about her memories of her father. Ana's facial expression became somber as she said that she did not have any fond memories of him, because he had "vanished" from her life after he separated from her mother and moved to a distant town. She remembered again the image of his burning her with an iron to teach her it was not a toy when she was 4 years old, looking at the scar on her hand as she described her pain and fear.

The clinician made a link between past and present, asking if, when Martin "*vanished*" from her life, his leaving brought back memories of her father's abandonment. Ana seemed surprised by the connection, and said after a pause that she had not thought about it. After another silence, she said in a sad voice that maybe Martin was like her father in the way he first vanished and now hurt her when they got back together. The clinician answered that, although this was an open question, Martin showed important forms of commitment because he had asked her to come to the United States to marry him, he wanted their daughter to join them once they were better established, and he was willing to participate in the therapy with her. The clinician added, "*As I listen to each of you, I think that you are both showing that you want to give your baby a different life than what you had.*" Ana seemed reassured by this hopeful response, and said quietly but intensely that she really wanted Martin to be present in her children's lives and that she would work hard to make it happen.

## MARTIN'S STORY: PAST AND PRESENT

The individual session with Martin showed his profound ambivalence about his relationship with Ana, repeating the statement he made during the joint session that he felt trapped by Ana into becoming a father. When the clinician asked him how he had decided to ask Ana to come to the United States to marry him, he responded, "*Guilt. But I also hoped to have a new beginning. I was lonely and she told me she loved me and that we should be together for the sake of our daughter.*" The clinician responded that those were powerful reasons, and asked how he felt now about his decision. He responded that he wanted a family, but that Ana created trouble between him and his sister, who had raised him and was the only person he could trust for many years since he emigrated to the United States.

As the conversation unfolded, it became clear that Martin was torn between his hesitation to disclose personal information and his urge to talk about the pressures he was facing. In response to the clinician's supportive responses and open-ended questions, he revealed a childhood history marred by IPV between his parents, his father's early death when Martin was 11 years old, and his mother's relationships with multiple abusive boyfriends. His contempt for his mother was the most salient theme in this session, as he practically spat while describing what he called her libertine lifestyle. This derision toward his mother was balanced on the other hand by his admiration of and gratitude to his older sister for taking on the maternal role and becoming his protector. As he spoke, the clinician started to understand his attraction, at age 35, to a virginal 18-year-old Ana when they first met about 12 years earlier and his flight from commitment once she became a mother. He held a polarized image of women as either fallen or saintly, and he reenacted this internal battle in the present through his conflicted relationship with the two women who claimed priority in his emotional life.

Seeking to both normalize the family conflict and promote reflectiveness about its underlying dynamics, the clinician supported Martin's wish for a family and commented on the difficulties that new couples routinely encounter when they bring their partners into their families of origin. She added, "*You and your sister have a very close relationship, and her children are like children to you. Do you think that Ana and your sister might each worry that you have to choose between the two of them, that you cannot love both of them at the same time?"* Martin thought for a moment but quickly dismissed this possibility, blaming Ana entirely for the stresses in the family. He then started using derogatory comments to describe Ana, saying she did not keep the house clean, did not shower regularly, constantly misplaced the house keys, and asked stupid questions. His contempt for Ana paralleled his contempt for his mother. The clinician held this in mind, but chose to focus on the immediate challenge facing this couple, commenting, *"I think you asked Ana to marry you before the two of you knew each other well. Most couples find things they deeply dislike in each other once they start living together. I think the job ahead for you and Ana is to find if there are enough things that you like in each other to keep you together in raising your baby."* Martin nodded as if pondering this message, and the session ended with an agreement for a joint session the following week.

### SPEAKING THE UNSPEAKABLE: MODULATING MARITAL RAGE

The following joint session became the stage for Ana and Martin to give full expression to their angry dissatisfaction with each other. They were 15 minutes late, and Martin apologized profusely for their tardiness, and said that Ana had misplaced the house keys again and that they spent a long time trying to locate them. Ana responded that Martin criticized her for everything, and added that in the morning he had scolded her for the way she prepared breakfast, called her food *"unsanitary,"* and refused to eat what she had prepared. Martin listened silently as her voice rose and her complaints escalated, until she touched on a particularly sensitive topic when she blamed his sister for putting ideas in his head in order to ruin their relationship. She then went on to blame both Martin and his sister for the miscarriage that preceded this pregnancy.

Ana's blame became a turning point for Martin, who became exasperated and said angrily, *"I'm so tired of this! Ana is always late for everything; she forgets the apartment keys and I have to leave work to let her in the house; when I get home from work, she hasn't cooked or cleaned our room. She is a good-for-nothing, slow, and dumb! She doesn't understand a thing of what you tell her."* Pointing to his head, he added, *"She is sick in the head, that's why she is coming here. . . ."* Looking at the clinician, he asked, *"Isn't she sick? You can see it! A normal person wouldn't act that way, right?"* Ana, who had begun crying, replied, *"I'm tired of living with someone who is always making me feel bad about everything I do! Someone who does not appreciate me! Someone who is constantly calling me names! I cannot live like this anymore!"* Ana burst into tears, sobbing uncontrollably and blowing her nose as she tried to stem the flow of tears.

This exchange was difficult to witness, but it also signaled that both Ana and Martin felt safe using the session to give expression to their rage and despair. The clinician remained quiet, trying to regulate her feelings before responding. She realized that she joined Ana in perceiving Martin as abusive, but she was also aware of the impact on Martin of Ana's accusation that he was to blame for her miscarriage. During this pause, Martin said, *"I don't even know why I am coming here. She is the sick one, not me! She is the one who needs help. She is crazy! Look at her and the way she is acting right now!"*

The clinician realized the importance of helping both parents become more aware of the power they had over each other and how vulnerable they were to the other's criticism. She needed to hold the pain that each of them felt and show them how their anger was a way of expressing their pain. She decided to bring them back to the present moment and reflect on the intense emotions each of them was having. Starting with Martin, she turned to him and asked, *"How do you think Ana is feeling right now?"* Martin shrugged his shoulders and replied, *"I don't know."* The clinician said, *"Look at her . . . Look at Ana and tell me what you think she is feeling right now."* Martin looked away and replied, *"I don't know . . . I guess she is upset."* The clinician replied, *"Yes, she is very upset because of what just happened."* There was another pause, and then Martin replied, *"That's the way I talk to her when I get angry, when she gets on my nerves, when she drives me up the wall!"* The clinician slowly began repeating the name-calling done by Martin a few minutes earlier, saying *"You called Ana stupid . . . dumb . . . good-for-nothing . . . sick in the head. . . ."* Ana listened intently as Martin shuffled uncomfortably in his chair. Turning to Ana, the clinician asked whether she would feel comfortable describing how she was feeling. Ana said, *"I'm angry, sad, hurt . . . how can someone who supposedly loves me treats me that way and say those things to me?"*

Martin looked deeply embarrassed, and the clinician asked him how he felt listening to Ana. Looking at the clinician, he answered, *"I did not realize what I say hurt her so much. That's how I am when I get angry. I am sorry."* The clinician said softly, *"Do you think you can tell Ana how you feel?"* Glancing at Ana, he mumbled that he was sorry for what he said. The clinician asked him, *"Do you remember when you got so angry at Ana that you started calling her those names?"* After a very long silence, Martin answered, *"When she blamed my sister and me for her miscarriage. I am not a murderer."*

This was a stunning message, and both Ana and the clinician were indeed stunned. Ana recoiled with an appalled look. The clinician thought immediately of Ana's comment during their first meeting that Martin had been in Special Operations in their country during a period of civil war and received a discharge after a severe injury. Martin himself had not mentioned this part of his past during his individual meeting with the clinician, but the mental association he made in response to Ana's blame raised the possibility that his combat experiences still haunted him. His response during the session put in context the multiple factors fueling his rage at Ana, whom he perceived as a relentless accuser who constantly confronted him with his shortcomings after trapping him with two pregnancies he did not plan or want.

"*How to respond?*" the clinician thought to herself. She then turned to Ana and commented that she looked appalled. Ana responded, "*Of course he is not a murderer. That is not what I meant.*" The clinician asked Ana to tell Martin about what she meant. Crying, Ana said to Martin, "*I don't think you are a murderer. But all the tension in my body from all the fighting made me have a miscarriage.*"

Still seething with anger, Martin replied, "*Your body could not carry the baby. Don't blame me for it. You had that miscarriage in the second month, when you were barely pregnant. You got pregnant again right away, and now you are carrying this baby just fine although we continue to fight just as much as before. You just need to blame me for everything that doesn't go the way you want.*"

The clinician mediated between Ana and Martin, saying that it is hard to say what makes a miscarriage happen because they are common in the first weeks of pregnancy, and asked whether they had a chance to grieve for the loss. They seemed surprised by the question, as if they had never considered it. The clinician went on to explain that people often don't give themselves permission to mourn after a miscarriage, but the sadness comes out in unexpected ways in the form of anger, depression, or blame. She said that both Ana and Martin had difficult lives with much sadness and fear. This was the time, she added, to think about how they were using those feelings now against each other. She added that this was also the time to join in thinking together about what kind of family they wanted for their baby. The session ended in a quiet, sad, reflective mood as the clinician's words traced their anger back to its source in previously unexpressed pain.

FEEDBACK SESSION: THE FORMULATION TRIANGLE AND TREATMENT PLAN

The following week involved a recapitulation of what had happened during the previous sessions to help the parents create a shared narrative of their present situation and what they needed to accomplish to feel ready for their baby. The clinician started by asking what their experience of the meetings had been, and if they had learned anything new about themselves or each other. Ana said that she had more trust that Martin would not run away from this baby the way he had ran away from his older daughter. Martin responded, *"Here she goes again. She is relentless. I don't know what I need to do to atone. I could simply have never returned her phone call, I could have disappeared from her life, but I didn't. I asked her to marry me, and we will bring our daughter here. But she cannot forgive me, and she needs to punish me by taking me away from my family."* Here again was the stark formulation of their mutual blame.

The clinician commented, *"Martin, I hear what you are saying. Ana is so hurt by the 10 years of not knowing where you were and raising your daughter alone that everything reminds her of it. When she talks about it, you get so upset that you did not hear her say just now that she now has more trust in you. When you think about what we did together until now, what comes to mind?"* Martin responded, *"The main thing I learned is that you don't need to be crazy to come to counseling. I am trying not to call her names now that I know that hurts her."*

Ana confirmed that Martin was indeed stopping himself from using insulting words to describe her, and that in turn made her less angry with him. The clinician used this positive development to ask if they wanted to hear what she had learned about them, and they agreed. The clinician then said, *"Remember that when we first met I told you that what happens to us when we are growing up stays with us when we are adults, and it shapes our moods and our relationships with our partners and our children?"* Ana and Martin nodded. The clinician went on to say, *"Both of you lost your fathers when you were young. Martin, your father died when you were a young child. Ana, your father left you when you were little, and before he left he hurt you so badly that he left a scar that you still carry on your hand. What happened to each of you leaves a deep wound in the heart of a child. Martin, you did not have a trusted man who could teach you how to be a husband and a father. Ana, I think that when Martin left all the memories of your father leaving came back to you, and you still worry that it is just a matter of time until it happens again. When you get mad with each other now, you are getting mad also at the people who were supposed to be there for you but were not."*

Martin and Ana listened silently, seeming very much in tune. Then Ana asked, *"What can we do?"* The clinician responded, *"We can think about that together. I believe that you can learn how to be less angry with each other if you remind yourselves that your anger comes from far back, from things that frightened you and hurt you when you were little and you had a right to be kept safe. You can practice here how to talk about what upsets you without making each other so angry that you hurt each other. That will help you to be happier and will also teach your baby to trust you and to feel safe with you."* Martin said, *"I am willing to do that, but I will come more often after the baby is born. I have too much work to do right now, but I will come every other week or at least once a month."* Ana smiled and responded,

*"That is OK with me. I want some time here for myself. Can I come every week?"* The clinician answered that she certainly could, and the parents and clinician agreed to continue treatment.

REFLECTIONS ON THE FOUNDATIONAL PHASE WITH ANA AND MARTIN

This clinical example with a high-conflict couple illustrates the importance of an active clinical stance from the very beginning. The foundational phase blurs the conventional boundaries between assessment and treatment. P-CPP clinicians use these initial sessions to gather assessment information in a clinically informed manner that introduces the parent-to-be to the clinician's therapeutic style. Clinicians then use the assessment interventions as immediate ports of entry to guide in-the-moment interventions, which may include all the P-CPP therapeutic modalities in order to assess which modalities are most effective in creating positive change. In the case of Ana and Martin, the clinician used unstructured developmental guidance, psychoeducation, and emotional support as the primary modalities, with some insight-oriented interpretations linking their childhood experiences with their current emotional challenges. The progress they made in their self-understanding and their empathy for each other, although modest, reinforced their motivation to work together on behalf of their baby and made possible their agreement to continue treatment.

# Core Treatment Phase

The core treatment phase builds on the knowledge co-created during the foundational phase, as the clinician helps the parents expand and deepen the clinical themes that emerged in the process of getting to know one another. New themes and disclosures emerge with the client's growing trust in the clinician and familiarity with the treatment process. This treatment phase takes into account the increasing proximity of childbirth and encompasses labor and delivery, the postpartum period, and the inclusion of the new baby into treatment. The clinician interweaves the concrete interventions described in the following sections with the therapeutic modalities that are clinically indicated.

## Preparing a Birth Plan and a Checklist of Needed Items

The clinician assists the mother in developing a birth plan. The birth plan is a handout that the mother receives and completes together with the help of the clinician during one or more sessions. As she completes her birth plan, the mother reflects on her wishes for the actual birth and the level of support she has in place for childbirth and the post-partum recovery.

Active involvement with primary care is an important component of this phase. The clinician encourages the mother and/or the parents to get information from the OB/GYN health care providers about her options for the childbirth process. This conversation prepares them to make informed decisions if the actual birth does not go as planned (e.g., whether to accept an epidural if it is recommended, when to consider a cesarean section, or what types of medications may be used for labor and delivery—an especially important topic if there is a family history of opioid overuse) and enables them to be clear about their wishes for the baby's care (e.g., whether or not to circumcise if the baby is a boy). The clinician takes this opportunity to assess maternal functioning, and begins implementing different interventions to help the woman manage her mood and trauma-related symptoms as appropriate. Here are the questions included in the "My Birth Plan" handout:

1. "When I am ready to go to the hospital to deliver, I will call. . . ."
2. "I will have the following person(s) at my birth delivery, which may include a birth doula. . . ."
3. "I want my delivery to be like. . . ."
4. "I want the following person(s) to visit and be at the hospital with me. . . ."
5. "The following person(s) will take me home. . . ."
6. "I will have the following person(s) help me during the first few days after birth. . . ."
7. "If I have a baby boy, I will want him to. . . ."

Two checklists list the items needed to prepare for the baby's birth: the hospital bag checklist and the newborn baby checklist. The woman can either complete these checklists with the clinician during a session or take them home to complete on her own. The first checklist includes things the woman needs to pack for her hospital stay, including a change of clothes and personal care items. The second checklist includes a list of essentials needed for the baby, such as baby clothes, diapers, and an infant car seat. These checklists help assess the family's capacity to meet concrete needs and make referrals when needed to community agencies that provide emergency assistance with basic needs.

## Psychoeducation about Caring for the Newborn

Starting in the third trimester and depending on clinical needs, many P-CPP clinicians start incorporating DVDs, magazines, and books about meeting the physical and emotional needs of newborn infants. The goal is to enhance the mother's sense of self-efficacy in caring for and mothering her newborn infant. This psychoeducation and support around newborn care is particularly important when working with first-time mothers; recent immigrants; women with severe symptoms of depression, anxiety, PTSD, or other conditions; and/or those at risk for mood disorders. The more knowledge the woman has about her infant needs and the more prepared she feels about meeting those needs, the more likely she will be to establish a healthy relationship with the baby. The clinician presents daily caregiving routines (e.g., feeding, diapering) as one of the main vehicles to strengthen the mother–infant relationship and promote effective parenting. Fathers are actively encouraged to participate in these preparations, although clinical experience shows that both women and men often prefer this aspect of treatment to be woman-centered, with women attributing to themselves the primary caregiving role.

### Preparing for a Postpartum Break in Treatment

Most mothers request a break in treatment of anywhere between 2 to 4 weeks in order to recover from giving birth. To ensure the continuity of treatment and prevent early termination, the clinician begins to plan for the break in treatment as the due date draws near. The clinician and the woman discuss and reach an agreement on different matters pertaining to treatment continuity.

### Planning for Contact during Labor and Delivery

As the woman's due date approaches, the clinician and the woman coordinate how the woman will let the clinician know that she has delivered and whether she wants the clinician to visit. The woman may make a phone call to the clinician herself or give written consent to the social worker to call. Safety needs to be considered in these decisions. A visit to the labor and delivery ward by the clinician may not be appropriate if the woman is involved in a violent relationship and/or her partner does not know that she is receiving treatment.

### Contact Following Birth

It is also during the late pregnancy phase that the clinician and the mother reach an agreement on how they will remain in contact after discharge from the hospital and as she begins recovering from birth and adjusting to the demands of caring for a newborn. In some cases, weekly phone calls are sufficient until the mother is ready to resume treatment. In other cases, home visits may be more appropriate, such as when the woman has no support system in place, is depressed or becoming depressed, and/or is recovering from a cesarean procedure.

If the clinician and the woman agree to stay in contact by telephone, the clinician needs to be flexible when scheduling phone appointments in order to convey the message that the main priority is for the mother to take care of herself and the baby. The clinician and mother also agree ahead of time on the content of the telephone sessions or home visits. The clinician discusses her role within the woman's support system as well as the kind of supportive guidance she will provide during this time. For example, the clinician explains in nontechnical language that she is available during the phone calls to provide self-care advice (e.g., *"answering questions you might have about your body as you recover from childbirth"*); individualized developmental guidance (e.g., *"think together about questions you have about your baby"*); mood management techniques (e.g., *"talk about how you are feeling and think of ways to increase your energy or lift your mood"*); and different activities conducive to the mother–infant relationship.

## Assessment of Cultural Practices during and/or Following Birth

The clinician assesses whether the woman follows specific postpartum-care-related practices and provides support as appropriate. Different cultures have different traditions following childbirth, and different generations within a specific cultural group may differ in their degree of observance. The clinician is attentive to these issues in order to play a supportive role when feasible.

For example, many Latina mothers practice *la cuarentena,* the postpartum rest period supported by values of familism and collectivism (Lefèber & Voorhoeve, 1998; Stern & Kruckman, 1983; Taylor, Ko, & Pan, 1999). Although there are *cuarentena* variations across different Latino groups, shared characteristics include observing 40 days of rest and seclusion following childbirth, receiving help with household chores from female relatives, eating special foods and abstaining from others, modifying some hygiene habits such as bathing and hair washing, and protecting oneself from cold air. Among those who value these rituals, noncompliance is believed to put the mother's and baby's health at risk. At the same time, adherence to these rituals can create stress when it puts immigrant women in conflict with expected behavior in the host culture.

## Addressing Reproductive Health Plans and Practices

The P-CPP clinician first raises the topic of reproductive health and practices in the latter part of the pregnancy, tailoring her approach to the values and practices the woman described during the foundational phase. The clinician asks about the woman's ideal family size and spacing between births; explores links between her current romantic situation, contraceptive practices, and a possible future pregnancy; and inquires about her perception of her partner's attitudes and wishes about having another baby. When the woman is willing, the clinician presents family planning options so that she can make an informed decision about the kind of family planning method that is most appropriate for her. Collaboration with the OB/GYN staff is pivotal, especially when working with women who have a history of unplanned pregnancies and/or lack knowledge about the different contraceptive options. The woman's partner participates when appropriate, including during conversations about attitudes and options regarding male birth control.

## Postpartum Period

The early postpartum period ushers drastic changes and adjustments for both the new mother and her newborn infant. While the new mother begins her recovery from the arduous physical task of giving birth or having surgery in the case of a cesarean section, the newborn baby begins a journey of survival in a world beset with unpredictability and novel sensations. Once the woman delivers, the clinician visits her and her infant in the labor and delivery ward; she also collaborates with other service providers where service coordination is appropriate. After the discharge from the hospital, the clinician follows the plan that she and the mother made regarding contact while she recovers from childbirth. During telephone calls or visits (as per the mother's request), the clinician provides self-care advice and psychoeducation about infant development, particularly around how newborns communicate their needs. The clinician also continues to monitor maternal mood and implements interventions to help the woman manage her stress and mood as appropriate.

The clinician also begins to assess the quality of the mother–infant relationship, particularly whether the mother shows evidence of being in a state of "primary maternal preoccupation" (Winnicott, 1956). In this state, which Winnicott saw as crucial to the healthy development of the infant, the mother is able to adapt her own needs to those of the baby. The clinician observes the mother's quality of attunement to the infant and her ability to read the baby's cues, helping the mother when needed to find a guilt-free, comfortable balance between self-care and care of her infant.

### Including the Baby: Supporting the Foundation of a Secure Attachment

Although the baby has been consistently present and held in the clinician's mind as she provides treatment prenatally, the actual birth is a turning point in the clinician's work with the family. The real baby is no longer primarily the recipient of each parent's wishes, fears, and fantasies, but a person who needs to be understood and responded to as a unique individual. The "good enough mother" described by Winnicott (1956) is able to respond to her baby's actual needs and demands most of the time, rather than responding to projected desires and demands that have their source in the mother's reenactment of her own conflicted early relationships. The same hold true for the good enough father. P-CPP interventions during the period immediately following the birth of the baby seek to prevent these reenactments by helping parents perceive their babies through a lens based on developmental knowledge and present reality rather than conflicted memories.

The baby's physical presence during the therapeutic sessions has concrete repercussions for what happens during these sessions. In addition to remaining receptive to the parent's individual and interpersonal experiences, the clinician maintains a steady focus on the baby and on the parent–baby relationship. Emotionally supportive, unstructured developmental guidance fosters reciprocity through the interventions described below.

1. Help the parent notice and understand the baby's responses to environmental stimuli to promote a sense of wonder in the baby's capacities.
2. Help the parent notice and respond to the baby's interpersonal bids to promote intimacy.
3. Help the parent recognize when the baby becomes a trauma reminder and find ways of redirecting the traumatic response to its original trigger in order to free the baby from the parents' distorted attributions.
4. Consolidate parental affect regulation skills in relation to the demands of early parenthood.
5. Guide the mother and the father toward collaborative co-parenting by highlighting their shared joy in the baby,

identifying shared and competing parenting values and goals, and promoting adaptive problem solving.

6. Assess the health needs of the baby and the parents and implement concrete assistance to establish and maintain developmentally recommended primary health care.

## Clinical Vignettes of the Core Phase with a Single Mother and Her Baby: Susan and Albert

Susan's core treatment phase expanded on the history of abuse and neglect that emerged during the foundational phase. Susan went back and forth between different themes that involved her childhood experiences, her relationships with her sons' fathers, and her current efforts to give her sons a better life in the midst of difficult circumstances. Her father remained an idealized figure, as she continued to describe loving memories of him, and the clinician looked for ports of entry that would clarify the links between her positive childhood experiences of her father and her choice of abusive men as partners. She seemed to need to protect her father from any negative feelings, with her anger and disappointment invariably directed at her abusive mother and sisters.

### BRINGING REALISTIC NUANCE TO THE IDEALIZED FATHER FIGURE

In a pivotal session, the clinician listened to yet another scene of Susan feeling frightened by her older sister's abuse, legitimized her experience, and then asked, "*What do you think made your sisters behave in such a nasty way toward you?*" Slowly and painfully, Susan described that her father became physically abusive toward her sisters and her mother when he was drunk, and she witnessed these scenes with a mixture of fear and relief that she was not the target of her father's anger at those times. The clinician commented, "*Your feelings make so much sense. What else do you remember about those times?*" Susan thought for a while and then said very quietly, "*I felt guilty because my mother and sisters blamed me for being my father's favorite. After he left, they used to make fun of me when I asked when he was coming back. They said he forgot about me. They hit me when I cried, telling me that they would give me something real to cry about, that he was a bad man and I didn't know how lucky everybody was that he left.*"

As Susan continued to talk about her father, mother, and sisters, she started sharing fragments of conversation that she overheard among the adults that provided a counterbalance to her positive memories of her father. She recalled suspicions that he might have been involved in drug trafficking, and the mystery surrounding his absence made her worry that he was among those killed every time she read or heard accounts of gang violence. In this context, a possible meaning of Susan's choice of men who became violent when drunk could be an unconscious enactment of her conflicted experience of her father through a split between her images of her father as loving toward her, as violent toward her sisters, and as a possible criminal.

The clinician made this theme a central focus of the treatment, linking Susan's contradictory male images with her challenges being the mother of two sons and the soon-to-be mother of a third son. She introduced the topic by saying, *"Do you think that your relationship with your father and your partners has an effect on how you raise your sons?"* This question became an organizing theme for Susan, who answered with a question of her own: *"Do you think my sons will be like their fathers?"* These two questions placed the unborn baby boy within the framework of his imagined relationship with his brothers. The clinician's efforts were directed at creating a psychological environment in which males could be raised to be loving and to express negative emotions in safe ways, so that the baby and his brothers could be free from the pressure to reenact the relationship that Susan had with her sisters while growing up.

### LABOR AND DELIVERY: REFRAMING THE REEXPERIENCE OF EARLY TRAUMATIC MEMORIES

Susan telephoned the clinician to let her know that she was at the hospital's childbirth center and was in labor. The clinician visited her briefly and found Susan in good spirits, accompanied by her older children's godmother. While in the ward, the clinician met with the social worker from the birth center to coordinate postpartum service delivery.

As the day went by, it became clear that Susan was embarking on a long and arduous childbirth process that eventually lasted 45 hours and involved induced delivery due to fetal distress. Baby Albert was a healthy 9-pound, 3-ounce baby. The medical file noted the long and difficult labor and a third-degree tear during delivery as the only complications.

Soon after the delivery, the neonatal social worker called the clinician to request a visit because Susan was crying inconsolably; the staff had been unable to help her calm down. The clinician found Susan tearful in bed and the baby sleeping in a heated crib next to her. The clinician briefly congratulated her on the arrival of baby Albert, handed her a tissue, and asked how she was feeling. With tears rolling down her cheeks, Susan answered, *"I'm exhausted and sore all over . . .*

*giving birth to Albert was one of the worst experiences I ever had in my life!"*
The clinician responded in an empathic tone, *"You sure did have a very
long and difficult labor . . . no wonder you are exhausted and sore. Did something else happen?"* Susan then began talking about her angry feelings
toward the medical staff, whom she described as *"cold and inconsider-
ate"* with her. She added, *"Instead of helping me, they made things worse
for me and my baby!"* She went on to recount that at one point there
were four nurses and two doctors in the delivery room, and that all of
them were telling her to push harder. Wiping her tears off her face,
she said angrily, *"I was exhausted. I had no energy, and they were all asking me to push! I honestly couldn't push any harder. I just couldn't!"* The
clinician validated Susan's feelings and normalized her reaction to the
medical staff's request given how physically exhausted she had been. In
an almost whisper, Susan said that something very embarrassing had
happened, and went on to disclose that at one point she had pushed
so hard that she had defecated. When this happened, Susan said, she
saw from the corner of her eye that *"one of the young doctors was smirking
and squinting in disgust."* When she saw the doctor's reaction, Susan felt
flooded by feelings of shame and guilt. She added that she was glad
that a different doctor had stitched her third-degree tear.

The clinician responded by normalizing Susan's loss of bowel
control and expressing regret that the young doctor did not yet have
the professional maturity to expect it as a frequent occurrence during
childbirth. She added, *"You were trying as much as you could to comply
with what the doctors asked you to do, and instead of praise you saw disgust."*
Susan nodded, still sniffling but calmer now. The clinician then said,
*"You told me you were ashamed and very sad when this incident with the
doctor happened. Do you remember having those feelings in the past?"* After
a pause, Susan, who had stopped crying by now, said, *"Now that you
mention it . . . you know when the doctor did that . . . when he looked at
me that way, it reminded me of when I was about 6 years old and my sister
scolded me when I had accidents. One time, I had bad diarrhea and had an
accident. My sister undressed me in front of everyone, even the neighbors, who
began laughing at me. She told me in front of everyone that I was dirty and
smelly."* The clinician responded, *"I can only imagine how you felt when
she said that and did those things to you. You were such a young child."* Susan
replied, *"I felt really bad . . . ashamed of myself . . . dirty and smelly like she
said, and embarrassed because she said it in front of everyone."* The clinician
said that it is so wrong when parents and caregivers humiliate young
children who are just learning to control their normal body functions
like defecating. Susan added, *"You know, when I pooped I felt like I was a
little girl all over again, especially when I looked at that doctor's reaction. I
got so angry at him!"* The clinician said, *"It's understandable because what*

*happened revived in you painful memories and feelings.*" As Susan continued to remember her feelings in the past and in the present elicited by this embarrassing moment, she started to entertain the possibility that the young doctor's reaction might have been due to his inexperience and then said that she might have misinterpreted it. The clinician used this opportunity to assess Susan's feelings about her baby after the difficult birth. Susan, smiling at her baby who was still sleeping, said in a soft voice, "*It's not Albert's fault. He was trying very hard to come out. I feel blessed that that he was born so healthy.*"

During the second day of Susan's stay at the hospital, the clinician met with the social worker and the medical staff for service coordination. None of the service providers expressed concern over Susan's ability to care for her newborn. They commented that Susan responded very lovingly when the baby cried. Once discharged from the hospital, Susan continued to have weekly telephone contact with the clinician, who provided self-care recommendations and developmental guidance. The clinician also made sure that Susan attended all the medical appointments for herself and the baby, including an appointment to talk about family planning and choose a form of birth control that was agreeable to her.

### REFLECTIONS ON THE CORE TREATMENT PHASE WITH SUSAN AND ALBERT

The therapeutic work that unfolded during the foundational and core phases resulted in a significant decrease in Susan's depression, anger, and traumatic responses after her son's birth. Baby Albert was a big, strong, and healthy baby who quickly acquired organized sleep–wake cycles, communicated needs clearly, and calmed quickly when Susan responded to his crying. Her older sons expressed some annoyance about the changes in daily routine and decreased maternal availability, but they were primarily excited about becoming "big brothers" and delighted when baby Albert started following them with his gaze and smiled in response to their antics.

The clinician realized that the best predictor of the baby's healthy development would be Susan's success in changing her pattern of quickly falling in love and becoming pregnant from her relationships with men she hardly knew, who felt trapped by her pregnancies and responded with violence and abandonment. The clinician's therapeutic stance involved empathy with Susan's longing for unconditional love, insight-oriented exploration of the childhood roots of her resignation to abuse and expectation of abandonment, and reflective developmental guidance about how to protect herself by bringing a more mindful state of mind to her relationships with men. Candid conversations

about her fertility and reproductive choices were an integral component of these interventions.

### Clinical Vignette of the Core Phase with a High-Conflict Couple and Baby: Ana, Martin, and Rosa

Ana attended 16 individual sessions before the baby's birth. Ana and
the baby, Rosa, attended 26 mother–infant therapy sessions. Martin
participated in 14 therapy sessions. There were a few cancellations due
to illness, bad weather, and a crisis in the clinician's life, but the family
always participated in scheduled sessions. The sessions were in Spanish
at the hospital-based program.

The bitter fights between Ana and Martin were a recurrent theme
during the core phase, interspersed with periods of contrition, emotional closeness, and vows to continue their efforts to curb their insulting mutual recriminations. The clinician understood their emotional
volatility as an entrenched component of their respective personality
structures. She targeted her interventions at helping them become
increasingly conscious of how their early experiences of abuse and loss
had shaped who they became as adults. She also encouraged them be
more aware of their tendency to respond with uncontrolled rage when
displeased by the other. She helped them practice conscious behavioral self-restraint by breathing, lowering their voices, and agreeing to
end arguments until they were calmer. Conflict resolution techniques
proved very useful during these times. Both during the pregnancy and
after the baby was born, the clinician spoke directly to the fetus/baby
about how he or she felt while witnessing the parents' angry exchanges.
This therapeutic approach invariably had the effect of calming the parents, who both wished to provide a family environment for their baby
that was safer than the one they had growing up.

In an individual session after the feedback session, Ana reported
that she was having a baby girl, and she and Martin had agreed on
calling her Rosa because this was Ana's favorite flower. The clinician
offered congratulations and asked Ana whether it would be all right if
she called the baby by her name. Ana smiled broadly and, while caressing her belly, said that she had never thought about doing that, but she
liked the idea and would start calling the baby by her name as well.

During the following sessions, Ana talked openly about her grief
over her separation from her older daughter, her conflicts with Martin,
and her symptoms of depression and anxiety. Among other interventions, the clinician modeled for Ana how to talk to her unborn baby
about her "*strong and difficult feelings.*" While looking at Ana's belly,
the clinician said, "*Rosa, your mom is feeling sad today. She is telling me*

*how much she misses your sister who is in Colombia with your grandma.*" In another session, Ana arrived to her appointment very upset because of a heated argument with Martin earlier that day in which he had insulted her. After giving space for Ana to describe and process the incident, the clinician, while looking at Ana's belly, said, "*Rosa, your mom is very upset right now because she had an argument with your father. When your father gets angry, he uses hurtful words . . . and that makes your mom feel sad and angry with him. Your mom and I are trying to figure how to help her feel better. We are also trying to see how to help your father not to do this anymore, so when you come, you won't have to listen to scary fights between them.*" As she spoke, the clinician alternated between looking at Ana's belly and looking into Ana's eyes, making sure she spoke to both mother and unborn baby. The clinician interspersed these interventions with intervals of helping Ana track her somatic reactions and engage in diaphragmatic breathing and grounding exercises. Ana responded positively to these strategies.

During this phase of treatment, it became increasingly clear that Ana and Martin were in different stages in the process of adapting to a new culture. Martin was at ease operating in a bilingual and bicultural milieu, while Ana was a recent immigrant struggling to learn a new language and understand the intricacies of daily living in a foreign country. Ana described several episodes of Martin becoming angry when she made comments about missing her country, talked about the differences she noticed between Colombia and the United States, or asked questions about using public transportation. By Ana's report, Martin also laughed and ridiculed her when she spoke in English, saying, "*You are so stupid, slow, ignorant.*" These reports gave new impetus to the importance of including Martin in the sessions once again, but Martin became evasive and said that he was too busy earning the money they would need to support the baby.

As the due date drew near, Ana's lack of familiarity with childbirth medical practices in the United States called for including preparations for the birth as a focal point of therapy. The clinician assisted Ana in drafting a birth plan that included her wish for Martin to take time off from work to be by her side during the delivery and immediate postpartum period. She also made it clear that she did not want her sister-in-law to visit at the hospital, a point of contention with Martin that was easily resolved when it became clear that discharge would occur within 48 hours after delivery. The neonatal social worker helped Ana arranged the services of a Spanish-speaking doula who would provide support during labor and delivery. The clinician also gave Ana useful handouts in Spanish listing the things she would need for herself and the baby at the hospital and on her return home.

In response to Ana's anxiety about labor and delivery, the clinician helped her visualize the different stages of the process, describe how her body responded, and practice breathing and relaxation exercises. The clinician also raised the topic of family planning. Ana was so embarrassed at first that she stammered when she answered that she did not want to get pregnant again for at least a few years. She remained clearly embarrassed while the clinician described the different birth control options available for both women and men. As the conversation continued and with the clinician's support, she became increasingly self-confident as she articulated her reactions to each specific form of birth control. She eventually said with considerable conviction, *"Martin keeps complaining that I get pregnant. Now I will show him that I can have control of my body."*

## ROSA IS BORN

Ana called one late afternoon to let the clinician know that she had gone into labor. The following day, the clinician received a voicemail from Ana giving her the news that *"Rosa arrived."* The clinician called Ana to congratulate her and ask her whether this would be a good time to visit. Ana welcomed the idea and said that Martin was there as well. When the clinician arrived, she found Martin holding the sleeping baby and congratulated the parents. Ana said with a smile that she was feeling tired but happy, and that everything had gone well because she had practiced the breathing exercises and Martin had supported her during the birth. Looking at Martin, she said eagerly that now he could start joining the therapy more consistently, as he had promised to do after the baby arrived. Martin looked subdued but agreed, restating that the sessions would need to be on his day off. The conversation then turned to Rosa, who was healthy and weighed 9 pounds, 2 ounces. Ana said proudly that her labor lasted only 7 hours and attributed the easy delivery to having Martin and the doula by her side during the entire process.

## EARLY POSTPARTUM SESSIONS

During the following 3 weeks, the clinician checked in with Ana by telephone. During these weekly telephone conversations, the clinician checked on Ana's mood and provided guidance about rest, nutrition, keeping postnatal medical appointments, and following through with the family planning decisions that she and Martin had agreed to. Ana derived much joy from the baby and reported that she and Martin were getting along well. She reported on Rosa's likes and dislikes and her tendency to cry for prolonged periods in the late afternoon. She described her own ease with breastfeeding and her efforts to implement a feeding and sleeping routine. Everything seemed to be going well for baby, mother, and the triad with Martin.

## THE ESSENTIAL TRIAD IS TENTATIVELY ESTABLISHED

As Ana had hoped, Martin came to the first therapy session 5 weeks after the postpartum break in clinic-based sessions. After a brief feeding in the waiting area, Rosa fell asleep and remained asleep during the entire session. Martin seemed low keyed and cautious as he entered the playroom. The clinician welcomed them, adding that she was glad Martin was able to join them. He smiled nervously and said, "*I am coming again because Ana asked me to . . . and because Ana is now coming with Rosa.*" The clinician commented on how Rosa had grown since the last time she saw her. Ana and Martin looked at each other, and both nodded in agreement. Martin then said that Rosa was also a very smart baby. The clinician asked him to tell her more about it. Ana said, "*Rosa likes to be held upright against my shoulder when she is ready to go sleep.*" Martin added that Rosa had a big appetite and that she used her "*powerful cry*" to let them know when she was hungry, and calmed down fast after she was fed. The clinician complimented them on how well they knew their baby given the short time she had been living with them. Martin agreed, saying that things were going well with the family, especially now that the baby was born and they were living by themselves in a new apartment. Ana agreed that things had changed for the better since Rosa's arrival. The rest of the session unfolded quietly, with the parents taking turns harmoniously in describing the baby and their new routine co-parenting her.

## MARITAL CONFLICTS REEMERGE

This close and collaborative partnership was disrupted when Rosa got sick with a cold at 10 weeks, which Martin attributed to Ana's incompetence in caring for the baby. Ana reported during a dyadic session with the baby that Martin had told her, "*You don't know how to take care of our baby. It is your fault that Rosa caught a cold. Look at the way you dress her. Do you think you live in Colombia? You know nothing about babies! What kind of mother are you? You are a good-for-nothing!*" When asked how Martin's comments made her feel, Ana began crying and said that she felt very upset and angry with Martin. The clinician acknowledged how hurtful Martin's words had been and validated Ana's feelings. After she calmed down, Ana added, "*When we argue, I get so angry at him and I say things to his face. I remind him that I was the one who raised our older daughter, not him! He left us and vanished from our lives! What kind of father is he?*" She added that these arguments frequently escalated into verbal fights about Martin's disappearance from her life and about her accusations against him and his sister of provoking her recent miscarriage. The gains they had made during the foundational phase in addressing these topics seemed to have dissipated under the stress of shared parenthood.

When the clinician asked Ana where Rosa was during these arguments, she reported that Rosa was usually in the room with them, either asleep or awake in her crib. She then said that she was worried about arguing with Martin in front of Rosa, because Rosa had awakened a couple of times because of the yelling and had started crying inconsolably. The clinician turned to Rosa, who was in an active alert state, and said, "*Your mom notices how scary it is for you when you hear your mama and papa yell at each other. . . .*" She paused and noticed that tears had begun rolling down Ana's face. She continued by saying, "*Your mommy is very upset right now . . . She is telling me how scared you were when they woke you up with their yelling. We are trying to find ways of protecting you from that because your mama knows that this is hard for you.*" As the clinician handed Ana the tissue box, she told Rosa, "*Your mom is crying because she is sad . . . she is worried about you and wants these fights between her and your father to stop.*" As on previous occasions, these interventions made Ana calmer, and she held the baby closely while looking at her with a loving expression.

Before the session ended, the clinician conducted an IPV risk assessment that revealed no imminent risk of physical abuse. The clinician also observed how Ana interacted with Rosa, and asked whether her symptoms of depression were affecting her mood and energy in taking care of Rosa at home. Ana responded that "*no matter what*" she was always attentive to Rosa's needs. Ana's behavior during the session corroborated this assertion. For example, Ana was able to read and respond to Rosa's cues of distress and soothed her successfully when she became fussy. At the end of the session, Ana stated feeling a little better after talking about the incident and said that she was going to ask Martin to come to the next session. Martin indeed came uninterruptedly for the following 4 weeks. The following session represents a turning point in the treatment.

RESTATING THE UNSPEAKABLE TO CREATE RAPID CHANGE

Ana, Martin, and 4-month-old Rosa arrived 20 minutes late to their appointment. Ana appeared as if she had been crying because her eyes were puffy and red. Martin was polite but very serious when he greeted the clinician. As in an earlier session, he apologized profusely for being *"so late"* to their appointment, and added that he did not like being late for anything. Rosa, who was very alert, smiled when the clinician greeted her.

The parents and the clinician sat down on the carpet. Ana was sitting cross-legged and had placed Rosa in a supported sitting position on her lap. Rosa was playing and exploring the toys that Ana had brought for her. She was grabbing and mouthing a colorful giraffe and a teething toy. Sensing the tension between Ana and Martin, the clinician asked how they were doing and whether something had happened on their way to the clinic. Ana remained silent while looking down as she continued handing the giraffe to Rosa, who seemed immersed in holding, banging, and dropping the toy. Martin said that they were *"OK."* Ana said angrily, *"Maybe you are OK but I am not!"* Martin looked at the clinician as if he did not know what Ana was talking about. The clinician asked Ana to describe how she was feeling, and Ana responded with a contorted facial expression that she was very angry and upset. There was an awkward silence, and the adults looked at Rosa, who was chewing on her teething ring. Martin interrupted the silence by pointing out that they were late today because Ana was *"too slow this morning, as she always is."* He added that they had had an argument about it before arriving to the clinic and then, his voice rising, listed in an accusatory tone all the things that in his opinion Ana had done wrong that week.

The clinician listened attentively, trying to gain an objective sense of Ana's ability to negotiate everyday activities in a new country. The actions that most aggravated Martin involved Ana's overly casual approach to housekeeping. She did not do the laundry, so he found at the last minute that he did not have a clean shirt to go to work; she left the dirty dinner dishes from the previous evening in the sink overnight; she did not bathe the baby daily; the house was dusty. Martin's voice kept rising as the list of chores left undone grew in his narrative of daily life in the household. He finally said, *"She is impossible to live with—she is dirty and lazy, and all she does is complain. She is not even a good mother. She thinks that loving the baby is enough, but look at the cold Rosa got because of the way she dresses her."* At this, Ana burst into tears, and Rosa followed as if on cue.

The clinician thought to herself that Martin had a consistent pattern of demeaning Ana that had diminished over the course of recent sessions but continued to flare up in ways that were deeply detrimental to Ana and Rosa and represented a threat to the family. She decided to take a risky course of action with the hope of shaking Martin into a recognition that his words were crossing a boundary. Looking at Martin, she told him in a respectful but firm voice, *"What just happened in the room has a name . . . it is called emotional and verbal abuse because you are frightening your wife and your daughter. In this country many people would even call it domestic violence."* Martin stopped talking and stared down at the floor.

The clinician then turned to Rosa, who was still crying, and said, *"You are telling your parents that you are scared . . . that you get frightened when you see your father get angry at your mother . . . yelling at her, saying hurtful words to her . . . it's so scary for you."* Martin then said, *"I grew up listening to my father saying much worse things to my mother . . . I don't hit Ana!"* He paused for a few seconds, as if reflecting on what he just heard, and then asked the clinician with a tone of disbelief, *"And you are calling that domestic violence?"* The clinician replied, *"Yes, many people would call it that."* There was a long pause, and then Ana said to Martin, *"You have no idea how much it hurts me when you say those things to me. . . . You never give me a chance to tell you how I feel! This is how I feel when you treat me like that!"* Martin said, *"I never thought I was abusing you. I thought this is just the way couples argue. I'm sorry."*

The clinician asked Ana if there was anything in Martin's complaints that made her think of ways she could make life easier at home. Ana answered that her way of getting back at Martin when she was angry with him was not to do the things he expected of her in managing the household, such as doing the domestic chores. She said he always praised his sister for keeping an immaculate home, and the comparison was so offensive to her that she responded by wanting to be the opposite of his sister as payback.

The clinician commented, as she had in an earlier session, that each of them had grown up with parents who fought with each other, and children learn from what they see happening around them. Much as their parents' fights frightened them, they also learned that fighting was the way to express what they did not like. She then engaged Martin and Ana in a conversation in which they practiced saying in a neutral tone what they wanted from each other. Martin said he wanted a tidy, predictable household; Ana said that she wanted Martin to speak kindly to her. The clinician asked whether they sounded like reasonable wishes to each other, and they both agreed that they did. They also agreed that they would try to remember to give the other what he or she wanted, and they would remind each other when they failed, trying to speak without yelling.

As the session ended, the clinician commented that this had been a very difficult session for all of them, and summarized the session and its outcome. She then thanked both Ana and Martin for being open to discussing their feelings and trying to change patterns that annoyed the other. When it was time to say good-bye, the clinician said to Rosa, who had calmed down by then, *"Today was very scary for you because the two people you love the most got angry and yelled at each other. Your parents are trying very hard to learn to talk to each other in ways that are not hurtful and to give you a safe place to live where there are no scary fights. That is why they are coming to see me. Your father now knows his words sometimes can be very hurtful for you and your mommy, and your mommy knows that sometimes she does things that make your daddy mad."* Martin held Rosa in his arms and nuzzled her neck as they left.

## Recapitulation and Closing Phase: Consolidating Treatment Gains

The process of ending treatment presents rich clinical opportunities to work through feelings of abandonment and loss, revisit and celebrate gains made, and anticipate how the parents will cope with future challenges. Trauma-informed treatments call for specific attention to the frequent overlap of interpersonal trauma with experiences of loss, because family violence frequently involves the rupture of family ties, separation from at least one parent, or the death of a primary caregiver. The termination phase invariably evokes painful conscious or unconscious feelings of abandonment, rejection, and loss, but these feelings can promote reflection, provide opportunities for repair, and support growing self-understanding long after treatment ends.

P-CPP usually ends when the baby turns 6 months old on the assumption that traumatic interference with the parents' emotional involvement and their capacity to protect the baby can be resolved in a significant proportion of families during this interval of time. However, much depends on the character structure of the parents and the severity and chronicity of their mental health problems. If clinical needs remain when the baby turns 6 months old, treatment continues along clinically indicated lines.

Raising the topic of length of treatment and the planned termination date during the foundational phase has considerable value because it provides transparency about the expected course of treatment. During the first or second session, the clinician informs the parents that as a rule treatment lasts until the baby is 6 months old, and goes on to explain that they can decide to end treatment sooner, or they may request to continue treatment if they find they continue to need it. During the core treatment phase, the clinician periodically reminds the parents about the expected termination date and elicits their feelings about ending treatment. Anticipating termination as an integral part of treatment helps the parents mobilize their anticipatory coping resources to minimize feelings of abandonment and loss.

The closing phase involves a continued focus on the relevant clinical themes as well as an appreciation and acknowledgment of the positive changes the family has made. The clinician comments on the parents' trajectory from the initial session until the present moment, helping them reminisce about their frame of mind and emotional state when they began treatment, revisit transformational therapeutic moments, and celebrate the baby and their new role as parents.

A few weeks before the baby turns 6 months old, the clinician invites the parents to respond to the same structured questionnaires that the parents filled out during the foundational phase. The clinician explains that the parents and clinician can look together at the similarities and differences in how the parents described their mood, attitudes toward their baby, and feelings about becoming parents at the beginning and now the completion of treatment. The pre–posttreatment review with the parents provides a concrete way of reflecting on improvements, assessing continued challenges, and deciding on plans to end treatment, continue it, or make referrals to other appropriate resources.

Termination can have a celebratory tone when both the parents and clinician see the treatment as successful. There might be sadness about saying good-bye, but there is also a feeling of pride in the accomplishments and joy at seeing the baby thrive and the parents rejoice in the baby. In different circumstances, terminations may have a somber or painful emotional feel. This is particularly the case if treatment is ending for external reasons (e.g., the clinician leaving the agency, the parent moving out of the area, the agency enforcing time-limited treatment, financial considerations, or other reasons). In every case, it is important to acknowledge the positive gains together with the challenges that remain, because the integration of positive and negative feelings into a manageable ambivalence is one of the hallmarks of emotional maturity.

Regardless of the circumstances for ending treatment, the clinician always endeavors to build a bridge to the future by helping parents anticipate and practice adaptive coping responses to challenges they will inevitably face going forward. Helping secure access to needed resources can add a positive note to the closing phase. It is also important for the clinician to express genuine appreciation and to convey best wishes for the future of the parents and the child. A realistic positive regard on saying good-bye affirms the parents' dignity and is protective of both the parents and the child.

*Clinical Vignettes of the Termination Phase*

Termination proceeded smoothly both with Susan and with Ana and Martin. Both families filled out the structured assessment forms a few weeks after their babies turned 6 months, and in both cases there were significant improvements in adult clinical symptoms, parenting stress, and commitment to the baby.

Susan reported feeling a new sense of acceptance about her father's disappearance. She said it grieved her not to know whether he was dead or had started a new life without her, but she felt resigned to not knowing unless something unexpected happened to inform her of his fate. She reported joy in mothering Albert, felt a new tenderness toward her older sons as she watched them rejoice in the new baby, and was less worried that they were destined to become the aggressive males their fathers were. She also discovered in herself for the first time a sense of serenity in not having a partner. She said that, at age 29, she had time to wait for the right person to come along and until that happened she had her children, her church, and her friends.

Ana and Martin used their shared commitment and love for the baby as a vehicle to manage the dissatisfactions that continued to flare between them. They adopted the clinician's method of speaking to Rosa directly after a fight, telling her they were sorry to have frightened her and showing her that they were now friends. They made themselves join with each other in playing with Rosa, and found that joint play made them feel the commonality of sharing in the baby's pleasure. In playing, they also rediscovered singing—including remembering popular songs from Colombia that they were now singing together to the baby. They rejoiced in Rosa's healthy development, and told themselves and each other that the determination to give their daughter what they did not have was their impetus to overcome the waves of resentment that continued to wash over them unexpectedly. Each of them reported wishing they had a different childhood, with more love and protection and less fear and loss. At the end of P-CPP, they started couple therapy at a community mental health clinic to continue repairing the relationship between them, both for themselves and for Rosa.

# Section III

# Implementing P-CPP
## *Extended Clinical Cases*

This section consists of four extended clinical cases that illustrate how P-CPP was implemented with four women who each presented a different configuration of traumatic experiences within an overall context of great adversity. The detailed case descriptions have the goal of describing each clinician's reasoning in implementing the specific therapeutic modalities chosen in response to a clinical moment. Each of us was the clinician in one of the cases to demonstrate P-CPP compatibility with different individual clinical styles. The treating clinician's initials are provided in each case the first time she is mentioned.

# Clinical Case 1.
# Learning to Become a Family: P-CPP with Parents Recovering from Substance Abuse and Violence

This case describes the treatment of Eva and Sean, a couple with a past history of substance abuse and violent criminal behavior. They reported intense fears that they would relapse into their previous lifestyle under the pressure of caring for a baby after a few years of hard-earned but still fragile recovery. As treatment unfolded, it became clear that the unborn baby was being drawn into unresolved parental conflicts and had become the target of traumatic triggers, distorted perceptions, and negative parental attributions that stemmed from the parents' childhood experiences of abuse and neglect. Treatment focused on the disturbing childhood memories evoked by the pregnancy, fantasies of the unborn baby, fears and wishes about the baby's place in their lives, and the new meanings they could construct about themselves as individuals and as parents as they came to understand the connections between their early experiences and the trajectory of their adult lives.

## Referral and Presenting Problems

Eva was referred by her prenatal care team at the county hospital. The social worker making the referral described her as a European American 42-year-old woman who was 30 weeks pregnant with her first child and who had become antagonistic toward her physician when she disagreed with the treatment prescribed to treat her hypothyroidism. Eva had refused the medication and wanted to treat herself with herbal infusions, which the physician considered ineffective. A tense stalemate between mother and physician had been reached following angry confrontations, and the staff at the Women's Clinic offered Eva the opportunity to speak with "experts in mothers and babies" as a way of affirming that Eva's refusal of medication reflected an underlying ambivalence regarding her pregnancy, and hoped that we could help her accept the physician's advice. Eva welcomed the referral.

The conflict over medication had been resolved by the time of Eva's first meeting the clinician (A. F. L.). Eva opened the first session by saying that she had agreed to follow the physician's advice and take the medication as prescribed, but added bitterly that it took an altercation to get a mental health referral. She went on to explain, in a heated tone of voice, that for several months she had been telling the OB/GYN social worker about her ambivalence about her pregnancy, her fear of not being able to love her baby, and her sense of feeling trapped into becoming a mother because at her age she no longer had the choice of waiting until she was ready to have a child. The health system, she complained, did not take these feelings seriously enough to offer a mental health referral. She added, "*It was only when they worried about the baby that they offered me help. In their eyes, I only counted as a baby carrier.*" This statement was the first manifestation of a theme that would recur during treatment: Eva's experience of being resentfully secondary to the baby. As the clinician listened, she asked herself what unconscious factors might have prevented this clearly intelligent and resourceful woman from taking the initiative in seeking out therapy for herself. As Eva's history unfolded, the theme of being secondary became the expression of a long-standing experience of being displaced and superseded by her younger siblings, waiting in lonely and futile expectation for her parents to notice and take care of her. The implications of this experience for Eva's transference to the clinician were clear: It would be crucial to balance attention to the baby with attention to the mother for treatment to be effective in promoting a secure attachment and supporting the mother's and the baby's mental health.

## Starting Treatment: The Foundational Phase

The foundational phase is designed to assess different facets of functioning, develop an initial clinical formulation, and create the first stage of a treatment plan. In this sense, the foundational phase merges assessment and the initial steps of treatment. The clinician elicits information and uses carefully timed clarifications, trial interventions, and close monitoring of the parents' responses to form impressions about their ability to use reflection, establish a working relationship with the clinician, and open themselves to possible links between their difficulties with the pregnancy and their baby and their own emotional experiences as individuals. Eva's commitment to psychological growth and readiness for treatment became quickly apparent in the eagerness with which she spoke about her inner world, described her life history, and responded to initial interventions during the foundational phase. When the clinician asked at the beginning of the first session about her reasons for finally agreeing to take medication for her hypothyroidism, Eva replied, "*I had a vision of the baby. It was beautiful and perfect, and made me feel that I did not need to take medicine, that the baby would be all right. But my husband said that in the vision I could not know whether that was the way the baby looked because I took medicine or in spite of my not taking it. That made me realize I had a responsibility both toward my husband and toward the baby. So I agreed to the treatment.*" She then quickly returned to the theme of her worries about not loving the baby by adding, "*But I feel nothing toward the baby, no excitement, no love, no nothing. There is a block inside me that does not let me love my baby. And I want to love it.*" Taken together, these statements and her agreement to a treatment she did not want were powerful expressions of Eva's commitment to her husband, Sean, her desire to join him in protecting the baby, and her longing for a healthy, perfect baby. The clinician had the clear sense from this exchange that Eva would be an effective partner in her own treatment.

At the same time, the first session also raised questions about Eva's character structure and the possibility of a thought disorder. She said she had several cats and two dogs, and added casually that if the baby turned out to be allergic to them she would have to give the baby away because she had the animals first. She then commented that she worried that Sean would object to her giving the baby away, and then she would have a difficult choice to make between Sean, the animals, and the baby. She went on to speak with delight about the animals, describing in elaborate detail her pets' penchant to plot practical jokes on her, pretend surprise if she returned home earlier than she had told them she would, defy her by doing the opposite of what she told them to do, and laugh about her among themselves. All this was described in a jovial tone, as if Eva were speaking of pesky but lovable creatures.

The jovial tone changed abruptly and became angry when Eva spoke about the baby as tying her down because, unlike what she did with the animals, she could not leave the baby alone if she wanted to go out. As the clinician asked Eva about her ambivalence toward the pregnancy, she responded, "I am afraid that the baby will make my past return." She then spoke of her adolescence and young adulthood as a time of turmoil and self-destructiveness, describing herself as the "*momma*" of a notorious motorcycle gang, hooked on alcohol and amphetamines, involved in interstate drug trafficking, and always fleeing the police and the FBI.

Eva had been married to one of the gang's leaders, whom she described as a "drug fiend" who had abused Eva physically and mentally and inflicted deep wounds with a knife, and she bore severe scars that remained from this attack. He had also been involved in two automobile accidents so severe that both he and Eva had almost bled to death on both occasions. He threatened to kill Eva if she tried to leave him. For years, Eva wished that he would die in a shootout with the police, and imagined his violent death both as a form of revenge and as a means of liberation. He had indeed died, but not in an encounter with the police. He drowned in a swimming pool while stoned on drugs. Eva said that his peaceful death was a great disappointment to her, and that its discrepancy from her carefully nurtured fantasy of a violent shootout was so jarring that for a few days afterward she could not reconcile herself to his dying in a different way than she had envisioned. The intensity of Eva's murderous fantasy and her difficulty navigating a discrepant reality raised yet another source of concern about the intactness of her thought processes when under stress.

The death of Eva's first husband was indeed a source of liberation for her. She became convinced that she would also die unless she could break the cycle of using amphetamines during the day and alcohol at night. She left the gang, joined several organizations to treat her addiction, and finally succeeded in maintaining a stable recovery 7 years before becoming pregnant. Two years earlier she had married Sean, whom she described as someone with a troubled past who had also recovered from addiction to alcohol and drugs. Eva said that her present marriage was "*idyllic*" but she feared that the baby would shatter her relationship with Sean and plunge her back into addiction. Since becoming pregnant, she dreamed repeatedly that her first husband was not dead but had returned to claim her as his legitimate wife. Eva feared that these dreams were a portent of the danger she was facing, because becoming a mother would be so stressful that she would be tempted to drink and use drugs again. She reported that she often woke up at night crying, "*I don't want the baby.*"

As Eva and the clinician traced the origin of Eva's use of drugs and alcohol, she said that her mother used to give her whiskey, codeine, and paregoric when she was very little. Eva remembered liking the feeling these substances gave her. She learned to sneak into the liquor cabinet when she was still a young child, and by age 13, she was regularly drinking until she passed out. Her parents, she said, never noticed the steadily decreasing level of liquor in the bottles because they seldom drank. The clinician expressed amazement that her parents did not notice her passing out. Eva responded that her father was an extremely withdrawn although sporadically violent man, and that her mother was "*strange,*" "*out in a world of her own.*" When a few years earlier Eva told her mother that she had just celebrated her fourth "*sobriety anniversary,*" the mother expressed mild surprise at her daughter's alcoholism, but showed no interest in pursuing the topic. For Eva this was a sadly familiar response: what Eva said "*never made any impact on her.*"

Eva's mother became a recurring topic in the ensuing sessions.

The oldest of five children, she lost her own mother at age 14, and her father subsequently abandoned the children. The four youngest ones were placed in foster homes by the state, and Eva's mother was sent to live with a maternal aunt. She dropped out of school and worked very hard to support her siblings and bring them out of foster homes. She could never realize her life's dream of becoming an engineer. She married an engineer instead and went on to have five children, just as her own mother had done.

Eva was the oldest, precisely her mother's position among her own siblings. Eva remembered her mother telling her that she never wanted any children, and Eva had to take care of her siblings from a very young age. Her most fervent wish as a child was to be alone, but she found herself constantly interrupted in whatever she did. If she read, her mother would call on her to feed one of the babies. If she played, she had to stop because another sibling needed changing. Not surprisingly, Eva reported that her happiest moments were when she was on her own. Although her mother did not work, Eva did not remember spending any time alone with her, except for occasional outings to the park.

Eva remembered wanting to grow up in a hurry in order to be autonomous, and proudly recalled her mother's saying that as a baby she learned to run before she walked. Yet growing up also became a trap. An example: as a young child, Eva had for some reason conceived of washing dishes as the ultimate symbol of being a grown-up. She confided this fantasy to her mother, who told her that she would be allowed to wash dishes when she reached a certain height. Eva eagerly awaited that day, measuring herself often and making marks on the wall. When she was finally tall enough, she was allowed to wash dishes as promised. But from that day on, washing dishes became her daily obligation. When she protested, her mother replied: *"You said you wanted to do it, now you do it."*

While Eva described her past, the clinician made occasional sympathetic comments, and observed her response in order to assess Eva's ability to use the clinician for the exploration and understanding of affective experiences. Although somewhat guarded in the overt expression of emotion, Eva was able to acknowledge some of the pain she had experienced as a young child and was receptive to the possibility of a link between those experiences and her present difficulties. One example stands out. After Eva enumerated her many chores as a substitute mother to her siblings, the clinician commented on the burden of having to take care of children when she herself was a child. Eva nodded her agreement and remained silent for a while. She then made the connection the clinician was implicitly suggesting. She asked, *"Do you think that is why I now have mixed feelings toward my baby?"*

Eva herself offered the answer to this question. She spoke tearfully about her parents' lack of involvement in her life and about the complete absence of rules that might help her decide what was right and what was wrong. Her mother told her that she did not bother to set rules because her children would disobey them anyway. Eva remembered her longing to have firm answers to her questions about issues, such as when she should be home from a date, but her parents' answer was invariably *"Whenever you think it's right,"* and Eva looked at her friends' parents for guidance in these matters. She bitterly said, *"I guess that kind of childrearing is all right if you can survive it."*

This early wish for clear guidelines about right and wrong was particularly intriguing given all the basic moral, legal, and social rules that she had broken for so many years as a member of a criminal gang. Although the clinician never pursued this line of inquiry in the course of treatment, Eva's ability to leave that lifestyle firmly behind and become a substance abuse counselor was a tribute to her ability to find and uphold her commitment to what was right.

### Feedback Session, Clinical Formulation Triangle, and Offer of Treatment

Remembering the past with deep emotion was making a difference in Eva's experience of the present. During the third session, Eva announced that for the first time she had been able to buy some clothes for the baby. She revealed that she was elated because, although well advanced in her pregnancy, she previously had been unable to prepare in concrete ways for the baby's birth. Shyly, she said, *"So you are curing me."* The clinician asked how Eva thought the cure was happening. Eva answered that she was not sure, but thought that talking about things that had bothered her for a long time but had remained unspoken was helping. Again, this was an indication of Eva's intuitive understanding that the root of her present problems lay somewhere in the past. The clinician remained concerned about the possibility of a thought disorder, but Eva's capacity for introspection and her emotional intelligence suggested that the problem might be either circumscribed or linked to Eva's intense anxiety about her pregnancy. Treatment was certainly indicated, and Eva seemed ready for it.

The clinician was aware of Eva's fragile self-esteem and her reparative need to be the focus of treatment rather than marginalized by the baby. As she extended the invitation to treatment, the clinician said, *"We have met for three sessions and are getting to know each other. You are an experienced counselor, and you have been remembering how the way your parents treated you as a child affected you and could have an effect on how you imagine yourself as a mother. Today you told me that remembering the past is helping you prepare for the baby, and you said you are very happy about that. Would you like to continue meeting weekly for as long as treatment seems useful?*" Eva's eyes moistened with tears, and she said, "*Yes. I am ready to be counseled, now that I got used to the idea.*" Sensing the underlying ambivalence and remembering Eva's earlier confrontation with her physician as a possible indication of her dislike of authority, the clinician asked her how it felt to be a counselor being counseled. There was an instant flash of acknowledgment in Eva's eyes as she replied, "*Tough!*" She went on to explain that she had been a detoxification counselor for 5 years, and had recently resigned her position to become a homemaker and a mother (a situation that in the clinician's eyes paralleled that of Eva's mother). There were few counselors as experienced and well regarded as she was, Eva said, and she missed her work and the feeling of being valued that it gave her.

While the clinician was aware of Eva's possible competitiveness and envy, she chose to address the incipient negative transference from a different angle. She said, "*Is it hard, being such an experienced counselor, to come see another counselor about whom you don't know very much?*" Eva immediately agreed with visible relief. She went on to say that counselors are the worst patients, that they play games, and that they "*beat their counselors at their own game. That way they stop you from getting close to them and hurting them.*" The clinician replied that sometimes people put up barriers when they feel the counselor says too much too soon and when they need some protection until they feel ready to listen. Eva nodded in agreement, seeming very much in tune. The clinician then said, "*If you ever feel that you are playing games with me or that you have to put up barriers because I am saying things that bother you, will you please tell me? Then we can look at what is happening and try to understand it together.*" Eva promised to be a ruthless critic, and went on to talk warmly about a dear friend who had the same surname as the clinician.

As the feedback session was wrapping up, the clinician asked Eva if she would be interested in Sean joining the treatment at some point. This invitation posed the risk of making Eva feel marginalized, but the clinician believed that the open-ended wording and an emphasis on Eva's agency in making the decision would mitigate this risk and introduce for Eva the importance of the partner as a presence both in the mother's life and in the baby's life. As if on cue, Eva said, "*I will give it some thought, but he is really happy with the pregnancy. I am the one who's not.*" This response made clear that Eva perceived the invitation to Sean as a possible intrusion in her relationship with the clinician, with the prospect of becoming secondary yet again. The clinician answered, "*You know best, and you decide. This is your treatment.*" Eva smiled widely as she said good-bye. The threat to the emerging therapeutic bond had been averted. Giving Eva a feeling of control over the treatment process and an invitation to partnership rather than competition with the clinician had helped negotiate successfully the first barrier to treatment.

The foundational phase gave the clinician a start in understanding Eva's situation, which was important in formulating guidelines for treatment. It was evident that Eva was emotionally neglected as a child. Eva's much-resented obligation to be her siblings' caretaker was superimposed on an inner emotional depletion and unfulfilled longings to be cared for while growing up. Given the severe physical abuse that she experienced with her first husband and her description of her father as having periodic outbursts of rage, violence in her nuclear family was also a possibility, perhaps in the forms of domestic violence and/or child physical abuse. When the clinician asked about it, Eva remembered the terror she experienced when her father hit her and her siblings with a belt, while her mother did not intervene to protect them. Eva's response to her upbringing seemed to be an identification with the aggressor that had many layers of meaning. As an addict involved with a violent motorcycle gang, Eva had simultaneously defied her neglectful and abusive parents, lived a lifestyle consistent with her low self-esteem, expressed her rage at her abuse and neglect by inflicting abuse on others, and tried to fulfill her unsatisfied needs through drug and alcohol abuse.

It was unclear how Eva had rescued herself from the addiction, violence, and lawlessness that filled her past, but it was clear that the unborn baby had rekindled the impulses that had led to that earlier lifestyle in the first place. The unborn baby had become the representative of those earlier sibling babies that, in Eva's childhood perception, were guilty of harassing her, depleting her, and robbing her of her childhood and converting her into a precocious, unwilling, and angry mother. The clinician's task would be to understand the mechanism that linked the present unborn baby to the earlier ones, and to help Eva reexperience the earlier feelings in connection with their legitimate, original recipients, her parents and her siblings.

## Core Treatment: Deepening the Work

### Being Left Out, Feeling Unloved

The clinician's open-ended offer of including Sean in the treatment seemed to have an effect on the content of the next session, in which the predominant theme was Eva's fear that the baby would destroy her relationship with her husband and make her lose all the gains that she had made in overcoming her addiction and starting a new life. As the clinician probed these fears, Eva spoke of her conviction that she would feel "*left out*" whenever her husband spent time with the baby. Her husband, she said, was ecstatic over her pregnancy, and she had only agreed to have a baby because of her deep love for him. She now feared that he might not be able to love both her and the baby at the same time and would be so enthralled with his baby that he would have little time left for his wife.

Exploring the feeling of being left out led to increasingly intense memories, first of the recent past, and later of her childhood. Eva spoke of how her first husband had brought a young lover into the marital bedroom, and how the three of them had slept together in the same bed. Eva remembered feeling very much left out. She then remembered vividly her suspicion that this girl was a police informant. "*I hated her so much that I told her I would kill her when my husband was not around.*" The girl believed the threat and disappeared forever, much to the husband's annoyance. When the clinician asked Eva if she really intended to kill this girl, she replied, "*You bet.*" This was a chillingly ego-syntonic response that raised new questions about Eva's character structure, but the clinician chose to address it as the only defense available to Eva's impoverished ego in a moment of profound despair. This therapeutic choice led to insights that might not have been possible with a non-psychodynamic approach.

The clinician commented on Eva's anger that somebody had come between herself and her husband, an anger so intense that it had made her want to kill. The clinician then asked whether Eva had experienced those feelings before. After thinking for a long time, Eva spoke about how angry she had been at her mother when she was pregnant with her fifth child. She said, "*It was terrible. When my little sister was born, I was 13. I wanted to kill my mother, and I wanted to kill my baby sister by cutting into my mother's stomach. When the baby was born, I could not look at her for 2 weeks, I refused to be in the same room with her for 2 weeks. Later on, when I was 15 and my little sister was 2, I was supposed to take her to the beach. I remember all these cute guys, and I was walking, trying to look good, and my little sister used to call me mama. I yelled at her to shut up, that I wasn't her mama.*"

Again, as before, the clinician sympathized with the burden of having to take care of a child when herself a child, and went on to restate the connection between Eva's early experience and the present prospect of taking care of another baby as yet unborn. Eva replied thoughtfully that she really did not feel that she was 42, that psychologically she felt quite young, certainly not at the age where she would like to have a child. The clinician commented that Eva was only now beginning to enjoy the freedom she had not had before. As a child, she had to do things that were beyond her age, and then she had spent many years locked in a marriage and a lifestyle that were painful for her. The clinician added that she could well understand Eva's fears that her baby's birth could put her back in a situation where she was not in control of her actions. Eva agreed with tears in her eyes.

The theme of being left out was continued in the following session, which Eva began by complaining about her inability to fix up the baby's room. She could not even walk into the room, she said, let alone buy furniture or make drapes. The clinician asked what Eva felt when she thought of fixing up the baby's room. She thought for a while, and said, "*It feels just like moving.*" She then went on to talk about what moving meant for her: rootlessness, constant pursuit by the FBI, being forever suspicious of friends and acquaintances who might denounce her, and the danger of trafficking drugs across state lines. As she spoke, she again went on to talk about the violence, about guns and shooting and people killed, both by the police and by other drug dealers. She again remembered her husband's lover, whom she had wished to kill.

The clinician commented in response that when Eva had first talked about wanting to kill this woman, she had also remembered that she had wanted to kill her baby sister even before she was born. Eva seemed receptive to this analogy, and the clinician enlarged the analogy by pointing out that this baby sister was somebody else who had come to change things for Eva in painful ways, just as her first husband's lover had changed things for her by coming between her and her husband. Eva thought for a while, and said, "*You know, I always had this fear that I would squish a little puppy, or a little kitten, or a baby, squish them real hard and kill them. I have always been scared of that impulse, for as long as I can remember. I think that what terrifies me is that I might feel like doing that to my baby.*" The clinician said, "*And you really want to protect your baby from that impulse that you are so afraid of.*" Eva said yes. She then remembered that once her girlfriend had asked her to hold her baby. Eva had agreed, but as she held the baby, she became increasingly scared of harming him. She ended up panicking, and screamed to her girlfriend, "*Take this thing, take this thing.*" The clinician commented that Eva was trying very hard to protect the baby from the impulse that she feared so much. Eva said, "*Yes. I knew that the baby was innocent, that he hadn't done anything to me. Like maybe there was this baby 3 weeks ago that did something wrong to me and I felt like killing him, but I didn't want to transfer that feeling to this baby here right now, who didn't do anything to me.*" The clinician said that perhaps there was a baby that, in her view, had "*done something wrong to her,*" not 3 weeks ago, but perhaps a long time ago, when she was a little girl. Eva looked very thoughtful. The clinician added, *"Perhaps you don't want to transfer those feelings to the baby that you are carrying right now, the baby who is innocent of the things that happened to you then."*

Eva looked very sad, and said that she had been trying to remember what happened when her mother was pregnant with her first brother, and her parents had promised her that this baby would be a gift to her. Eva believed this promise. But when the baby was born, the parents took the baby into their bedroom, and left Eva all alone in her room. The clinician said, *"It must have been awfully lonely to be in that room at night, knowing that your baby brother was with your parents in the grown-ups' room."* Eva said yes. The clinician then made the connection with the present by adding, *"No wonder it is so hard to go into the baby's room right now."* Eva answered, with tears in her eyes, *"I never thought of that. Maybe you're right."* She then went on to talk about how little attention she had received after her baby brother was born.

When the clinician inquired about Eva's feelings for her little brother, Eva said that whenever she thought of him, she could only remember her fear of smothering a little chick or a puppy or a kitten. She added, *"Maybe when I was little, I accidentally smothered some animal, and that's how the fear started."* The clinician said that young children confuse wanting to do something with actually doing it, and are afraid that feeling something is equal to doing it. She added that maybe Eva had been so upset at her baby brother that at times she felt like smothering him, even though she never did it. Eva's eyes filled with tears. She sobbed for a few minutes, and then spoke again about the loneliness and the disappointment of her brother staying in her parents' bedroom and getting all the attention she once had. She then said in a choked voice that maybe she had been so angry that she had wanted to kill her brother. The clinician said, *"Maybe the feeling, when it comes, is so very scary because it almost feels like it is going to become an action."* Sobbing, Eva blew her nose, and said, *"Maybe that's what makes me so panicky about having this baby."*

The clinician asked what Eva meant. Eva said, *"I think I'm afraid that this baby will be so much trouble that I'll feel like smothering it too."* The clinician said, *"Maybe the feelings that you had toward your brother are now coming back and are making you afraid of hurting this baby. And you want to protect this baby, you do not want to hurt it."* Eva cried for several minutes. She then said, *"It is such a relief to know that I am afraid of hurting this baby because I really want to protect it. That means that I really love it."*

In later sessions, Eva and the clinician were able to link Eva's fear that the baby would come between herself and her husband with the early experience of feeling displaced by her brother in her parents' affection.

How can we understand what happened? In the supportive context of treatment, Eva had been able to remember and examine her murderous impulses toward her first sibling, who had displaced her from her parents' affection. Being left out resulted in the catastrophic reality of being unloved. The clinician then made explicit Eva's unconscious equation of that first sibling with the baby she was now carrying. Most crucially, the clinician helped Eva to understand her fear of her murderous impulses as an effort to protect her unborn baby and, hence, as an indication of her love for it. In siding with Eva's embattled and perhaps impoverished ego, the clinician was providing her the kind of supportive, ego-building experience she had lacked in her childhood and adolescence, when the absence of clear and caring parental guidelines had left her unable to counterbalance her aggressive impulses with loving, nurturing ones. The clinician's intervention reassured Eva that she was capable of experiencing love and that she had the desire to protect and nurture her baby. The relief clearly experienced by Eva was eloquent proof of her agony in thinking of herself as capable only of rage.

As is apparent from the process notes excerpted above, there were many alternative approaches to interpretation. The clinician could have used Eva's anxiety about her murderous impulses to explore further into her past—for example, to delve into the possible oedipal implications of her parents' promise that the sibling would be Eva's own baby, or into her perception of the parents' breach of that promise. Such an approach would no doubt have been fruitful in the context of individual treatment for Eva. Instead, the thrust of P-CPP was to understand the intricacies of Eva's psychological conflicts as they pertained to how they stood in the way of her becoming a mother with a positive emotional investment in her baby. This therapeutic goal informed clinical decisions about what material to seek and what interpretations to make. The clinician chose to focus on the material that seemed promising for helping to resolve the conflicts that Eva experienced around her baby and her role as a mother. This goal supported the technique of linking the emerging experiences and feelings from the past with the feelings that Eva reported toward her pregnancy, her unborn baby, and her role as a mother.

### Eva's Husband Joins the Treatment: Addressing Rage, Preparing for Labor and Delivery

Until the emergence of the material linking Eva's murderous impulses toward her siblings to her inability to love her unborn baby, Eva's husband Sean had not joined any of the sessions despite the clinician's open-ended invitation. The clinician understood his absence as a sign that Eva needed to work through her conflicts about being left out and being unloved before she could bring her husband into the treatment. Each of Eva's siblings had left her feeling empty and displaced in her mother's affection. The clinician believed that Eva could safely invite Sean in only after these feelings had emerged and become conscious. Indeed, as anticipated, Sean came in for the first time after this session.

Sean's presence changed drastically the affective atmosphere of the treatment. He was a tall, profusely tattooed man with long red hair and a full unruly beard who filled the initial session with a mixture of bravado expressed in four-letter words, a recital of his many virtues and grandiose plans for the future, and finally a touchingly timid confession of his fears and of his physical disabilities due to a recurrent disc problem that caused sometimes immobilizing pain. Eva seemed half-embarrassed and half-amused as he monopolized the first part of the session by explaining in painstaking, self-absorbed detail the financial difficulties and interpersonal complexities of his job as a delivery truck driver.

After the first hour of a very long first joint session, Sean finally broached a topic that was clearly of great concern to him: Eva's labor and delivery. He initially presented his own role as an auxiliary one: he would be there simply to assist Eva, and his feelings were of no importance since the delivery was not "*his trip*." As both Eva and the clinician reassured him that this was a "*joint trip*" and that his feelings were important, he started talking about his guilt for putting Eva in a situation that she wanted only partially and in which she would have to endure physical pain. He explained that Eva had agreed to have a child because he wanted one, and he now felt guilty because Eva was having so many mixed feelings, and he did not know what would happen. Eva hastened to remind him that she had also been actively involved in the decision to have a child, and assured him that, although she had not wanted children in principle, she did want a child with him. "*I would not have a baby only for you, not even for you, dear,*" she said playfully but tenderly.

Sean then went on to speak about his fears of being present in the delivery room. He talked about his discomfort in situations where he was not in control and had to defer to authority figures. He wanted the delivery to go smoothly, but when he was uncomfortable, he said, he became angry, and when he was angry, he often resorted to physical attack. The clinician asked whether he was afraid that this would happen during the delivery. He said yes. He was afraid that if the nurses or doctors were bothering Eva or "*ordering her around,*" he would first ask them nicely to leave her alone, but if they did not obey he might "*punch their noses or crack their heads."* The clinician sensed that this response was simultaneously a confession of Sean's fear of his own aggression and a test of the clinician's capacity to tolerate the potential for danger without herself becoming afraid. She chose to side with the real-life implications of the behavior that Sean feared in a way that she hoped would not elicit Sean's defenses. With this in mind, the clinician commented softly that this would certainly have the opposite effect of what he wanted—to help make the delivery go as smoothly as possible for Eva. Both Eva and Sean agreed.

As Sean spoke about his fear that he would attack the doctors or nurses, Eva also began to express her own fear that she would react violently if she felt out of control. For both Eva and Sean, who had lived for years outside the law, violence had long been the customary way of responding to frustration, anger, and fear. They had worked hard to find alternative modes of expression, but feared that under the pressure of the delivery they would fall back on their most familiar response.

The clinician then addressed both the real-life challenges and the psychological stress the couple was feeling by saying that they had two tasks ahead. One was to plan for the practical aspects of the delivery so that the doctors, midwives, and nurses were aware of Eva's and Sean's wishes, and had an opportunity to negotiate alternatives should the parents' wishes run contrary to the usual hospital practices. This procedure would ensure that the parents and the medical personnel knew each other's positions and agreed on a delivery plan, thus minimizing the chance of unpleasant surprises for the parents and the possibility of angry outbursts at the staff. The second task was to work with Eva's and Sean's feelings, so that once they were in the delivery room they would find it easier to remember that a bossy nurse was nothing more than that, not an awesome authority figure in control of their lives. Eva and Sean laughed and found this plan quite congenial.

At the end of this first joint session, with his hand on the doorknob, Sean revealed the very concrete reasons for his fear of his own violence. Noting that the entrance door to the program was kept locked, he asked, *"Did you have any break-ins?"* When the clinician answered that there had been a few, Sean remarked in an offhand manner, *"That's what I went to jail for the last time."* Still with his hand on the knob, Sean spoke for 15 minutes about his various experiences in jail. *"One night in jail my buddy and I got loaded, and I went crazy. I tried to kill him with a chain saw. I got transferred to San Quentin for that. Six months. That was really awful. Lousy food. The guards steal your food and beat the shit out of you to keep you in line. Just like on the outside. When I was outside, I was working for this drug king. I had to take care of the guys that were giving trouble. Knocking heads, if you know what I mean. I'm glad I got out of that. Eva and I are in another space now."*

While it might be true that they were in *"another space,"* it was also clear that both parents were struggling with the encroachment in the present of a violence-laden past. The clinician felt enormous responsibility to remain alert to this danger and not be lulled by her positive feelings and the strong therapeutic alliance that was being formed with each as individuals and both as parents.

## Joint Work with the Parents: Tracing the Roots of Rage to Create a Safe Present

In the next few sessions, Sean continued to talk a great deal about his life. He spoke about the years of being a *"dope fiend,"* constantly on the run. He would decide one day that he had had enough, take a suitcase, and leave everything and everybody behind to start the same lifestyle again somewhere else. *"I could leave everything, because I did not care about anything or anybody, I only cared about myself."* He talked about betraying people, about being betrayed, about not trusting anybody, and about not being trusted in return. He talked about making a lot of money and using it all in his arm, *"shooting up"*; he also talked about being so abjectly poor that he made detailed plans to kill the drug dealer he was working for and make off with his money. Eventually Sean gave up on this idea because he was convinced he would be discovered and sent to jail *"for good."* He decided instead to go straight and asked his landlord, who took a special interest in rehabilitating people, for help. This man lent Sean some money, got him a job, and helped him get in touch with Alcoholics Anonymous (AA) and other similar organizations. It took a long time. Sean said, *"Now I find that the straight life is much easier. Even when things are difficult, it is much easier. For one thing, people trust you."* Eva agreed, saying, *"If you are sleazy, nobody trusts you, and that is hard."*

Sean could speak at length about his life, but time was of the essence because Eva was quickly approaching her delivery date and the danger of the parents' aggression becoming unleashed in the delivery room continued to loom large. Looking for a tactful way of bringing the baby into the conversation, the clinician commented that the past seemed to be coming back with great force, and added that having a baby often did that: it forced people to remember their past because they needed to prepare for the future. This comment focused Sean on the immediate issues facing him and his wife. He said thoughtfully that he had been thinking a lot about becoming a father and, he added, there was some news that made him think even harder. During the prenatal visit the day before, they found out that the baby was in a breech position and that a cesarean section might be needed unless the baby turned around. *"I keep telling that little asshole to get his ass in gear or I'll kick the shit out of him."* The clinician said in a soft voice that, with that kind of warning, it would not be surprising if the kid was too scared to even move. They laughed, and Eva said, in an overly sweet voice that betrayed her fear, *"I tell him it's either the cesarean or his bicycle, that we don't have money for both."*

The defense against fear of body damage had emerged in the form of aggression against the perceived perpetrator, who this time was not the doctors but the baby. It was clear that in spite of the laughter this was a very serious topic, and that these parents might easily resort to violence as a way of disciplining their own child. Although this reality was not yet immediate, it was an important topic to pursue, partly because it reflected the parents' perception of the unborn baby as willfully inflicting pain on them and partly because their comments opened the door for preventive intervention before violence actually occurred.

The clinician asked directly what they thought about physical punishment, and both parents said it was the natural way of teaching a child not to do what he was not supposed to do. The clinician answered, *"I actually don't agree with you. Were you physically punished when you were growing up?"* Both parents said yes. The clinician asked them to remember how they felt at the time. Both said they could not remember. The clinician said that this was quite understandable, that when children were hit they felt so much resentment and fear that they tried very hard to forget those feelings when they grew up. After a long silence, Sean turned to Eva and said, *"Maybe that is why I feel the way I feel toward my parents, honey."*

Slowly, Sean started talking about his parents. They were both *"lightweight,"* and he did not respect them. His mother was a *"sniveling bitch"*; his father was an alcoholic who was *"Mr. Nice Guy"* to everybody but Sean, whom he beat often and for a long time. Sean then remembered an episode that had occurred when he was 9 years old. He and his friend were throwing dirt clods from a hill onto the highway below. At one point, a car was passing by and Sean did not see it because he was further back, but his friend enticed him to throw a dirt clod right then. The clod fell on the car's windshield and shattered it. Sean ran away, but the driver caught Sean's friend, who led the man to Sean's house to speak with Sean's father, who went out with a tree branch in his hand to find his son. When they met, the father held Sean by the arm and dragged him home, while hitting him in the leg with the branch until Sean's leg was bloody. Describing the scene, Sean said, *"At first I cried, but then the pain turned into hatred and I stopped crying. I did not want to show any feeling. My father started yelling at me, saying, 'Cry, for God's sake.' But I refused to cry. That is the last time I remember crying in front of anybody. From then on, I only felt rage. He didn't even let me explain."*

Sean remained silent for a while, his eyes reddened, trying to compose himself. He then said, *"I don't understand why I was so scared at first, and then I could only feel anger."* The clinician commented that it is usually easier to be angry than to be scared. *"You were so frightened, and there was nobody there to help you feel less scared. So you had to help yourself, and used your rage to protect yourself from that fright."* Sean's eyes filled with tears, and he sobbed for a few minutes. He then said, *"And I've been carrying that rage inside me ever since. I could never do anything else with it."*

After he regained some composure, Sean looked at Eva and asked her how he had started talking about his childhood. Eva said that they had been talking about spanking their baby so he would get in the right position and Eva would not need a cesarean. There was a silence. The clinician then said to Sean, *"I can understand better how you feel about Eva having a cesarean. You have suffered so much, and now it's hard to think that the woman you love can be hurt like that and you can't protect her. Eva's pain makes you so scared that once again it's easier to feel the anger."* Sean's eyes filled with tears again, and he again sobbed for a few minutes. He then put his foot on Eva's chair, and Eva rubbed his foot gently. Eva then said, *"We will not let it happen, honey. That baby is still going to turn around."* They talked quietly with each other for a while, tenderly trying to reassure each other. The clinician then said, *"I think that you are trying very hard to find new ways of raising your child, to overcome your own childhoods and the way you were raised. You are trying very hard to raise a child that will not have the memories that you have and that you are still struggling with."* Sean sighed and said, *"That's exactly true. And, man, is it hard."*

The clinician responded that she knew it was hard and added that the important thing was that they had the courage to look at those feelings now, before the baby came, so they could prepare themselves to feel the feelings without hurting the baby. The clinician added that the feelings probably would still be there after the baby came, and the baby would reawaken other feelings, but they were already finding ways of handling them. The clinician also cautioned the parents that the intensity of the feelings they spoke about might make them want to stop talking about them for a while; they might even find that they did not feel like coming for the next few sessions. They might also find themselves upset at the clinician, because the feelings were so strong that they could spill over to her. This anticipatory insight-oriented explanation was necessary because time was of the essence, and the parents needed to be equipped with coping skills to anticipate and manage the impulse to flee from treatment if the intensity of their feelings frightened them. Both Sean and Eva denied firmly that this would happen, and said that they felt ready to continue working on their feelings.

## Preparation for Labor and Delivery: The Fear of Body Damage and Losing Love

Sean was present in two of the four remaining sessions preceding the delivery. Eva explained his absence in terms of his work schedule. However, it is also likely that he needed to maintain some distance from the highly charged affective material that was emerging. There was also an unspoken understanding between him and Eva that Eva would continue to have individual treatment sessions. The clinician accepted the situation without making an effort to explore the reasons for Sean's absence because both parents were using the sessions quite effectively to come to grips with the strong emotions that were threatening to flood them.

### ADDRESSING FEAR OF BODY DAMAGE IN THE NEGATIVE ATTRIBUTIONS TO THE BABY

The material that emerged in these sessions revolved around two main issues. The first issue was Eva's fear of how she would react to seeing the baby immediately after birth. The second issue, described in its essentials in the previous section but reworked again in the course of the two sessions in which he was present, was Sean's fear that seeing his wife in pain would trigger in him an irresistible impulse to attack the medical staff. These two themes were linked by a concrete concern: the possibility of a cesarean should the baby continue in the breech position.

Both parents perceived the baby as willfully refusing to turn around. Eva, in particular, believed that the baby knew what the parents expected it to do and was too stubborn to do it. When asked to elaborate on this perception, she said airily, "*My pets know what they are expected to do. Sometimes they do it and sometimes they do precisely the opposite, just to show us that we can't order them around. Why should a kid be any different?*" (Not since the first session had there been such worrisome evidence of the possibility of a thought disorder.) This comment was among many others that reflected Eva's perception of the baby as stubborn, willful, and determined to have its way. This perception triggered in turn Eva's wish to retaliate. "*If the kid cries at night, I will feel like sticking it in a closet so it will learn that I won't be manipulated.*" The clinician speculated that the possibility of a C-section was mobilizing in Eva a profound fear of body damage, which in turn elicited rage and the wish to punish the perceived cause of this damage, namely, the baby.

The clinician's effort to explore Eva's possible fear of body damage led in some fruitful directions. Eva revealed that for many years she had been unable to experience pain. For example, she had burned herself while ironing, but did not know it until hours later, when she happened to glance at the burn. *"I guess I learned to turn off my dopamines when I was little,"* she said. Eva went on to talk about being beaten by her father with the buckle of a belt until she bled whenever she did something wrong, and recalled trying to *"live through that by pretending it did not hurt."* These memories led to her recalling many violent scenes with her siblings while she was growing up. Eva remembered that on one occasion she had raised a knife over her brother during a fight. She said the scene was still in her mind *"as a dream,"* devoid of emotion. Yet she knew herself capable of experiencing deep rage. The clinician asked whether she also knew herself to be capable of acting on that rage. Eva said yes. Bringing the theme of anger back to the imminent delivery, the clinician said, *"I can understand why you are so worried about the delivery. You experienced violence all your life, and you learned to defend yourself using violence because that is what you were taught. And now you are facing a situation where violence will not protect you, a situation where you have to submit your body to somebody else and hope that that person will not hurt you."*

This interpretation, repeated many times with slight variations, led in an unexpected direction: Eva responded by talking about her lifelong fear of dependence, a theme that she had alluded to in earlier sessions when she spoke of her wish to *"grow up in a hurry."* Now she described episodes in her past in which she had gone to great lengths to avoid asking for help even in tasks that she clearly could not complete unaided. She remembered crying with frustration because she could only reach to within a quarter-inch of the ceiling where she wanted to hang a planter, and straining for hours to bridge the gap so that she would not need to resort to a taller person for help. She also recalled spending half a morning moving a huge rug from one end of her room to another, a little at a time, again in order not to ask for help.

FEAR OF DEPENDENCE, FEAR OF LOSS

The clinician asked how Eva explained to herself her reluctance to depend on others. Eva talked at first at a rather intellectualized level about her mother's unavailability and her loneliness as a child. She then said, almost casually, *"As a matter of fact, I used to confuse my mother with my aunt who lived with us. I used to call that aunt 'Mom.' And sometimes when one of them came into the room I did not know who it was, whether my mom or my aunt."* As one memory led to another, Eva spoke poignantly about this aunt, who took her everywhere, read her stories, and allowed her to help in the kitchen. Then, when Eva was 4, this aunt decided to move to another city. She left and never came back, leaving only a box of books behind. Years later, Eva still liked to look at the books while thinking about her aunt. Remembering, she said sadly, "*Maybe that is why I learned to read when I was 4.*"

The clinician sympathized with the feelings of loving and losing somebody, and added that such an experience could have made Eva feel as a small child that she did not want to rely on anybody for fear of losing that person again. It was easier to be an independent grown-up; this way, she could hope to avoid the sadness of being disappointed in her love. Eva agreed thoughtfully. She then began to speak of her dog, Clarissa, who, according to Sean, was restless whenever Eva was gone and moaned softly next to the door while waiting for her. Eva wished Clarissa could be content with Sean's presence and not miss her so much. The clinician said, "*It's hard to need somebody, and it's also hard to be needed.*" Eva replied sharply, "*She doesn't really need me. She's just laying a trip on me so I will feel guilty and not leave her. I bet she's not next to the door all the time. I bet she's doing her thing, and as soon as she hears me she rushes to the door and pretends that she has been there all along.*"

The clinician commented that it was easier to think that Clarissa was playing a game because Eva loved Clarissa so much that it would be painful to think of her as really suffering while Eva was gone. Eva replied, with much feeling, "*Well, I would not want to leave her if I knew she suffered. And I don't want to be trapped, never going out by myself even for an hour just because I don't want her to suffer.*" The clinician asked, "*Does it have to be either that Clarissa is only laying a trip on you, or that she suffers so much that you can never leave her?*" Eva considered this for a while. Then she said, "*No. I tell Clarissa when I'll be back by tapping on the table, once for every hour I'll be gone. Then she knows what to expect. And she stays with the cats, or with Sean, so she knows she'll be well cared for until I come back.*" The clinician said this was a very thoughtful way of handling separation. Eva then spontaneously made her implicit worries quite clear: "*But will it work for the baby?*" The clinician responded with some developmental guidance, speaking to the issue by linking Eva's easy intuition regarding her care of the pets with the needs of a baby: making separations gradual, helping the baby understand what would happen through clear greetings and departures, and providing familiar and trusted substitutes. When coached in the language of what her pets needed, this information became less frightening to Eva. She was clearly relieved that babies were not mysterious organisms, that they were not very different from her pets.

Using the pets' feelings as a launching point to explain a baby's needs proved fruitful in releasing Eva's empathy for her unborn child.

In the following session, Eva said, "*You know, I thought that I would just leave the baby in its room and let it cry at night if I felt too tired to get up, but now I feel differently. The whole family sleeps in the master bedroom: Sean, me, Clarissa, the cats. Why should the baby be any different? I'll put the crib in our bedroom for the first few months so the baby doesn't feel left out.*"

From identification with the aggressor, casting the baby off to a lonely room the way she had been cast off by her parents when her brother was born, Eva had progressed to an empathic identification with her unborn baby. The infant had joined the family.

## Preparation for Labor and Delivery: Concrete Plans and Liaison with the Medical Staff

At the same time that insight-oriented work with the parents was taking place, the clinician also took concrete steps to minimize the chances of violent parental behavior during the delivery. The clinician spoke to Eva and Sean about their wishes, fears, and fantasies about the medical procedures and about the midwives' delivery practices. Unlike some mothers, Eva had no objection to intrusive medical procedures should these prove necessary. She did have very strong feelings about some of the practices midwives use to enhance early parent–infant bonding. She particularly disliked the idea of having the baby placed on her stomach: "*All that artsy-craftsy bonding stuff gives me the creeps.*" She also disliked the use of dim lights: "*Please ask them not to have dim lights. Dim lights drive me nuts. I know that's supposed to be good for the baby to come in with violins in this wonderful semidarkness resembling the womb, but I need bright lights to keep my sanity.*" Most emphatically, she did not want pain-killers even in the event of a caesarean, because she was afraid they might trigger her addiction again. When the clinician suggested that she could consult with the doctors about a painkiller that contained no addictive substances, Eva's face took on a pained expression as she said, "*You don't understand. When I worked as a counselor, these addicts would come in with prescriptions given to them by their doctors. I would look at the chemical components in the* Physicians' Desk Reference, *and invariably there were potentially addictive substances. Most doctors don't understand how vulnerable ex-addicts are to most substances.*" Eva also wanted to have only local anesthesia in the case of a C-section. "*Total anesthesia freaks me out. I am afraid of breaking down if I have it.*"

Sean concurred with his wife's concerns, and added his own. He wanted the staff to consult with them before "*taking over.*" He also wanted to be told what would be happening before people began "*handling Eva and doing things to her.*" Serious consideration was given in these sessions to the question of whether Sean would be present or not in the delivery room should a C-section be needed. Both parents preferred to defer a decision, and to see how they were feeling at the time.

With the parents' permission, the clinician met with the medical staff to discuss her own concerns about the possibility of parental violence and to apprise them of the parents' wishes and their reasons for them. The staff took seriously the clinician's account, and they had no objections to changing their management procedures to meet the parental requests, which seemed reasonable to them. The clinician and the parents wrote a delivery plan that was approved by the medical staff and placed in Eva's medical chart so that everybody present during the delivery would have ready access to the guidelines. Eva and Sean relaxed considerably after this task was completed, and anticipated the delivery with less tension. Their mood (and the clinician's) lightened considerably when in the weekly checkup before Eva's due date the physician announced that the baby had turned around and was now in position for a vaginal delivery. A C-section would be most unlikely. Eva and Sean greeted their offspring's move with a relief reminiscent of parents whose toddler agrees to end a tantrum. The clinician was grateful that an aggravating element was likely to be absent from the delivery situation, as parent–infant interaction was already at high risk.

### Reesa Is Born

Reesa was born 1 week after Eva's due date. She was a beautiful, placid baby of average weight and length and in excellent health. As the physician had predicted, the cesarean had not been necessary, although the baby was in a transverse position, and labor and delivery had been long and, by Eva's account, painful. One complication was that the placenta had not come out spontaneously, and Eva had screamed in pain and refused when the midwives attempted to remove it manually. *"I had reached my limit. I could not stand one more second of pain."* The midwives agreed to remove the placenta surgically, but this presented the problem of giving Eva total anesthesia, which she feared because she thought the experience might trigger her addiction again. The problem was resolved to Eva's satisfaction by the anesthesiologist, who induced a *"gentle sleep"* before giving her the substance that would make her experience a *"high."*

Eva sounded happy and relaxed on the phone when she called from her hospital bed to notify the clinician of Reesa's birth, although she spoke for 20 minutes about the delivery without mentioning the baby. She was particularly relieved that Sean had been *"wonderful"* during the entire process, remaining very attentive to Eva's welfare during the full day of the labor and delivery and negotiating nicely with doctors, nurses, and midwives. *"Things between us were fantastic. It was a wonderful experience between us, although I would like to forget all about the delivery.*" When she finally began to speak about the baby, Eva said, "*She's long, but she doesn't weigh very much. And she's actually pretty.*" To the clinician's question of what the baby was like, Eva replied, "*Pretty good, but greedy. She is hard to pry her off the breast.*"

During a hospital visit the next day, the clinician observed the parents and baby together for the first time. The scene when the clinician entered the room was a lovely one: mother, father, and baby cuddled together in the mother's bed. The parents were speaking softly and looking at the baby. Reesa was an unusually beautiful newborn who nursed well, cried seldom, and was easily soothed. She turned readily to the human voice and established eye contact with her mother when Eva spoke to her. She seemed like a rewarding baby who would not pose extraordinary demands on a mother's resources of patience and nurturance.

During the hospital visit, both parents seemed enchanted with the baby. They praised her looks and her temperament and expressed a quiet confidence that things would go smoothly for themselves and their baby. Even more impressive than their investment in the baby was their pride in themselves. Eva said, "*Even when I yelled at the midwife to stop trying to get the placenta out, I knew I was not going to lose my temper and kick her in the stomach.*" Sean admitted having had fantasies of "*kicking everybody out.*" He then said, "*I remembered what you said, that a bossy nurse was not a prison guard even if she reminded me of one. That made me feel calmer.*" Both parents praised the medical staff for their patience, understanding, and willingness to explain to them what was happening. The medical staff on their part praised the parents for their self-control. One of the midwives commented to the clinician: "*One could sense the potential for anger, but we all tried our best, and the parents really cooperated. And I tell you, it was a hard delivery.*"

In light of the real hardships of this delivery, the parents' ability to use their growing understanding of themselves to control their impulses was a very encouraging sign for their emerging relationship with their daughter. Yet Eva's initial comment about the baby's "*greediness*" sounded dangerously similar to the earlier perceptions of the unborn baby as willful and stubborn. Both before and after birth, Reesa was perceived as someone with murky motives and inclinations that Eva would have to grapple with.

## The First 6 Months: Negative Maternal Attributions Emerge

After Reesa's birth, most of the weekly sessions took place in the home. Sean continued to be present periodically, but it was clear that he wanted the freedom to come or not to come as he wished. His presence was always a sign that a joint issue between the parents and the baby needed attention. His absence allowed Eva to continue exploring her own difficulties with her baby, something that she was clearly reluctant to do freely when Sean was present. This arrangement seemed satisfactory for both parents, and the clinician saw no reason to interfere with it.

During Reesa's first month of life, the clinician observed that Eva's and Sean's interactions with their baby were unfailingly appropriate. However, Eva's descriptions of Reesa soon began to reflect increasing distortions in her perception of the baby. These attributions were both positive and negative in their content and affective tone. Eva believed, for example, that Reesa's motor skills, linguistic abilities, and capacity to make sense of the world around her far exceeded the capacity of other babies of the same age. She credited the baby with being able to turn over in her crib and crawl, to laugh at conversations between Eva and Sean, to reach for and grab appealing objects such as a little doll, and to throw away objects she did not like, such as the pacifier Eva sometimes used as a replacement for the breast. Eva was radiant with pride as she described these abilities.

Eva was particularly amused by what she called Reesa's sense of humor (something that she also delighted in when it came to her pets). She described in detail the "*jokes*" that Reesa played on her during feeding. In one of these instances, Reesa had stopped sucking and had her eyes closed. Thinking that the baby was asleep, Eva very gently tried to get her nipple out of the baby's mouth. Suddenly, Eva reported, Reesa opened her eyes with a "*big smile*." Eva interpreted this response as an "*I-fooled-you joke*" in which the baby was pretending to be asleep in order to catch the mother unawares. When the clinician asked Eva how she felt about this joke, she answered, "*Oh, I loved it. It is really funny to see what she considers to be a joke. It's like the fifth-grade joke about what is green and furry and had a hundred feet. Reesa and I laugh about that one a lot.*" Although distorted, these maternal attributions were harmless in themselves, and the clinician chose not to challenge them because they served a protective function for Eva, allowing her to enjoy what she considered a special bond with her daughter and serving as a counterweight to her ambivalence.

### HUNGER AND BEING FED: ADDRESSING A ZERO-SUM CONFLICT

Eva also gave negative attributions to Reesa that were more immediately worrisome. Several of them involved feeding, with the baby often perceived as a greedy and uninvited guest at the mother's breast. Eva believed that the baby pulled up her nightgown at night, nursed, and then pulled the nightgown down again so Eva would not notice that the baby had had a clandestine sip at the mother's breast. (Reesa was brought into the parents' bed for the 2:00 A.M. feeding and was often not returned to her own crib in the parents' room.) Once Eva even suggested that the baby had jumped from her crib to the parents' bed to help herself to the breast. Taken aback by this distorted perception of what a 3-month-old baby could do, the clinician asked what made Eva think that Reesa had done that. Eva responded nonchalantly, *"My breasts were very light when I woke up, and they are usually full of milk."* Choosing to test whether this distortion of reality was amenable to change, the clinician said in a lighthearted tone, *"Eva, could we think of other possibilities? Reesa is only 3 weeks old. Look at her. Do you think she has enough control of her arms and legs to jump over from her crib to your bed and back again?"* Eva responded jovially, *"Ah, you and your ideas about development! You have your academic beliefs, but I know Reesa. She doesn't need to do that now, but she can do that when she wants."* The clinician answered, equally jovially, *"Well, on this one we'll just have different ideas, but we can keep comparing notes."* This accepting therapeutic response seemed at the time the least likely to evoke Eva's resistance and interfere with addressing negative attributions when they emerged.

New, distorted perceptions involving the baby's aggression soon came up. Once, when the baby's hand lightly touched Eva's cheek, the mother said, *"Are you hitting me? I am not hitting you . . . yet."* On other occasions, Eva commented that the baby *"pulls hair real good"* and *"gets big handfuls of hair off my head."* She also complained that the baby had the *"temperament of a speed addict,"* with a few days of intense activity interspersed with a day or so of sustained quietness and prolonged sleep. Eva's tone in making these comments was initially either amused or flippant, as if to fend off any attempt on the clinician's part to offer an alternative point of view. However she became increasingly less tolerant of what she perceived as the baby's constant demands, and gradually her complaints became focused on feeding.

Eva's initial description of Reesa as greedy had been an early warning sign of feeding as an area of potential conflict, but she at first denied any feeding difficulty and spoke proudly of her abundant milk and sturdy nipples. Although she commented that nursing was more of a routine than a source of pleasure, her affect remained neutral whenever she spoke about this topic, and she seemed competent and self-assured when she fed Reesa in the clinician's presence.

Indications of trouble were at first indirect. In a session when Reesa was 4 weeks old, Eva persistently ignored the baby's fussing. She finally offered a pacifier, which the baby refused. Eva asked the baby whether she was hungry, but she did not offer the breast. The clinician asked when Reesa had eaten last, but Eva said only that she did not remember and did not elaborate. This sequence contrasted sharply with Eva's sensitive responsiveness to her baby in previous visits. It was clear that something was amiss.

Looking for a tactful way of addressing Eva's failure to remember the baby's feeding schedule, the clinician commented that maybe she had a hectic morning and could not remember what had happened when. Eva replied that she had not had breakfast herself that morning because things had been so hectic. The clinician commented that perhaps when Eva did not eat herself it was hard to remember about Reesa's eating. Eva laughed, and said that in the rush she could not remember anything. She then began to feed Reesa and changed the topic.

The clinician waited for an opportune moment and returned to the topic of feeding. This time she focused on Eva, commenting that Eva's not eating breakfast made her worry that Eva did not have the space to take care of herself. Eva responded in a sullen, angry voice that she did not have time to take care of herself. "*Meals are always being postponed. I never eat on time anymore. When I am getting ready to eat and Reesa starts crying, I feel that she's interfering with my well-being and threatening my health.*"

This forceful statement signaled a serious problem: Reesa was now the culprit in Eva's worries about her health. The clinician expressed concern for Eva's well-being and elicited some information about the daily routine of baby care and household chores. It emerged that Eva's own eating habits involved eating many snacks throughout the day instead of three main meals. Sleeping also involved many "*catnaps*" instead of one long stretch of sleep. Eva resented the baby's intrusion in her routine. She said that she could no longer eat in peace, because whenever she cooked the baby smelled the food and woke up crying for it. "*And when I am hungry, I have to eat right away, I can't wait because I get ravenous and get a headache and stomachaches. And there is that baby screaming and not letting me eat.*" The expression "*that baby*" was an eloquent sign of Eva's increasing emotional distance from her baby.

In an effort to see whether a simple behavioral intervention might be effective, the clinician asked whether Eva had ever tried putting the baby to the breast while she was having a meal. Eva said that she could not do that, because eating was something that she had to do alone and with intense concentration. She disliked to eat and talk, or even to eat and read. Anything that detracted from her complete absorption in eating was an unwelcome interference. Eva went on to explain that Sean felt the same way. It had taken them 1 year of strained politeness over shared meals, but they had finally confessed to each other that they preferred to eat alone. Now Sean ate in the bedroom watching TV, while Eva ate in the dining room thinking her own thoughts.

As Eva continued to speak about eating, it became increasingly clear that this activity was closely linked with her sense of self, and that she was fiercely protective of her privacy whenever she felt someone might interfere with her eating. She remembered that her first husband once tried to snatch a slice of pizza from her plate, and Eva pressed the prongs of her fork on the back of his hand and threatened to drive the fork through his flesh if he stole her food. He never did it again. She also remembered mealtimes at her parents' home, marked by angry yelling among the siblings. "*Sometimes I doubled up in pain at the end of the meal, I was so tense. And I was always afraid I would not get what I wanted, because somebody would take it before the platter came around to where I sat.*"

The clinician commented on the many kinds of hunger that Eva had experienced as a child, hungers that she had struggled with and that nobody had helped her satisfy. It made complete sense, the clinician commented, that when hunger came up now Eva had to satisfy it right away and could not tolerate delay. Eva answered sadly, "*There are all kinds of hungers I tried to satisfy in whatever way I could. That's why I used ·speed and alcohol and I don't know what else. I always was a compulsive eater, although I was always very skinny. I have always been ashamed of how skinny I was, but I could never gain weight. I guess I always had the metabolism of an addict.*" The clinician asked, "*Do you think that Reesa's metabolism is the same as yours?*" Eva responded, "*Sometimes I do, but it remains to be seen.*" The clinician responded, "*Maybe you'll think that it's me and my academic ideas, but metabolism is not destiny. You once told me that you thought your parents' approach to childrearing was maybe good if one could survive it. And you survived it in spite of your metabolism.*" Eva responded, "*Maybe you are right.*"

Sean was present in the next session and gave a new slant to the unfolding theme of Eva's hungers. Turning to his wife, he said, "*There are lots of hungers that you never talk about. Like when you told me yesterday that you had been horny the whole week and were waiting for me to start. How could I know?*" Eva's fear of dependence was so pervasive that she could not reveal to her husband that she was feeling desire for him.

The theme of sexuality thus made its appearance in the sessions. It emerged that both Sean and Eva had used drugs in their respective pasts to make sex "*more kinky,*" and their interest in sex had waned since they had stopped using drugs. Sean complained about Eva's lack of interest, but it was apparent that for both of them it was easier to attribute their sparse sexual activity to Eva's lack of interest than to

Sean's or to the relationship between them. As they spoke about their relationship, it was clear that this couple, both of whom had enormous difficulties controlling aggression, had resorted to elaborate rituals to protect each other from their anger. In the process of suppressing aggression they had also suppressed their sexuality, but this was an acceptable price to pay for the preservation of their relationship.

The clinician knew that addressing the dynamics involved in this situation was beyond the therapeutic agreement with the parents and beyond the therapeutic goal that had been set. Accordingly, the clinician limited herself to supportive intervention in this area, encouraging increased communication between Sean and Eva about their desire to have sex and about their likes and dislikes in lovemaking. Interestingly, 3 weeks later Eva commented that they no longer enjoyed eating separately; they were taking their meals together and conversing about the events of the day while they ate. Eva could not understand what had happened but welcomed it as "a new way of feeling close to Sean." In a later session, she referred obliquely and with much shyness to an improvement in the sexual arena as well.

## IMPULSE TO LEAVE, FEAR OF BEING LEFT: UNDERSTANDING TRANSFERENCE TO ADDRESS RESISTANCE

The focus on the marital relationship represented a temporary diversion from a direct focus on the baby, but the urgency of Eva's conflicts regarding her child made itself felt very soon again. In a sequence of individual sessions, she spoke of an intense desire to give Reesa away. She did not quite know how to do it and went over different alternatives in her mind, only to find that every plan had a drawback. If she yielded to fantasies of leaving home, she knew that she would leave not only Reesa but also Sean and the pets, and she felt unable to live without them. If she left Reesa on the doorsteps of a church or a hospital, as she often wished to, she feared that Sean would kill her for giving his baby away. (This fear had some basis in reality: Sean had threatened to kill her when Eva presented the plan to him in a moment of despair.) Eva found herself worrying also that nobody would understand the baby and care for her as well as Eva herself did. Hence, every plan to leave the baby ended in a paradox: Eva found it unbearable to relinquish the baby's care to somebody else, but also found it unbearable to carry on with it.

Searching for an understanding of these feelings, the clinician asked when the wish to leave the baby had started. Eva said that Reesa had lately become very fussy, and that she had episodes of screaming, getting purple, and thrashing about with her arms and legs. Eva complained that she had no patience for this behavior. The clinician said that she would like to understand more about the baby's behavior. Could Eva talk about the sequence of events that led Reesa to scream so intensely?

After much halting exploration, it finally became clear that, by Eva's own account, she was waiting *"anywhere from 1 second to half an hour"* before responding to Reesa's cries. The clinician asked if Reesa's most intense crying was occurring when Eva waited half an hour before responding. Eva readily agreed, and asked with some reluctance whether she should respond sooner. The clinician answered that half an hour was too long to wait for a young baby, and went on to offer some developmental guidance, saying that babies depend on the people around them for help with their needs and that crying is a way of signaling those needs. If they get no help, they get increasingly more desperate and cry more and more as the needs become more intense. The clinician added that unmet needs can make a baby feel lost and panicky, and that Reesa could well be having such experiences when she had to wait a long time before her cries were answered. With this comment, the clinician hoped to address Eva's own firsthand experience with the feelings generated by unmet needs.

Eva was silent for a few minutes, and then said that it scared her to think that her daughter was feeling panic. In a more plaintive tone, she then objected that she had things to do: take a shower, dry her hair, make dinner, and fold the laundry. She could not be constantly interrupted, and the baby needed to learn to wait. The resonance from the past was clear in her words. Eva's mother had forced her as a young child to stop what she was doing to attend to her siblings. As an adult, Eva was doing to her baby what her mother had done to her, using the defense of turning passive into active by forcing the baby to wait until her own needs were met. Eva's desire to give the baby away was perhaps an effort to escape a situation in which she was either a victim or a perpetrator: a victim if she postponed her own pleasures to respond to her baby, a perpetrator if she made the baby suffer by forcing her to wait. Either way, the memories of unmet needs reemerged inescapably either in response to her baby's frantic cries or to her own rage as she postponed getting what she wanted to respond to the child.

As the clinician tried to guide Eva into thinking of ways to accommodate both her own and her baby's needs, she met with unexpected resistance on Eva's part. With her eyes full of tears, Eva said, *"I know there is a painful childhood behind me; I know that I was never happy as a child and that I always wanted to grow up. But I don't know if I care about the connections and I don't know what I'm going to get out of it. All I know is that every once in a while I have this feeling that I am living a life that I don't want, that I want to run away. I think that it's almost like the three faces of Eve, that there is an Eve inside me that is not Reesa's mother and that is dead, and I'm mourning because I don't want her to die.*" The clinician heard this statement as a poignant protest against the treatment focus on Reesa's welfare and on Eva's feelings as a mother. Once again, as in many times in her past, Eva felt left out. This time the feeling was triggered by the clinician, who was listening not to Eva as a woman but only to Eva as Reesa's mother.

This had a profound countertransference impact on the clinician, who felt a flood of empathy for Eva's loneliness and guilt for not having noticed it earlier. The clinician spoke to this feeling, and Eva acknowledged with deep embarrassment her wish to have more of the clinician's attention. Quickly resorting to the flippant humor that served her well as a defense against pain, she then said, "*You are not giving me what I want, Mommy.*" Her free association then led her to speak about a previous therapeutic experience many years before. Eva was desperately seeking help for feelings of anxiety and worthlessness, but found herself unable to articulate these feelings to her counselor. After a few initial sessions, the counselor told Eva that he had a salary and did not need Eva's money, and that he was wasting his time because Eva was unwilling to face her problems and work on them. He then announced that he would stop treatment with Eva, because there were too many other people who could make better use of his help. Recalling the scene, Eva said, "*I was so incredibly hurt. I could not believe that he was throwing me out just like that.*"

The present clinician expressed shock and sorrow about this experience. She then said, "*Could it be that when you get angry at me for trying to find the links with the past, you are afraid that unless you are willing and ready to agree with me, I will also throw you out?*" Eva laughed and cried at the same time, and said, "*Yes. I was so happy when after the first few sessions you asked me if I wanted to continue. I was so grateful to you. I was afraid you would say to me that I was not ready for therapy, that you had your salary and did not need me and that you were going to use your time on somebody else.*"

This disclosure led to an exploration of transference feelings. Eva disclosed that she found herself waiting for the clinician to ask about her feelings, and felt forgotten when the focus of the sessions remained on the baby. This theme led back to Eva's intense fear of dependency and her determination to fend for herself instead of asking for what she wanted. The clinician suggested that she could make it a practice of asking Eva in every session if there was something personal that she wanted to talk about, and Eva gratefully agreed. The clinician then asked if Eva would also consider making it a practice to volunteer something about herself without being asked as a way of learning that asking for attention does not need to be dangerous or lead to rejection. As she explored and clarified these transference processes, Eva became better able to empathize with her daughter's experience when she waited to be fed. *"I hate to wait to eat; why should she like it?"* However, there was a limit to Eva's empathy. She still believed that if somebody had to wait, it should be Reesa.

## PARALLEL PROCESSES IN ATTACHMENT RELATIONSHIPS: MARRIAGE AND MOTHERING

The themes of waiting and of unsatisfied needs led to Eva's own dissatisfaction with Sean. She said that her present circumstances forced her to depend on him, but she was unsure about his reliability. He had been fired from his job for cursing over the truck's shortwave radio, and the financial situation was tight. Even more difficult for Eva was Sean's attitude toward the baby. He liked playing with Reesa, but took for granted that Eva should take over whenever the baby cried or needed feeding or changing. This made Eva particularly angry because Sean had promised her throughout the pregnancy that he would step in whenever she felt overwhelmed by the baby's demands. Learning about Eva's anger at Sean helped the clinician understand an addition meaning of Eva's fantasy of giving the baby away: it could be a way of retaliating against Sean's failure to live up to his promise.

It was very difficult for Eva to talk about her anger toward Sean even when he was not present in the sessions. For her, feeling was closely tied to action, and discussing feelings of anger and disappointment presented the serious risk of her taking impulsive action. Once again, as she had done during the pregnancy, the clinician reminded her that feeling and talking need not be translated into action. She also stressed that feeling angry did not negate her deep love for Sean. This permission for ambivalence was an important revelation for Eva, similar in its importance to her early discovery, during pregnancy, that fearing her impulses to hurt the baby showed the love underlying her anger.

## TRIADIC SESSIONS: ADDRESSING TRAUMA TRIGGERS TO DECREASE THE RISK OF CHILD ABUSE

Once again, as during the prenatal part of treatment, Sean started attending the sessions after Eva had found some resolution of her inner conflicts—in this case, her ambivalence toward her dependence on him. Once again, Sean became the center of the ensuing sessions by speaking about his problems with impulsiveness, rejection of authority, and violence. The clinician helped Sean feel in his body the difference between the feeling of wanting to curse and the action of cursing, which was the reason for his dismissal from his job. She also talked with him about the different expectations he encountered in the white-collar world he was now seeking to enter and the world of *"dope fiends"* he had once frequented, and encouraged him to find new ways of expressing his anger. Here, too, as in the work with Eva, Sean's negative feelings toward the clinician had to be monitored and sometimes explicitly elicited. The clinician's role as an auxiliary ego helping Sean with his reality testing implied that she often had to say unpalatable things. Although the clinician phrased these unwelcome messages in respectful ways, she had to gauge the impact of her remarks to ensure that they did not elicit a violent response. To his credit, Sean was remarkably candid. Once, for example, he referred obliquely to fantasies of breaking the clinician's jaw. The clinician responded, *"Thanks for telling me. That would cause a lot of problems for me and for you. The whole point of our meeting is to help you avoid that kind of trouble, and you are finding words instead of actions to tell me how you feel."* Sean replied, *"I'm so relieved that you are not scared of me. If you were scared, I would really feel like hitting you."*

This exchange confirmed that Sean had enough ego strength to "speak the unspeakable" without collapsing, and opened the way for a deeper exploration of the link between feeling rejected and reacting with violence that was started during the prenatal phase of treatment. Now Sean revealed that he had an intense impulse to hit Reesa when he could not console her immediately if she cried. It was at times when this happened that Sean gave Reesa back to Eva: it was an effort to protect his baby, but Eva had no way of knowing that until he spoke about it during the sessions. The clinician responded to this revelation by asking Sean to let himself feel in the moment what it was like to attempt to soothe Reesa without success. Sean responded with a choked voice, *"She is telling me that I am no good."* The clinician asked, *"Is that a familiar feeling?"* Sean answered, a little sharply, *"You know it is. It is what my father told me all the time."* The clinician asked, *"Forgive me for pushing you a little, but do you think maybe Reesa becomes your father at those moments?"* Sean breathed deeply for a few moments without answering. Then he nodded "yes" wordlessly. The clinician said softly, *"That is what we call a trauma reminder. Your father hit you so much, and you decided that you would hit instead of being hit. Now Reesa's crying takes you back to that time, and your body remembers and wants to fight back."* What followed was a conversation about ways of "listening to the body." The clinician praised Sean for his intuitive listening to the body in giving Reesa back to Eva before yielding to the impulse to hit her. She then asked whether Sean could bring himself to an awareness of his wish to hit and instead see Reesa as a helpless little baby who was overwhelmed by her own intense body sensations that she could not manage when she cried so much. Sean, looking deeply moved, mumbled that he would try.

Revealing to each other their fears of being overwhelmed by their anger and helplessness helped this couple find solutions for helping each other. Eva became more tolerant of Sean's sporadic withdrawal from the baby. Sean, in turn, became better able to offer concrete assistance to Eva. This was particularly evident in the stalemates that occurred between Eva and Reesa when both of them were hungry at the same time. Sean said that he could not eat anyway when Reesa screamed, and suggested that in such a situation he would give Reesa a bottle until Eva finished dinner and felt ready to offer the breast. Eva was at first afraid that Sean's offer to feed the baby would contain an implicit criticism of her mothering, but she finally agreed with relief to the plan.

In ensuing sessions, the parents reported that this system was working smoothly. Reesa's screaming declined, and Eva no longer mentioned any desire to leave the baby. Sean said, "*It helped me when Eva told me about your saying that Reesa could be disorganizing. We know all about that, and we don't want Reesa to find out about it.*" He added a familiar comment that showed there was still reason to be worried about the parental perceptions: "*Reesa has the temperament of a speed addict.*" Eva readily agreed, and said, "*We want her first words to be 'beer' and 'Valium.' That way, if someone asks her what she wants, she won't answer that she wants speed, like we did.*" Even this comment, worrisome as it was in its implications, was said in a light and accepting tone that was very different from Eva's earlier complaints about the baby as malevolent and willful.

Reesa was present throughout these sessions. Her presence enabled the clinician to assess both the accuracy of the parents' perceptions and the adequacy of the child's development. The observations yielded no evidence that Reesa had an unusually "*intense*" temperament, as the parents believed. She was a baby with unusual sending power, whose signals of pleasure and distress were clear and who was readily satisfied once her needs were met. She remained a beautiful baby, with sparkling eyes and a ready, contagious smile. During the period when Eva complained of the baby's fussiness, the clinician did note an increase in the baby's irritability and some frantic tone in her search for the mother's breast, which she often used for comfort. This could be a response to Eva's unpredictability. Since by her own account Eva would either respond immediately or wait as long as half an hour, it is likely that the baby had difficulty developing reliable expectations about her mother's availability. However, Reesa's frantic search for the breast as a means of comfort proved short-lived. This behavior declined as Eva became better able to respond more promptly and consistently to the baby.

## REFLECTIONS ON THERAPEUTIC MODALITIES DURING PREGNANCY AND AFTER REESA'S BIRTH

The clinician found that there were marked differences in what happened during treatment before and after Reesa's birth. During pregnancy, Eva's fears that the past would return led seamlessly to an exploration of her childhood experiences, which emerged with remarkable ease. After Reesa's birth, Eva spoke less often or directly about her childhood, and she was more open to understanding her difficulties with Reesa through the prism of her transference to the clinician and her ambivalence toward Sean.

It is possible that this shift was due to the very real challenges posed by the care of the baby. Eva's fears during pregnancy that she would harm her baby were traced to the rage she felt as a child for having to become the mother of her mother's children. After Reesa's birth, the baby's claim on her meant that she might not have enough time and energy for herself. In order to protect her baby, she needed to rely on the clinician's and Sean's availability, a need that in turned triggered her fear of dependence. As Eva was reassured again and again of both her husband's and her clinician's availability, negative attributions to the baby occurred more and more rarely. When they did arise, their appearance usually signaled the presence of negative feelings toward either Sean or the clinician, which when explored and understood could be readily detached from the baby.

The importance of the transference during this period illustrates a delicate technical problem in relational approaches to psychotherapy, including P-CPP: the need to balance the treatment focus on the baby and the baby–parent relationship with an awareness of the parents' emotional needs as individuals. In parents with a relatively sound character structure, the commitment to the baby usually supersedes the conflicting feelings of resentment at sharing the clinician. In parents with histories of chronic and severe deprivation and trauma, on the other hand, the triggers for internalized "fight, flight, and freeze" early responses—withdrawal, aggression, dissociation—can be pervasive and overpowering. In these cases, treatment might paradoxically depart from the focus on the baby's well-being in order ultimately to serve the baby best. In the classical "ghosts in the nursery" intervention (Fraiberg, 1980), the identification with the aggression needs to be traced to the repressed affective experience of childhood terror and helpless rage in order to free the baby from becoming the target of these repressed affects.

## The Second 6 Months:
## Addressing Distorted Positive Maternal Attributions

The decline in negative attributions to the baby led to a shift in the focus of treatment. Now there was an increase in Eva's claims that the baby was capable of reasoning, ideas, and behaviors that, in our present state of knowledge, are considered to be beyond the capabilities of an infant. In themselves, these distorted positive attributions seemed harmless. They involved, for example, Eva's conviction that Reesa could recognize letters, thought that TV commercials for sugar-frosted cereals were reprehensible, and got excited when she overheard her parents talking about a possible trip to the zoo. These distortions were worrisome nonetheless because they involved a faulty interpretation of Reesa's behaviors—the attribution to her of thought processes and motivations she realistically could not have. The concern was that, as Reesa began to acquire the capacity for symbolic representation, she might incorporate these maternal misinterpretations into her own thinking, leading to distortions in her own symbolic representations and sense of self.

This was a thorny therapeutic challenge. How do we tell a mother that she is wrong in attributing a preciously rich inner life to her baby, particularly when these attributions serve a protective function against ambivalence and rage? Before deciding on a course of action, the clinician tried to gain an understanding of the specific psychological meaning that these distortions served for Eva. Through careful listening and observation, the clinician hoped to understand the areas of Reesa's behavior most commonly involved in maternal positive distortions and the effect that these distortions had on Eva's interaction with her.

The process of watching, listening, and waiting led to an important discovery. Eva registered the baby's behavior accurately and responded to it appropriately, but assigned to it a communicative intention it could not possibly have. Although numerous, the distortions could be understood in every case in terms of a basic underlying process: they negated the baby's helplessness and attributed to her communicative skills that, if real, would in effect give Reesa the power to tell Eva how to take care of her. For example, Eva described an episode in which Reesa started to cry without apparent reason. When Eva looked at her, she noticed that the baby kept stretching her head in the direction of the crib, which was next to them. Eva concluded that the baby was sleepy and was telling her that she wanted to be in bed. Eva put her in the crib, and Reesa, satisfied, fell promptly asleep. There were many similar examples. At 8 months, Reesa was credited with pursing her lips for "yes" and rolling her eyes for "no" when asked if she was hungry. Eva thought that she complained about a tummy ache by fussing while tapping her stomach with her hands. These attributions were remarkably similar to the attributions that Eva made to the behavior of her beloved pets. They were also in line with Eva's childhood wish to grow up in a hurry to escape her sense of helpless dependence on others. Just as she wanted to do things that were beyond her age when she was a child, she now perceived her baby as capable of doing things that she was too young to do.

In some ways, Eva's attributions were also similar to the working hypotheses that ordinary parents use to guide their ministrations to their preverbal babies. The difference was that ordinary parents rely on their empathy and on their knowledge of their babies to make educated guesses that they acknowledge as guesses. Eva could not give herself credit for owning her educated guesses: she relinquished responsibility for her own decision making to her baby. Perhaps she feared the blurring of boundaries that is inherent in the empathic response, and she needed to affirm her separateness from her baby by clear role assignments in the communications between them. The intriguing feature in this situation was that Eva could respond with empathy, but she could not acknowledge this to herself.

This clinical formulation laid the foundation for the ensuing course of treatment. One important decision was not to address those distortions that facilitated Eva's empathic response, such as the examples noted above. Instead, the clinician focused only on those distortions that might lead Eva to expect a premature self-reliance on the baby's part, because they were based on Eva's own conflicts over neediness and dependence.

Eva provided many opportunities to work with these distortions. She reported, for example, that Reesa's face had a disgusted expression whenever somebody affectionately called her "*baby,*" but she beamed with joy when she was called a "*big girl.*" Eva also believed that Reesa looked bored whenever she was told that other babies would come to visit, but was positively ecstatic when told she would play with a 4-year-old. Other reports involved Reesa's perceived frustration when her mother attempted to feed her solid foods, because being fed made her feel "*like a baby*" and she wanted to eat by herself "*like a big girl.*" In the second 6 months of Reesa's life, Eva often preceded anecdotes about her daughter by talking about the times "*when Reesa was a baby.*"

The clinician addressed these maternal distortions in a variety of ways. When Eva's claims about her baby's self-reliance were particularly preposterous, the clinician showed surprise and mild skepticism, which she explained in terms of the departure of the mother's descriptions from "*what we currently know about children's development.*" The clinician also asked Eva to show her the baby's behaviors the next time they occurred so that the clinician could understand better what the mother was describing. This approach often took the form of good-natured banter between mother and clinician, in which the mother teased the clinician for working with children yet not believing in their hidden powers, and the clinician replied lightheartedly that she needed empirical data to be convinced. This teasing enabled Eva to save face by preserving her self-protective view of herself as a counselor speaking to another counselor. At the same time, the mild and respectful skepticism expressed by the clinician enhanced Eva's reality testing, and many times she acknowledged that she was reading too much into her child's behavior.

At a different level of intervention, the clinician responded to Eva's description of Reesa's adultlike responses by sympathizing with her desire that the baby grow up and by cautiously offering links with Eva's own early wishes to become an adult. Eva readily acknowledged her wishes that the baby become more self-reliant, and saw similarities between her baby and herself in this regard. Still, Reesa's adultlike qualities remained for Eva an uncontestable reality. She could not acknowledge to herself that she wished Reesa would outgrow infancy and become less dependent on her. At the same time, Eva remained remarkably respectful of Reesa's own pace of development. She encouraged her to achieve locomotion but was not inappropriate or intrusive in doing so. She remained attuned to the baby's signals. Most interestingly, she continued to breastfeed until Reesa spontaneously lost interest in the breast at 15 months—a clear demonstration that the earlier conflicts around feeding had been resolved.

During this period, Sean's participation in the treatment continued to be sporadic. He usually came to the sessions when he was concerned about his performance at work or when there were marital tensions triggered by his tendency to let Eva do all the household work and also take care of Reesa. He was playful with his daughter and liked to roughhouse with her, but did not mind avoiding the caregiving routines. This gave rise to periodic tensions with Eva, which were usually discussed in joint sessions. Once the tensions decreased, Sean stopped coming again. His was a task-oriented approach to treatment, and Eva seemed to accept this well.

### Reesa at 14 Months: Developmental Assessment

The clinician's ongoing observations of Reesa showed that she was developing adequately in all areas. She was an ebullient baby with a radiant smile and laughing, mischievous eyes. She showed a clear preference for her mother, whom she sought out both for social exchange and for soothing with a readiness that denoted her confidence in Eva's availability. She was also clearly attached to her father, approached him often, liked to play with his beard, and responded with bellyfuls of laughter when he played "horsie" with her on his shoulders.

Reesa had taken her first step at 11 months, and cheerfully marched throughout the small apartment seeking out the pets, finding minuscule wonders on the floor, and delighting herself with discoveries, such as the possibility of playing with the toilet water. She ate well and liked to feed herself, but she was also very interested in breastfeeding throughout the first year, although her interest declined progressively thereafter. Breastfeeding stopped smoothly at 15 months. She expressed anger and frustration unambiguously but responded well to her mother's firm limits. A very likable aspect of Eva's socialization practices was her sense of humor in doing it. By setting rules for her daughter, she seemed to be undoing the disorienting and anxiety-producing lack of parental direction that she had experienced as a child.

The only area of temporary concern was Reesa's sleeping. Throughout the first year, she slept in her crib in the parents' small bedroom, very near to their bed. Both Sean and Eva went to sleep well past midnight, and talked, watched TV, and played with the pets on their bed until then. Reesa was expected to join in the fun, and as a result her sleeping schedule was very erratic. This did not worry Eva, who saw no particular virtue in a predictable cycle of sleep and wakefulness. However, this casualness had to end when Sean decided to attend a community college during the day and then work until 10:00 P.M. to support the family. Nights were then for sleeping, but Reesa had not had an early chance to learn it. For several nights, she woke up crying and seeking to play. Finally, Eva and Sean decided to move the baby's crib out of their bedroom and into the baby's own lovingly decorated room. Reesa's problems with sleeping stopped 2 days later.

At 14 months, Reesa's performance in the Bayley Scales showed an alert, friendly, and expressive baby whose language and fine and gross motor skills were entirely age appropriate. Her developmental quotient showed that she was performing 1 month above the expectations for her chronological age.

## The Last 6 Months of Treatment: Violence Revisited

As Reesa achieved locomotion, Eva's perception of the baby became increasingly more accurate. She showed remarkable skill in supporting secure base behavior, giving Reesa freedom to explore and welcoming her return for solace and refueling. She read Reesa's communications accurately and responded to them appropriately. There was a noticeable decline in Eva's need to explain Reesa's behavior in terms of the child's desire to become an adult. As these changes occurred, there was a concomitant decline in Eva's anxiety about her competence as a mother. Eva often consulted with the clinician about aspects of Reesa's behavior that puzzled her, but did so with a tone of relaxed curiosity rather than with anxious self-doubt. The sessions took on a relaxed, chatty tone. Everybody had fun watching Reesa. The clinician began to consider moving toward ending treatment.

This mood was interrupted by Sean's dramatic return to the center of the sessions. He had begun college after dropping out of high school 15 years earlier, and was combining studying with nighttime work to support his family. He was under stress, unsure of himself, feeling he might not be *"smart enough to make it."* He expressed his stress in an outburst of violence in the classroom: he threatened to hit a female teacher with a chair for criticizing him and then fled the classroom, vowing to drop out of school.

The ensuing 3 months focused on working with Sean on this crisis while continuing the format of home visits with Eva and Reesa present. The result for Sean was successful. The college allowed him to return to classes, and he ended the year with high grades and with renewed insight into the mechanisms that triggered his aggression. He also renewed his attendance to his substance-abuse recovery group, which had lapsed because of his very hectic schedule. He and Eva decided that attending Saturday sessions was more important at this time than having a free day.

After the crisis was over, the clinician spoke about Eva's and Sean's self-confidence as parents and about the fine job they were doing raising Reesa. Eva replied, *"You know, I've been thinking the same thing. I enjoy seeing you and will be sorry to stop, but I think we can now do it on our own."* The old need for self-reliance was reasserting itself, but now it had a solid base supporting it.

## Reflections on the Therapeutic Process

The therapeutic process in this case can be divided into four fairly distinct phases, each characterized by a different focus within the overarching principles of P-CPP.

The prenatal period, which lasted 11 weeks, was marked by intense maternal anxiety over a pregnancy that although planned, was now perceived as unwanted. Eva sensed that there were profound psychological reasons involved in her fear of becoming a mother, and expressed this unconscious awareness in a beautifully succinct formulation: her fear that the pregnancy would bring back the past. Articulated in this way, the conflict offered the clue to its own resolution: the exploration of the past, because the dread of its return could only be understood by bringing to awareness forgotten but still actively painful secrets.

The process of uncovering early experiences was guided by the clinician's specific goal of bringing insight into the unconscious conflicts underlying Eva's ambivalence about her pregnancy and her unborn baby. This goal imparted a particular direction to the clinician's interventions. By linking the emerging experiences and feelings from the past with present feelings about the pregnancy and the unborn baby, the clinician sought to bring understanding to Eva's fear of becoming a mother. Other symptoms and conflicts, although perceived by the clinician, were not pursued in treatment unless there was a compelling link with the conflict over mothering. To do otherwise would have run counter to (and hence diluted) Eva's explicitly stated therapeutic goal of coming to love her child.

It is quite likely that Eva's remarkable ease in recalling and reexperiencing the affect of early events was due to the developmental crisis brought about by the pregnancy (Benedek, 1970). It was only during this period of enormous psychological turmoil that Eva was able to seek insight through the exploration of her childhood experiences. It was a remarkable coincidence that the baby's birth followed soon after a pivotal session in which Eva recalled and reexperienced her early murderous impulses toward the brother that, in her view, deprived her of her parents' undivided affection. After this session, the urgency of Eva's self-exploration diminished noticeably and never regained its former momentum. It is possible that Eva unconsciously strove to solve this fundamental conflict before her baby's birth in order to protect her daughter from murderous impulses rooted in the past. Once this task was achieved, Eva's psychological functioning gained stability. The treatment might well have enabled Eva to fend off psychological collapse by relieving her of displaced murderous impulses toward her daughter, relegating those feelings safely to the past, and reassuring her of her present ability to love.

The second phase of treatment was ushered by the baby's birth. This phase involved a decline in Eva's motivation for self-exploration and an increase in negatively charged attributions of the baby's motives. Eva was clearly resistant to recognizing these distortions as expressions of her ambivalence toward the baby. All attempts, however tentative, at suggesting that this might be so were met by flat and persistent denials. Even when planning dramatic moves such as giving the baby away, Eva refused to look inside herself for clues about the meaning of these fantasized actions. The presenting conflict over mothering, alleviated through the earlier treatment, was superimposed on what seemed like a developmental trauma disorder that was rooted in the neglect and abuse she had experienced as a child, manifested in her marked distortions and the danger of explosive acting-out behavior reminiscent of her past lifestyle.

The only avenue for broaching the feelings of ambivalence proved to be a supportive exploration of Eva's negative transference toward the clinician and her feelings of being betrayed by Sean, who had not kept his promise of rescuing her when she felt overwhelmed by the baby. A focus on these relationships allowed Eva to speak plaintively of her own needs. She was able to express her feelings of being ignored, because of the clinician's focus on Reesa and her husband's prevailing interest in his own pursuits. As powerful longings to be cared for and protected emerged, the dilemma that Eva faced became clear. In responding to her baby, this mother had only two roles available: victim or aggressor. Responding to her baby meant postponing her own needs, and she became a victim. Alternatively, choosing to ignore her baby to attend to herself instantly converted her into the aggressor she both feared and longed to be. Her child's helplessness triggered in Eva unbearable feelings of panic and disorganization. This psychological dilemma made any viable reciprocity with her baby quite impossible.

The approach to treatment in this phase consisted, in essence, in utilizing the transference to reassure Eva of the clinician's interest and availability and in developing concrete safety mechanisms to ensure Sean's psychological availability in periods of stress. The repeated emergence of negative distortions of the baby's behavior was met with an exploration of Eva's disappointment or anger with regard to the clinician or Sean. The distortions invariably declined as these feelings were explored, but the link between these two phenomena could never be explicitly addressed. Intrapsychic exploration had been replaced, in this phase of treatment, by emotional support, sympathetic acknowledgment of Eva's negative feelings toward the clinician and Sean, and the reassurance that anger need not destroy love.

The third phase of treatment coincided approximately with the second half of Reesa's first year. During this phase, the negative distortions gave way to the predominance of positive distortions centered on what Eva perceived as Reesa's unusually precocious attributes. These distortions served to relieve Eva of any awareness of the empathy she needed in order to understand her child. Eva equated empathy with a sense of merger and loss of identity. As a result, her remarkable accuracy in reading her child's signals had to be disguised as stemming not from her own sensitivity but from Reesa's precocious communication skills. An overdetermining factor was Eva's need to negate her child's neediness and to perceive her as autonomous and self-reliant. The treatment approach in this context consisted primarily of nondidactic developmental guidance, imparted in a light, collegial manner that could enable Eva to listen without losing face.

The fourth phase coincided with the onset of Reesa's locomotion. In this phase, there was a dramatic decline in the number and intensity of positive distortions and an almost complete disappearance of negative ones. This welcome development was probably due to the combination of two factors: the beneficial results of treatment and, quite crucially, Reesa's ability to alleviate her mother's fear of merger and helplessness through her own self-reliant mobility. Sean's participation in the treatment was sporadic but crucial. By coming to grips with his own violence as a response to rejection, he was able to become a more available father and a more supportive husband to a mother much in need of support.

The versatility of intervention techniques was a key feature of this treatment. The insight-oriented technique used during the pregnancy had to be adapted to the new stresses the parents experienced after Reesa's birth. Even for parents with a sound personality structure, the concrete demands of a real baby have a different psychological impact than the fantasized changes anticipated during the pregnancy. For Sean and Eva, who had painstakingly reached a tenuous psychological balance, the baby's presence and her demands constituted a constant reminder of their vulnerability to violent acting out. As a result, intervention during the postnatal period had to be responsive both to the realistic possibility of violence and to the rigid psychological mechanisms that the parents employed to protect themselves and their baby. Nondidactic developmental guidance, emotional support, and judicious use of the transference predominated over insight-oriented psychotherapy during this period.

Despite the varying modalities of the interventions, the baby and her welfare remained at the center of treatment both before and after her birth. This unwavering focus represents the unifying link in the variety of methods employed in the course of P-CPP, which envisions the infant–parent relationship as the most efficient vehicle for promoting the infant's overall health and well-being, but does not consider the quality of the attachment relationship as an end of itself. This priority on the baby's health and well-being, both in the present and in the future, provides for a flexibility of options when the parents are not able to utilize treatment to protect and nurture the child—something that fortunately was not the case with Eva and Sean.

## Epilogue: Follow-Up 10 Months after Treatment

Ten months after termination, Eva phoned to say that Reesa's second birthday was approaching and that she wanted to thank the clinician for having helped her to enjoy her daughter so much. Interestingly, the phone call took place in the same month that treatment had begun 2 years earlier. Reesa's second birthday was still 2 months away.

The clinician had the distinct impression that this was an anniversary call, and surmised that Eva might want a brief reencounter with the clinician. This impression was reinforced when Eva lingered on the phone, asking questions about the normal development of 2-year-olds in an easygoing manner, as if the contact with the clinician was more important than the answers to her questions. The clinician responded by inviting her in for a visit, with the intention of offering a gift for Reesa's second birthday, and suggested that a videotaped assessment of Reesa might be a good way of talking about 2-year-olds. Eva accepted the invitation with delight.

A two-session encounter was set up. The first session involved listening to Eva talk about herself, her daughter, and her marriage and doing a videotaped developmental assessment of Reesa. The second session, with Sean present, involved viewing the videotape, discussing Reesa's performance and her overall development, talking about Sean's career accomplishments since the termination of treatment, and discussing plans for the future.

The family was doing remarkably well. Sean had received governmental loans to finish college, and the financial worries of the past were at least temporarily relieved. He had good grades in school and planned to pursue a career in acupuncture after finishing college. He spent much time away from home because he studied, worked, and had a strenuous schedule of physical exercise to help his ailing back. This was a source of tension between Eva and Sean, but they managed the conflict in ways that protected the stability of their marriage. Eva was planning to return to work on a part-time basis. She believed that Reesa could now stand a few hours away from her without undue stress, and felt the need for more contact with adults after 2 years as a mother and homemaker.

It was quite clear that Eva had continued to think about herself and her past since the end treatment. She reported that she had become very close to one of her brothers, and they often talked with each other about childhood memories. Eva was surprised at the similarity between her brother's perception of her parents and her own. *"They were never there for us. We really needed to make it on our own. No wonder all of us had trouble of one sort or another while we were growing up."* She spoke with a gentle sadness, as if regretting the past yet coming to grips with it. She seemed to have the same attitude toward the present. She was aware of the limitations in her relationship with Sean: his self-absorption in his pursuits and his tendency to panic when she spoke of her dissatisfactions, so that she needed to keep many of her feelings to herself. She expressed acceptance of the situation as one that reflected both his and her personalities, and felt relatively at ease with the present balance in their relationship.

Most impressively, Eva had become a mother comfortable with herself and with her child. She was able to negotiate mutually acceptable solutions in conflictual situations and to use humor as an adaptive way of coping with stalemates when she and Reesa could not reach a compromise. She was firm yet matter-of-fact in enforcing rules. She seemed like a veteran mother, largely unruffled by the trials and tribulations of her role. She did get very angry at times, and occasionally slapped Reesa when she was at her wit's end. She always explained to Reesa afterward that she regretted doing so, and that hitting was not a good way of dealing with anger. (Reesa herself seldom used hitting when angry or frustrated.) Eva expected Reesa to understand and follow rules, and was proud of what she called *"grown-up behavior"*— Reesa's ease in interacting with other children and adults, her firmness in defending her toys, and her lack of clinginess. Eva often described Reesa as more *"grown up"* than older children with whom she played. It is difficult to know how true this was. However, Eva's earlier massive distortions in her perception of Reesa's behavior had largely disappeared. The only trace of distortion the clinician could detect was a tendency to overestimate the sophistication of Reesa's speech, particularly sentence length and complexity of grammatical structure. Reesa spoke like a regular toddler, and Eva had no difficulty in interpreting accurately and responding appropriately to her communications, but here again, as in the past, Eva needed to attribute the success of their exchanges to her daughter's skills rather than to her own.

Reesa herself was blossoming. She was a gentle, smiling 2-year-old who showed delight in her parents and friendly interest in the clinician, and who had a wonderful ability to engage in rich representational play. She cooked for the adults and ceremoniously served dinner, complete with after-dinner coffee; she took good care of a doll, cuddling her, feeding her, and putting her to sleep; she made pies and cooked them in the oven. Her parents reported that she had an imaginary friend named Reggie, who lived in the attic and who was responsible for strange noises and misplaced toys.

Reesa had a full range of affect and could be quite forceful in making her wishes known. She had tantrums, which were not long lasting or frequent and which the parents tended to manage by timing out, reasoning with her, or sometimes by teasing her for being "*a baby.*" Reesa's performance on the Bayley Scales was approximately 3 months above her chronological age. She was cooperative and enthusiastic throughout the testing, but tended to give difficult items back to the clinician, with the implicit message: "*You do it for me.*" This may have been related to Eva's emphasis on promoting grown-up behavior. Although Reesa was largely able to comply with the maternal demands, it seemed that sometimes she coped with the pressure by declining to try. Interestingly, Eva tended to accept Reesa's requests for help and responded to them in a good-natured way.

In summary, the picture emerging from this follow-up was that of a well-functioning family unit, with a thriving child and growth-promoting relationships between Reesa and her parents. The strains and stresses they experienced were well within the range of expectable difficulties in living and did not pose a danger to the child's development. The changes facilitated by treatment had endured many months after its termination, offering hope that they would remain stable.

# Clinical Case 2. Healing Chronic Traumatic Stress: Treatment at the Intersection of Domestic Violence, Immigration, and Historical Trauma

This case illustrates the treatment of Zazil, a recently emigrated pregnant woman of Guatemalan Indigenous descent who had experienced relational violence starting in childhood. The compounded impact of chronic childhood physical abuse and of witnessing domestic violence permeated fundamental aspects of her social–emotional development, including the infiltration of abusive patterns in her adult relationships in the form of IPV perpetrated by her husband. These patterns of interpersonal violence unfolded in the context of centuries of historical trauma, wholesale massacres, and institutionalized discrimination and oppression perpetrated against indigenous peoples. The treatment of Zazil and her family incorporated simultaneous attention to the psychological imprint of victimization by attachment figures and the matrix of internalized oppression generated by early and repeated experiences of humiliation and maltreatment for their ethnic identity and cultural heritage.

## Referral and Presenting Problems

Zazil, a 25-year-old pregnant, Mayan (K'iche') and Spanish-speaking Indigenous Guatemalan woman, was referred for mental health services by the Women's Health Center social worker owing to suspicion of IPV in her relationship with her husband, Pedro. The social worker reported that Zazil, 4 months pregnant with her first child, had arrived at her prenatal appointment with unexplained bruising on her face and arms. When questioned about these injuries, Zazil explained with averted eyes and a halting tone of voice that her injuries were the result of having slipped in the bathtub the day before. When Zazil met with the social worker, she emphatically denied any type of violence in her relationship with Pedro, and stated that she and her husband "*had nothing more serious than verbal arguments and misunderstandings, usually related to money problems.*" A medical chart review revealed that Zazil had had a miscarriage in the first trimester after an alleged fall 5 months earlier, raising suspicion about the veracity of her accounts of her first miscarriage and this more recent alleged fall. Zazil also presented with pregnancy-related medical problems. She was diagnosed with pre-eclampsia early in her pregnancy and was suffering from recurrent urinary tract infections, both of which required regular monitoring at the clinic. She had low weight gain, and a nutritionist was seeing her regularly to help improve her weight gain.

Although Zazil was regular in her attendance at follow-up prenatal appointments, both the social worker and midwife expressed frustration over her disinterest in her prenatal care and specifically her lack of compliance with basic recommendations in the treatment of her preeclampsia and lack of weight gain. The midwife reported that Zazil skipped meals whenever she was not hungry and did not seem concerned about the severity of her pregnancy complications, which could potentially lead to a miscarriage. She had also not followed through with referrals for supportive services to improve her basic living situation. Reaching an impasse in their efforts to provide effective prenatal care to Zazil, both the social worker and midwife decided to include a mental health professional to support treatment adherence, to assess the current risk of IPV, and to serve as a cultural mediator to support communication between Zazil and her medical providers. Collaboration among service providers was essential because of Zazil's high-risk presentation.

## Creating a Conceptual Frame: Clinical and Sociocultural Considerations

The referral information made clear that Zazil was not inclined to welcome treatment. She had vehemently denied any violence in her relationship with her husband, revealing only *"I suffer from nerves"* [*padezco de nervios*], an embodied cultural expression of distress. She had also disclosed to the social worker and midwife that she felt frustrated and overwhelmed by the demands of the service providers who were managing her high-risk pregnancy care plan. The early prognostic indicators painted a dire future for this mother and her developing baby. If left untreated, these risk indicators could result in a worsening pregnancy prognosis, continued vulnerability to victimization, and disturbances in the mother–baby dyadic relationship that could endanger the baby's developmental trajectory through the intergenerational transmission of trauma effects.

The clinician (M. A. D.) used the information provided by the referral sources to implement a culturally informed and emotionally supportive foundational phase approach with the goal of engaging Zazil in treatment. The clinical framework conceptualized Zazil's life circumstance of becoming a mother in the context of recent immigration (i.e., starting a new life while carrying a new life) as a potentially transformative developmental process that, if supported, could lead to psychosocial maturation as an individual and as a mother, with important ramifications for maternal and infant health. The clinician viewed the circumstances in Zazil's life as providing a port for entry for therapeutic efforts to transform her inner landscape, to foster the mother–infant relationship, and to use the therapeutic process to promote safety and reciprocity in her relationship with her husband.

Due to Zazil's exposure to historical trauma and personal history of racial and cultural discrimination, the clinician used a biopsychosocial approach that simultaneously considered the cultural, social, psychological, and biological dimensions that shaped Zazil's inner life. This culturally grounded approach took into consideration both the Western psychological paradigms and the cultural, historical, and social experiences of Latinos with *mestizo* heritage—that is, a person with both indigenous and Hispanic legacy (Flores, 2013). In this worldview, health is understood and experienced as a state of balance and interconnectedness of the body–mind–spirit, a belief held by indigenous groups prior to the Spanish conquest but still prevalent in many sectors of present-day Latin American cultures.

The clinician followed the cultural thread linking mental health to a "state of balance and interconnectedness" of central aspects of the self (*heart*/emotional, *mind*/mental, and *soul*/spirituality) with the external world (as experienced by the relational self). She hypothesized that Zazil was experiencing a state of imbalance and inner turmoil brought about by her current circumstances as a pregnant immigrant woman involved in a potentially violent relationship and experiencing acculturative stress in the context of intertwined personal and historical trauma.

In Zazil's case, collective or historical trauma consisted of the cumulative negative effects of racial discrimination and inequality systematically endured by indigenous people of the Americas from the time of the Spanish conquest and colonization to the present day. The experience of racial discrimination by indigenous people is a pervasive and persistent problem in contemporary Latin American societies (Telles, 2007). Frequently experienced psychosocial stressors include acculturative stress, poverty, language barriers, low education, inadequate social support, high-crime neighborhood residence, loss of habitat by encroaching powerful entities, and a history of racial discrimination driven by sociopolitical forces engendering inequality and social disadvantage (Abraído-Lanza, Echeverría, & Flórez, 2016). All these factors were clearly present in Zazil's clinical presentation.

Zazil's indigenous ethnic heritage as K'iche' Maya is associated with systematic cultural marginalization and persecution during and in the aftermath of a 36-year civil war in Guatemala that ended in 1996 when Zazil was 2 years old and affected millions of indigenous people, nearly half of whom live in extreme poverty (World Bank, 2003). A United Nations-sponsored report concluded that racism was a central component in the civil war violence that killed 200,000 Guatemalans, 83% of whom were Indigenous Maya (Commission for Historical Clarification, 1999). The Mayan population is also exposed to institutionalized racism within the justice and health care systems, an experience that engenders collective distrust in legal and health institutions, prevents them from receiving appropriate legal redress and adequate health care, and helps to explain their increased burden of disease and lower life expectancy (World Bank, 2003).

Belonging to a historically ostracized and oppressed indigenous group exposed Zazil to chronic stress and trauma throughout her formative years, shaping her sense of self, her social–emotional development, and her cultural identity, and creating internal representations of herself as bad, defective, and unworthy. Now settled in the United States, Zazil's status as an indigenous woman going through the acculturation process in an anti-immigrant sociopolitical climate placed her at increased risk of continuing to experience discrimination and other forms of social exclusion that negatively affected her physical and psychological health.

The clinician believed that the detrimental effects of racism and discrimination affected Zazil's ability to trust social institutions and posed a potential hindrance to the establishment of a therapeutic alliance. To promote trust, she diligently monitored Zazil's behavior and body language with the purpose of understanding her nonverbal communications as the basis to engage in culturally attuned reparative relational experiences. The therapeutic relationship gradually became a mutative factor through the clinician's role as a "new object" (Fonagy, 1998), with whom Zazil could identify as a partner who was allied with her collective identity.

The significance of nonverbal communications for the transference to the clinician was paramount in the treatment. Nonverbal relational exchanges integrate both perception and emotion, and profound interpersonal experiences—such as attachment, connectedness, empathy, and other emotional subtleties—are often expressed nonverbally rather than in spoken communication (Pally, 2001). Many indigenous cultures place great value on nonverbal communication, and privileging body language over spoken communication became a culturally appropriate way to provide Zazil with supportive relational experiences to promote self-acceptance and to counter vulnerability and shame. The clinician deliberately cultivated her own nonverbal signals (facial expression, posture, gestures, and tone of voice) as forms of communication and trained herself to monitor and respond in an emotionally attuned manner to Zazil's body language and nonverbal communications.

As treatment progressed, it became evident that Zazil's negative experiences had affected her threat appraisal and safety-seeking behavior. These areas of functioning became a focus of treatment to create safety in Zazil's relationship with her husband and to protect both her and the baby from ongoing victimization. Here too cultural considerations were paramount in the choice of intervention modalities. In Latino cultures the value of *familismo*—defined as unswerving loyalty, commitment, and dedication to the nuclear and extended family (Gloria & Castellanos, 2016) influences the early socialization of children, and girls are inculcated from a young age to be the guardians of family unity as the nucleus of society and the primary support system. The clinician knew that this cultural value in Latino couples experiencing IPV often reinforces the expectation that women will keep the family together, even if this means staying in an abusive relationship (Flores-Ortiz, Valdez Curiel, & Andrade Palos, 2002; Kelly, 2009). In this cultural context, simply telling Zazil that she should leave her abusive husband would not acknowledge her deeply embedded sense of her place in society. As a married pregnant immigrant woman with very limited financial resources and an inadequate social system, Zazil relied on her husband as an indispensable provider, and her dependence on him was reinforced by cultural values that encouraged loyalty and deference to the male of the family. In acknowledging these factors, the treatment incorporated a careful cultivation of the values of self-respect and protection of the woman and infant as complementary to the value of family unity, and incorporated Zazil's husband as an integral family member through his roles as breadwinner and father.

## Starting Treatment: The Foundational Phase

The foundational phase consisted of three 2-hour sessions followed by a feedback session in which the clinician extended an invitation to treatment. This phase allowed the clinician to learn about different aspects of Zazil's early experiences and social context while remaining aware that there would be more to learn as treatment progressed.

## Meeting Zazil

Although hesitant to accept the referral, Zazil agreed to meet with the clinician following the conclusion of a prenatal appointment with her doctor. The social worker who arranged the meeting introduced Zazil and the clinician and, following some culturally expected courtesy exchanges, the clinician walked with Zazil to her office in a different wing of the hospital. Zazil seemed shy and reserved, with her facial expression alternating between a worried look and a blank gaze.

Zazil was a small-framed young woman of significantly short stature. Her facial features clearly resembled a person of indigenous ancestry. Her long, straight black hair was neatly braided down her back, keeping her hair away from her face. She had a dark, flawless complexion and displayed an ample and soft smile that briefly curved up her lips during introductions. She was dressed in casual clothing, wearing lose-fitting pants and a midlength green sweater that covered her small, protuberant pregnant belly.

As Zazil and the clinician entered the office, Zazil respectfully waited by the door for the clinician to tell her where she could sit down. She had a constricted posture while seated, with her legs tucked inward and her arms folded together across her belly in what the clinician interpreted as a cautious, protective stance. She spoke Spanish with a subtle Mayan language accent because her native language was K'iche', the most common Mayan dialect in Guatemala. She had difficulty maintaining eye contact, and either looked away from the clinician or down at her fidgety hands. Noticing her discomfort, the clinician decided to start the session by asking very factual questions about demographic information, such as age, relationship status, gestational age of the fetus, race and ethnicity, the language spoken in the home, employment status, and so on. She hoped that demonstrating genuine interest would help assuage Zazil's anxiety and promote engagement with the therapeutic process.

Zazil indeed became calmer as she answered the questions in a low tone of voice. When her body posture became more relaxed the clinician asked simply, *"How are you? How is your baby?"* Zazil replied timidly that she was fine, but that the doctors told her that the baby was not. The clinician listened quietly, and while looking at Zazil and her belly, said, *"I am glad you are feeling fine, but sorry to hear what the doctors told you about the baby."* She chose not to state what she knew about the pregnancy because she wanted to hear Zazil's perceptions of the health of her baby and of the difficult interactions she had been experiencing with her prenatal care team. Looking down at her fidgety hands, Zazil said, *"Well, I'm not really fine. Lately, I've been padeciendo de nervios* [suffering from nerves]." She then went on to describe an illness associated with depression symptoms (deep sadness, problems sleeping, lack of appetite, and crying spells), and summed up her experience of this illness by gently touching her chest with her right hand with a very sad expression, as if she were experiencing physical pain in her heart.

The clinician silently held Zazil's feelings of sadness and emotional pain for a moment, and then said, "*I can only imagine what could be causing you so much ache here . . . ,*" as she put her hand on her chest and said, "*in your heart.*" The clinician thought that perhaps Zazil was referring to the health of her pregnancy and/or her volatile relationship with her husband. Zazil did not seem ready to elaborate on these themes. She said, "*I am tired of going to the clinic because they only make me worry about my baby. They ask me to do things that are not helping my baby, and at times make things worse for me and my baby. I'm tired of this.*"

This statement had a clear cultural meaning. Zazil was clearly overwhelmed by the medical providers' demands. She was also talking about her baby as if the baby was completely separate from her, in alignment with the Mayan belief that a pregnant woman is "two people," and as such she should be recognized and treated with greater respect and provided increased communal support (Menchú, 1984). Zazil continued by saying, "*That's why we never go to the hospital to give birth.*" She added with a sense of pride that a trusted *partera* (midwife) took good care of all the pregnant women in her community. The clinician validated the importance of the *partera* for the health and well-being of the women and their families in her community, and asked her whether she wished there were someone like that *partera* here in the United States. Zazil nodded her head with a yearning, sad smile. The rupture in Zazil's relationship with her service providers was now palpable to the clinician. The belief that "one should not trust the health care system because they do not understand or help you" was apparent from Zazil's statements.

A distinctive pattern began to emerge as the clinician continued eliciting information over the course of the sessions about symptoms and level of distress. Whenever Zazil was unable to elaborate on a given question, she apologized profusely, and said, "*I can never express myself well. I cannot communicate like other people can. No one can understand me; I try . . . but I can't. There is something wrong with me.*" The clinician initially normalized and validated Zazil's feelings of discomfort and uneasiness. She pointed out that her difficulty responding was understandable, because she was being asked to disclose personal information to the clinician as a stranger she had met only recently. Zazil denied that she was experiencing discomfort, and actually apologized to the clinician for making her uncomfortable. In her internal musings during these exchanges, the clinician wondered whether it was culturally inappropriate to talk about difficult feelings with a stranger, or whether perhaps Zazil's behavior was an expression of the internalized oppression in her interactions with people she considered as having power. Both possible explanations proved accurate as the treatment unfolded.

Following one of these exchanges, the clinician told Zazil, *"I hope that we can soon create a place where you can feel at ease being yourself, expressing yourself in ways that feel comfortable to you."* With a soft smile, Zazil replied that this would be difficult, because she felt the same level of discomfort wherever she went, no matter how many times she had gone to a particular place. The clinician asked whether this was something new that she was experiencing as a recent immigrant, navigating new environments and unfamiliar settings. Zazil replied that she had felt like this as long as she could remember, all her life. Sensing her shame and vulnerability, the clinician said in a comforting tone of voice, *"This must be so difficult for you."* Zazil replied simply, *"It is difficult."* The clinician asked Zazil whether there was somewhere where she could feel comfortable. She replied without hesitating, *"On the farm, among the people. Back in my community."* Zazil was clearly grieving for the cultural and personal losses associated with her emigration to the United States.

The clinician hypothesized in the course of this exchange whether Zazil's discomfort in so many places stemmed from her experiences of being "othered" for belonging to a devalued and ostracized indigenous group. *Othering* is defined as "a set of dynamics, processes, and structures that engender marginality and persistent inequality across any of the full range of human differences based on group identities" (Powell & Menendian, 2016, p. 17). This pervasive experience could most likely be traced back to Zazil's childhood and was deeply ingrained in her sense of self.

### *"Telling My Story"*

Zazil began sharing her early childhood experiences as the foundational phase unfolded. She was the oldest of eight children and was brought up in a Mayan farming community where she lived with her parents and siblings until she emigrated. Zazil's face lit up with joy as she talked about growing up on a farm surrounded by nature and animals. This joy contrasted with her sadness when she recounted the family's extreme poverty and the difficult times that she endured early in her life, including the times when her family did not have enough to eat and she had to go with her mother to the nearby town to sell fruit on the streets to make ends meet.

Noticing a dramatic shift in Zazil's affect and body posture when she spoke about these difficult experiences, the clinician said, *"Life must have been so hard for you, having to work at such a young age with your mother. I can only imagine the kinds of difficult things you and your mother experienced selling fruit on the streets."* Zazil teared up as she said, *"Those were bad times. The town's people were very cruel. They called us names and made fun of our Mayan accent when we spoke Spanish."* When asked who were the people who were making fun of them, Zazil responded, *"They were the rich people hanging out in the plaza. The adult children of well-to-do families who owned big 'fincas'* [states] *in the countryside."* She also recounted that her mother had worked as a housemaid in one of these states, but had to leave due to mistreatment by the mother of the children she looked after. When asked if she knew what kind of mistreatment her mother had endured, Zazil said that her mother never talked about it, but that one of her aunts had told her that her employers had beaten her mother up.

The clinician noticed Zazil's body language as she narrated these events, imagining the shame and confusion of a young child whose emerging identity was attacked and her sense of belonging devalued by rejection and discrimination. Zazil was clearly tense as she spoke, with her arms folded together across her belly as they were the first time she met the clinician. The clinician acknowledged how difficult it had been for Zazil to recount these very painful experiences, pointed out how tense her body seemed, and then asked her whether she would like to take a break. Zazil said that she had not talked about these memories with anyone before, and went on to say that she was upset with her mother every time the two of them got ready to sell fruit on the streets. The clinician understood that Zazil wanted to continue telling her story and did not press her on taking a break. Zazil said, *"I remember vividly like it was yesterday . . . I asked my mother time and time again for us not to wear our trajes* [traditional form of dress] *when we went to the main town plaza because we would stick out, but she insisted on it. She kept telling me, 'That's how our people dress. This is who we are. There are many people like us'."* She continued, *"She would scold me for saying that I did not want to wear my traje, and told me that a woman is not respected if she is not wearing her traje; it is sacred. I hated it!"* With resentment in her voice, she added, *"My mother knew we would get teased and even insulted, but she still dressed me up that way."* The clinician said, *"That must have been so hard for you. You were so young . . . you probably wanted to play rather than go with your mother to the plaza to sell fruit. Those people were very cruel to you and your mother. No wonder you didn't want to go."* The clinician was getting a glimpse of how Zazil had internalized the oppression and racism that she had experienced in her formative years. She could also hear her longing for protection and her conflicted feelings toward her mother, who could not protect her because to do so would have meant to deny their existence and the existence of their people. This unresolved ambivalence toward the maternal object resurfaced as a focus of treatment in later postpartum sessions.

As a young child, Zazil helped her parents in farm-related activities. She missed school consistently, especially during the harvesting season, and only completed the third grade of primary school. She recalled her father telling her and her siblings that *"School was not for us; we were not smart enough for school, but were really good at farming, being connected to the land, to where we came from, where our ancestors came from."* The clinician noticed the disappointment in Zazil's voice and her sad facial expression. She could have used this port of entry to explore what Zazil had hoped for herself in her early life, but instead chose to reflect on her affective experience and tie it to a wish for her baby's future. She said, *"It sounds like you felt differently than your father about attending school, and perhaps this could be something you may want to do differently with your baby."* Zazil listened quietly, shrugged her shoulders, and said, *"Maybe,"* as if this was something that would be still unattainable for her child in a foreign country with unfamiliar opportunities. The clinician wondered to herself whether Zazil's unresolved conflicts prevented her from separating her past experiences from the experiences she could envision for her baby.

Zazil then went on to describe her parents as being *"hardworking and very strict,"* particularly her father. She remembered a number of incidents when her father beat her with a wet rope for *"misbehaving, not obeying him, and not doing my duties and obligations on the farm."* She recalled her father telling her and her siblings that *"It was better to receive a bad beating from him than becoming the rotten fruit by not following the rules and getting into trouble."*

Zazil also disclosed that her father had served in the military before marrying her mother. The clinician hypothesized to herself that perhaps Zazil's father and his own ancestors had learned to use harsh corporal punishment to prevent their children from having problems with the law, because historically indigenous people have been treated unfairly in the judicial system. While considering this possibility, the clinician also imagined the level of trauma the father might have endured while fighting in the civil war. The clinician then asked Zazil whether she knew of anyone in her family who had gotten in trouble with the law and/or had died in the armed conflict in Guatemala. Zazil said that one of her paternal uncles was serving a long sentence, but she did not know the kind of crime he had committed, although her father said he was unfairly accused and sentenced. She added that a number of her relatives had vanished, most likely murdered by the Guatemalan armed forces during the war. She had also heard of women being raped during this time, a common occurrence during the war.

Zazil displayed a detached emotional stance as she spoke. She then went on to talk about the abuse she herself experienced at age 15 when she worked as a housemaid for a wealthy family in one of the *fincas* for a few months. She remembered that the adults and children called her "lazy" and made fun of her Mayan accent, short stature, and indigenous looks. She said, "*Like my mother, I was also mistreated by the family I worked for. They made me work long hours and at times didn't pay me. I lived with them, and some days I would only have one meal. I was quite young at that time. My grandmother came to visit me once and I told her how I was being treated. That very same day, she took me home with her. She rescued me from those people. I miss my ati't [my grandmother in K'iche']. I wish I could see her again . . . my abuelita . . . [my grandmother in Spanish]. She was always there for me, especially when I needed her the most . . .*" With a very sad tone in her voice, Zazil said that her grandmother had passed away the year before she had come to the United States. The clinician offered Zazil condolences for her loss, and told her that she could see how important her *ati't* had been in her life. Zazil went on to describe a close and loving relationship with her grandmother. She remembered hearing from her grandmother how special she was to her and how much she cared about her. Her grandmother also took Zazil and her siblings to her house whenever their father drank too much or when there was scarcity of food in their home. She added that her grandmother's passing gave her the courage to leave her family and emigrate to the United States in search of a better life.

To conclude this part of the interview, the clinician thanked Zazil for having confided such difficult experiences, and told her that getting to know her story, including the story of her family, was part of the process of supporting her on her path to becoming a mother. To conclude the session in a note of hope, the clinician highlighted the importance of Zazil's maternal grandmother as an ever-present protective figure in her life, rescuing her from harm's way and giving her refuge from family conflict, lack of food, and the maltreatment of strangers. As treatment unfolded, it became clear that although her grandmother was physically absent from Zazil's life, she would become a very present figure in her life and her healing process.

In the subsequent session, the clinician introduced the topic of possible domestic violence in her family of origin, hoping that this conversation could provide an opening to explore Pedro's suspected violence toward Zazil. When the clinician asked Zazil whether she had witnessed any violence between her parents while growing up, she described "*a few fights*" between them, but minimized the impact of these events on her and her siblings. The clinician then asked Zazil whether she could recall one such incident that was impactful to her as a child. Zazil quickly replied that she could not recall any such incident. The clinician understood that Zazil was not ready to talk about these experiences yet. She commented, "*These are difficult things to remember, to think about, to talk about because of how they might make us feel,*" and proceeded to make a general statement about how difficult and very scary it is for young children to witness the people they love very much, their parents, hurting one another. Zazil remained quiet, listening. She was clearly sending a message to the clinician: "*It is still too early to fully trust you with very personal family matters.*" The clinician remained attentive to other opportunities to explore this topic in future sessions.

## Immigration: Hope, Trauma, Dislocation, Loss

Changing the topic to talk about more recent experiences, the clinician asked Zazil about her immigration to the United States 2 years earlier in search of a better life. Zazil described her immigration journey as necessary at a time in her life when she needed to find a better way of supporting her struggling family and to forge a better future for herself, because in Guatemala she only foresaw a "*world full of hardships and suffering.*" Her tone of voice was somber when she said, "*Although I wanted to live and work in the United States, lately I have been questioning if all the sacrifices I made for this life by leaving my family behind and my friends, my country, the land . . . have all been worth it . . .*" She was clearly grieving the loss of her country, community, and family. She said that feelings of despair and hopelessness had settled into her heart, causing her pain and *nervios* (suffering, depression). *Nervios is* a traditional explanatory model described as "a physiological manifestation of interpersonal imbalance" caused by the person "not being true to her world (relational), not living in integrity, or experiencing discord within important relationships" (Flores, 2013, p. 53).

Zazil and a childhood girlfriend crossed the border with a group led by a *coyote* (human smuggler) who tried to rape Zazil twice during the trip. She became flooded with memories of the attempted rape, as she described how one of the older men who was also traveling with them defended her from the *coyote*. She described these attempted rape incidents as very traumatic, and said she felt helpless against the sexual advances of the *coyote*. She described having to walk all night across the desert while enduring freezing temperatures to avoid being caught by the border patrol officers and the relief she felt when they finally reached their destination.

The clinician had been observing Zazil closely and noticed that her body was showing a pattern of escalating tension as her shoulder muscles tensed up, her breathing quickened, and her hands began sweating. The clinician commented on how tense Zazil's body looked as she recounted these traumatic events, and added that she was showing that her body has stored the sensations of trauma and was now remembering how it reacted when these events occurred. The clinician then asked Zazil whether she thought of these traumatic events often. Zazil nodded in agreement, and said that she remembered these events *"at least three to four times a week, especially now that immigration was on the news so much."* She was visibly presenting with immigration-related trauma, while also dealing with the daily struggles and stressors faced by recent immigrants who carry the burdens of historical trauma as they also cope with difficult socioeconomic circumstances in the present. Her body was eloquent in showing the enduring presence of those experiences, and it was important to help Zazil learn strategies to help herself feel safer and become more regulated.

### Nature as a Benign Stimulus to Restore Bodily Regulation after Traumatic Triggers

The clinician paused for a moment as she thought to herself about how she could support Zazil in restoring a sense of bodily calm. Sensing a good-enough rapport, she decided to invite Zazil to take a couple of deep breaths with her and observe what would happen. Without much hesitation, Zazil followed the clinician's recommendation, and the two of them took two full breaths together. Then something remarkable occurred. Zazil briefly lifted her head up, perhaps as a way to avoid the clinician's gaze, and looked out the window of the office at the light rain falling in the cold morning. Suddenly, her affect shifted. In the next few minutes, she became collected and her body relaxed. Her facial tension dissipated, her spine straightened, and her stiff shoulders carrying tension softened in a downward movement. As if she had been transported to a different state of mind, with a soft smile on her face, Zazil stated factually, *"It's raining today."* The clinician had just witnessed how nature, in the form of rain, could quickly elicit changes in Zazil's body and affective state, bringing balance to her body and mind after being flooded by traumatic memories.

The clinician paused and asked Zazil whether she enjoyed the rain. Zazil replied with longing in her voice, *"It reminds me of mi tierra* [my land] *. . . it rains a lot this time of the year too, but it's never this cold. I miss it. It's very different there."* The clinician replied, *"I can see how much you miss it."* She then paused and remained silent for a few seconds, looking out the window herself. She then said that she too enjoyed the rain, and described how calming the drops of rain were falling from the sky, wetting the ground. Zazil added, *"I love the smell in the air after it rains. It's so fresh and clean! Water is sacred to us. That's why I like walking in the rain."* It was evident that Zazil had a spiritual connection to nature, her cultural legacy.

Following this calming and emotionally regulating experience, the clinician acknowledged how difficult it had been for Zazil to recount these traumatic events in her life and acknowledged how the rain had helped her relax. Zazil's quick smile conveyed to the clinician that her observation had been accurate and well received. The clinician then proceeded to provide psychoeducation about traumatic experiences and the ways the body remembers them. She also validated Zazil's experience of physiological arousal whenever she watched the daily news, because listening to news reawakened the trauma in her body.

This session showed that nature could become a potentially powerful tool for healing. Armed with this important information, the clinician made use of therapeutic strategies and mindfulness-based exercises that involved elements of nature, such as water, animals, and the sun that are highly valued and respected in Zazil's culture and could be harnessed to help her modulate her psychophysiological reactions to reminders of trauma and grief.

Life in the United States presented Zazil with many changes and transitions, including three housing moves in 2 years, an employment opportunity, marriage, and ultimately pregnancy and impending motherhood. She went to live with her maternal aunt, who had arrived a few years earlier, and met her husband at a family gathering. Pedro was also an immigrant from Guatemala who came from a Mayan village near Zazil's. After a 2-month romance, Zazil and Pedro got married in the neighborhood church, and moved in together to a room in a house they were renting with three other families who were relatives of Pedro.

Zazil described Pedro as *"a hardworking man whose only flaw is that at times he likes drinking too much."* She disclosed only one mild incident of physical violence before becoming pregnant, when Pedro shoved and pushed her to the bed following an argument about his drinking. Zazil emphasized that this happened when Pedro was intoxicated and that she did not get hurt. The clinician did not press Zazil for more details, because she sensed that efforts to explore this theme further would raise her resistance and endanger her emerging but still fledgling trust in the therapeutic relationship.

Drawing from her previous work with immigrant Latino populations, the clinician recognized that women involved in abusive relationships tend to adopt self-protection and survival strategies to cope with the growing anti-immigrant policies of recent years that has led to forced family separation as the result of deportation. Given the level of risk involved if one were to disclose a violent relationship to health care providers, women routinely withhold information about being involved in such a relationship for fear of being reported to local law enforcement and face deportation for themselves or their partners. The silence surrounding the likely violence in Zazil's relationship with Pedro represented a significant obstacle in working toward safety that the clinician hoped could become more amenable to intervention over time.

### Feedback Session, Clinical Formulation Triangle, and Offer of Treatment

The assessment revealed that Zazil's extensive history of historical and personal trauma was associated with severe symptoms of depression and anxiety and moderately high symptoms of posttraumatic stress. Although Zazil obtained high scores on a measure of maternal–fetal attachment, her behavior during the sessions was at odds with this finding, because she seemed to lack an affectionate bond with the fetus. For example, she displayed minimal affect when talking about the pregnancy and rarely touched or caressed her belly when experiencing fetal movement. Although this maternal behavior can be a risk factor for attachment problems in infancy, the clinician concluded that it was too early in the treatment to understand the meaning of Zazil's behavior given her cultural background, particularly because Mayan culture considers unborn babies to be separate individuals although they are still very much connected to their gestating mothers.

Zazil's regular attendance and the quality of her interactions with the clinician indicated that she found these meetings useful. Starting with the first session, the clinician had adhered to a predictable and carefully orchestrated greeting routine that conveyed respect and appreciation. Following one of these greeting rituals, Zazil revealed that this was the first time that she had felt a sense of ease about coming to an appointment. The clinician acknowledged this statement by saying, "*I'm glad to hear that you feel comfortable coming to see me.*" Given Zazil's experiences of invisibility and rejection, the clinician asked herself whether these therapy sessions were perhaps the first time that Zazil felt heard by someone who was genuinely interested in her life story, her situation as an immigrant, the health of her baby, and her relationship with her husband.

As she prepared to offer feedback and extend an invitation to treatment, the clinician kept in mind the stigma that surrounds mental health treatment in Latin American cultures. This was the first time Zazil was considering mental health services, and the clinician initially spoke about the negative connotation associated with seeing a clinician as meaning that *"one is crazy, mentally ill."* Zazil nodded her head in agreement. The clinician then posed Zazil a general question regarding what people in her community usually do when they have life problems, asking, *"What do women do in your village when they feel sad, upset, scared, hopeless, without a way out, in emotional pain, padeciendo de nervios* [suffering from nerves] . . . ?" Zazil responded, *"If it is something that can be solved within the family, then one talks to the older women in the family, like one's grandmother, mother, sisters, aunts, cousins, trusted neighbors—people who care about us."* She added, blushing and showing a tint of embarrassment on her face, *"When that doesn't help, we go see el chimán* [the shaman priest/healer], *especially when we are padeciendo de nervios* [suffering from nerves]." The clinician paused for a moment and said, *"It's great that people in your community have a healer to help them with such problems!"* Zazil seemed surprised by the clinician's approval of seeing a healer. The clinician then said, *"Although I'm not a healer like the one you see in your community back home, my work involves listening and helping women like you heal from difficult things they have experienced. I help them see whether there is a connection between what happened to them and what they are feeling in their hearts, what they are thinking in their minds, and what their bodies and spirits are telling them. I help them understand what is aching in their hearts. At times, I will be teaching you some exercises to calm your body and mind and to comfort your heart."* Zazil listened attentively, smiling at the clinician.

In response to Zazil's clear interest, the clinician said that she would like to have an open-ended conversation about ways of healing that were harmonious with Zazil's cultural values and belief system. Zazil seemed pleased with the clinician's proposal and responded with a clear statement of her hopes for treatment: *"I want to have a healthy baby!"* The clinician validated this very important wish, saying that together they could make sure that everything they did in treatment kept the baby's health and well-being in mind.

The clinician was pleased that the prospect of treatment seemed of value to Zazil. However, she still had the very important task of addressing Pedro's probable violence against Zazil and of co-creating with her a plan for addressing it in treatment. The feedback session presented the opportunity to accomplish this goal. Zazil's ongoing avoidance of the topic led the clinician choose a gradual approach. She started the conversation by suggesting to Zazil that they make safety one of the goals of therapy, saying, *"You shared with me your worries and the very difficult things you experienced in your life, and I thank you again for trusting me enough to tell me. I'm wondering whether we should make safety a goal for our work together. That means feeling safe.*" Zazil seemed initially puzzled by the clinician's statement, and replied immediately, "*I am safe.*" The clinician responded, "*I'm glad to hear that. Could you share with me what it means for you to feel safe? Or how do you think a person feels when she or he feels safe?*" Zazil remained quiet for a few seconds and then answered, "*The person feels good, protected, comfortable, calm, not scared.*" The clinician replied, "*Yes, you are right. The person feels all those warm, comforting feelings and so does the body, perhaps tranquil like the water in a lake, very calm.*"

Zazil's description of what safety felt like and meant for her had elicited a positive response in her body as evidenced by her relaxed posture. The clinician used this observation to inquire what it meant for Zazil to feel safe in different facets of her life, starting with areas that were not likely to arouse anxiety in order to maintain her engagement. She first asked how safe Zazil felt walking in her neighborhood. Zazil said that she felt quite safe walking in the daytime but not at night because of the high-crime rate in the area where she lived. The clinician commented, "*You know what to do to feel safe in your neighborhood.*" She then asked about work-related safety. Zazil said that she felt very safe, because her job was located in a quiet, low-crime neighborhood and her coworkers, mostly immigrants, were supportive and helped her feel comfortable when struggling to communicate with her manager, who spoke very little Spanish. The clinician then asked about safety when visiting the hospital where she received prenatal care. Zazil revealed that she felt safe and protected, because there was always security in the building. The clinician then said, "*It's great to hear you feel safe when you come to the hospital. What about when you go for your prenatal appointments?*" Zazil sat quietly for a moment, shook her head in frustration, and said, "*I don't like going there. I feel scared and nervous when I go to my appointments. I always worry about what they are going to tell me about my baby. The doctors tell me that they worry about my pregnancy, and I worry about my baby, especially about the things they are asking me to do. I get so confused with all the things they tell me to do . . . I don't even think those things can help my baby. I also worry about what they are going to ask me, like the last time when they said to talk to you, and how that's going to affect us.*" The clinician realized that Zazil was referring to the time when both the midwife and the social worker asked Zazil about the violence in her relationship with her husband and made the referral for mental health services. She responded, "*I can hear how much you want to make sure your baby is healthy and safe, and also how much you worry about it. I'm wondering whether I could support you during your visits to the prenatal clinic, just in case you need help when you get confused about what they tell you to do or when they explain things to you. Sometimes it helps when there is someone there for us, just for support.*" Zazil replied, "*Thank you. I don't do many of the things they tell me because I don't understand how they would help my baby inside of me.*" The clinician and Zazil then agreed to go together to her follow-up appointments.

After agreeing on a plan to ease her anxiety during her prenatal appointments, it was time to address safety in the home. The clinician asked Zazil, "*What about safety in your home?*" Without much pondering, Zazil replied, "*I feel safe at home, living with Pedro and his relatives.*" The clinician replied, "*I'm glad to hear that. What about when he drinks?*" Zazil looked down at her hands, and said, "*I guess . . . I do worry when he drinks, which he hasn't done in a while!*" Validating her concerns for Pedro's drinking, the clinician stated, "*You are right to worry when Pedro drinks too much because he can get scary at times.*" Zazil nodded in agreement, and went on to say that she was happy Pedro was no longer drinking but that she did worry he would do it again, especially once the baby was born. The clinician replied, "*It makes sense that you worry about something that happened before, and you don't know whether he will do this again. You are trying to protect your baby too.*" The clinician also conveyed to Zazil that she would be there to support her if "*God forbid something like that ever happens again, for your safety and the safety of your baby. Safety in the home is very important, especially now that you are carrying your baby.*" Zazil thanked the clinician and said that she hoped Pedro's drinking would never happen again. To close the session, the clinician thanked Zazil for having trusted her during the process of getting to know each other, and remarked that fathers are very important figures in their babies' lives. The clinician then raised the possibility of including Pedro in future sessions. Zazil seemed relieved by this suggestion, and responded that, although she and Pedro had had their share of problems, she loved him deeply and wanted him to be involved in their lives "*as a father should be, like my own father was.*"

Laying the foundation of a sound therapeutic alliance during this initial phase of treatment allowed the clinician to describe for Zazil the connection between her traumatic experiences and the impact of these events on her mood and behavior. In presenting the formulation triangle, the clinician explained that the many experiences of danger and resulting fear that Zazil had experienced since she was a child had taught her that the world could be a dangerous place, and that she needed to be always prepared for the possibility of being threatened or hurt. This readiness to protect herself, the clinician explained, made her body be in a constant state of alert and created anxiety, sadness, and fatigue—feelings that took energy away from preparing for her baby's birth.

Spirituality emerged as playing a pivotal role in Zazil's capacity to regulate her emotions during the foundational phase, and the clinician incorporated it as an integral component of the treatment plan. Mayan ancestral wisdom posits that good health derives from the harmony of body and soul—that is, the interconnection of the mind, body, and spirit. Zazil had a deep spiritual connection to Mother Earth (e.g., the different elements of nature, and animals), as reflected in her child-hood experiences in the highlands of Guatemala, as well as to the teachings of Catholicism that permeated her ancestral traditions and customs. Influenced by her mestizo heritage, Zazil followed the rituals and practices from both her Mayan ancestors and her Spanish colonial legacy as she was raised to embrace her traditional Mayan beliefs along with her Catholic faith. Rigoberta Menchú (1984) explained the relevance of Catholicism in the lives of the K'iche' Mayans, stating that "our people have taken Catholicism as just another channel of expression, not our one and only belief" (p. 9). Within this syncretic cultural frame, trauma and depression are seen as manifestations of imbalance. The clinician hypothesized that supporting Zazil's spirituality during the treatment could lead to restoring her mind–body balance. The clinician framed the treatment as a joint effort whereby she would support Zazil in pursuing her life goals in alignment with her cultural values and beliefs. Zazil's positive response to this frame held the promise of a productive treatment.

## Core Treatment: Increasing Self-Understanding and Opening a Space for Baby

As the therapy entered a new phase following Zazil's acceptance of the treatment plan, the clinician continued to cultivate the therapeutic relationship as a mutative factor in addressing her internalized oppression. As in the earlier sessions, the clinician's nonverbal behavior was carefully designed to convey respect for Zazil through facial expressions, body posture, eye contact, culturally appropriate touch, gestures, and tone of voice. Greetings at the beginning and at the end of the sessions became a powerful ritual that gave a message of predictability, reciprocity, and trust. The clinician hypothesized that the greeting rituals promoted changes in Zazil's self-representation through body-based messages of connection, as in *"we are meeting again," "I see you, you see me,"* and *"we will see each other again soon."*

The greeting ritual went as follows. Zazil often came 5–10 minutes early to her appointments and sat in the waiting area until the clinician came to meet her. As she approached Zazil, the clinician displayed a warm and friendly demeanor in the form of a nod, a smile, and/or an open-hands gesture. Leaving appropriate personal space between them, the clinician then shook Zazil's right hand using both hands to show respect and appreciation for "*us coming together again*." With a warm smile, an open hand gesture, and her head tilted to the side, the clinician motioned to Zazil, and said in a calming tone of voice, "*welcome, come into the office*." Once in the office, the clinician invited Zazil to sit and make herself comfortable. The clinician always waited for Zazil to sit down first before doing so herself as a sign of respect. These experiences, in all likelihood, diverged from what Zazil had previously experienced when greeted by others. The clinician thought that this mindful greeting helped the two of them reconnect with dignity in each session so their work could resume.

Four sessions after starting the core phase, Zazil announced that she had already picked a name for her baby girl, saying, "*We decided to name our baby 'Iris',*" and explained that the baby would be named after her favorite flower, which grows abundantly in her native land. The clinician asked Zazil if she could use the baby's name to greet her and talk to her or about her. Zazil answered with a cheerful smile that this was not usually done in her culture, but that it would be fine for the clinician to do it because the *baby was aware of the outside world,* a very important cultural belief that Zazil would later elaborate in the treatment. Following this session, the clinician began including baby Iris in the greetings, following a similar pattern as just described. The baby became an active participant in the therapy even while in Zazil's womb.

### Pedro's Violence Is Named

Zazil was running late for the next session, an unusual occurrence because she was always on time or early. After a 15-minute wait, the clinician phoned her to find out if she was all right and if she would be coming to the appointment. Zazil answered in a hurry, apologized, and said she was on her way to the clinic. She arrived 20 minutes later, and as she entered the clinic, the clinician noticed that she looked distressed and that her hair was in a ponytail, not neatly braided as it usually was. While greeting one another, Zazil apologized profusely for her tardiness as she entered the room. Her eyes were puffy as if she had been crying and/or had had a sleepless night. While the clinician waited for Zazil to sit down, she carefully scanned her face and extremities but found no visible injuries. She then asked Zazil how she was feeling. Zazil shook her head from side to side, frowned, and looked down, and her face became inundated with sorrow. The clinician asked if something had happened to her. Zazil remained silent. Realizing that it was difficult for her to talk about what had happened, the clinician said, "*Sometimes it's hard to talk about the difficult things that happen to us . . . especially if one is not used to doing this . . . or with someone whom one has recently met.*" Zazil nodded her head, and after a long pause said, "*I am just tired of the same thing . . . he is drinking again. More than sad, I'm angry at him.*" The clinician said, "*Oh . . . Pedro went back to drinking like you worried he would.*" Zazil said, "*Yes, he arrived home drunk very late last night. The smell of alcohol was so strong. It reminded me of when my father used to drink and came home late like that. I'm tired of Pedro wasting our money on drinking! I'm worried that we may not have money to buy the things we need for Iris, not even diapers, or even worse, that we may not have a place to live by the time she is born!*"

The clinician validated Zazil's anger toward Pedro and concerns about their financial situation, but chose not to pursue the reference to her father but instead explore the events of the night before to determine whether there were safety concerns. To assess whether Pedro had been violent toward Zazil during this incident, she asked, "*How did Pedro react when you became upset because he came home drunk?*" Zazil, looking down with a somber expression on her face, replied, "*He got angry at me. He insulted me and pushed me to the side as he was leaving the room.*" The clinician then said, "*It sounds like Pedro became angry and aggressive to the point of insulting and pushing you . . . even though you are pregnant.*" Zazil nodded in agreement, remained quiet for a moment, and then added, "*After he went to the bathroom, he came back to bed and fell asleep. I was so angry at him, I couldn't fall back sleep.*" Zazil denied that any more violence took place during this incident, but acknowledged that there had been times in the recent past when Pedro had acted like this toward her.

This was the first time that Zazil was disclosing Pedro's aggressive behavior during her pregnancy. The clinician then went on to inquire how she was feeling physically and how baby Iris was feeling inside of her after this very stressful and worrying incident. Zazil reported that she had had a rough night because baby Iris had kept her awake, "*moving all night!*" The clinician said, "*It sounds like you and Iris couldn't sleep last night. I wonder if you two got scared because of what happened with Pedro last night?*" Zazil replied, "*I think so. I told Iris about the hard things I go through to prepare her for life.*" This important statement offered a glimpse into her cultural beliefs and childrearing practices linked to her legacy of hardships. Still processing what had transpired after the incident, Zazil added that she took a nap in the morning and had overslept, and that's why she was late to her appointment. She added that she had woken up not feeling hungry, but forced herself to eat lunch as she had been instructed by the nutritionist, and that doing this had actually helped her "*feel better, less tired.*" The clinician rein-forced Zazil's protective behavior by simply saying, "*That's great! You followed the nutritionist's recommendations in spite of not feeling hungry, and it sounds like you and Iris are feeling better. You really knew how to take care of Iris and of yourself.*"

To assess risk of further victimization, the clinician asked Zazil how things were with Pedro in the morning. Zazil said that Pedro had talked to her before going to work, asking her to please forgive him for drinking too much, and reassuring her that he had the money for this month's rent. Heaving a sigh of relief, Zazil said that knowing that Pedro had not spent the rent money on drinking had made her feel less worried about becoming homeless. However, she added that she was still mad at Pedro and worried that he would become violent again. The clinician went over a safety plan with Zazil "*just in case Pedro drank again and became more aggressive.*" Zazil agreed to call the clinician for support, but she declined to take the telephone numbers of bilingual domestic violence shelters, saying that she could go to her aunt's house if Pedro were to drink again. Finally, the clinician used this opportu-nity to provide psychoeducation about IPV and its different forms. She also discussed with Zazil the negative consequences of violence expo-sure both for the mother and the unborn baby. Zazil's focused gaze and attentive expression during this explanation suggested that she was taking in this new information.

## IPV Appears

A month later, Zazil arrived on time to her therapy appointment, but the clinician noticed immediately while greeting her that she had a split lip and a light scratch on her right cheek. Alarmed, the clinician asked, "*How are you, Zazil?*" Zazil looked at the clinician and broke down in tears. In a soft but concerned tone of voice, the clinician asked, "*Did something happen to you? I noticed that you are hurt . . . your lip is split, and you have a scratch on your face . . . what happened?*" Zazil continued cry-ing and wiping off her tears as they rolled down her face. To help Zazil calm down, the clinician gave her a glass of water and asked her to take deep breaths to calm her body down. After taking a few sips of water and breathing deeply a few times, Zazil began recounting what had transpired over the weekend. Zazil said that Pedro once again arrived home drunk on Saturday night. Infuriated by Zazil's reproaches about his drinking, Pedro slapped Zazil so hard that he gave her a split lip. As Zazil attempted to leave the room, Pedro scratched her face. Pedro's cousin and his wife, who had been awakened by their arguing, got involved and took the intoxicated Pedro out of the room. Concerned about the physical well-being of both Zazil and her baby, the clinician asked Zazil whether Pedro had hit her in the stomach during the altercation. With a blank stare, Zazil replied, *"Not this time . . . ,"* and began sobbing, burying her face in her hands.

The clinician acknowledged how difficult it was for Zazil to talk about this recent incident because it seemed to be triggering painful memories of something similar in the past, alluding to her first miscarriage. After a long pause, Zazil, who was still crying but able to talk, said, *"This time I covered my belly. Last time when I didn't, drunken Pedro hit me so hard . . . that I lost the baby. We did not know that I was pregnant."* Zazil cried for a few minutes as she remembered this very difficult day in her life. Zazil then admitted that this was the first time that she had ever talked to anyone about what caused her to miscarry 5 months earlier. The clinician thanked Zazil for her trust, and held Zazil's feelings of deep sadness and sorrow as she continued describing what had transpired following the previous incident of violence. She said that Pedro had been jailed and later released, and added that she did not tell her OB/GYN doctor at the time how she had lost the baby for fear that Pedro would get into more trouble and risk deportation. She added that Pedro had been mandated to attend a 1-year domestic violence recovery program and an Alcoholics Anonymous (AA) group, but Pedro had attended the domestic violence classes only a few times and the AA group only once.

When the clinician asked Zazil what had happened following this latest incident of violence, she said that this time Pedro apologized the next day for hurting her, and promised that he would quit drinking for good and go back to the AA group. She also said that she had moved to her aunt's house *"until Pedro followed through with his promises."* Zazil added that her aunt understood and was supportive because she herself had been in an abusive relationship in the past. The clinician commended Zazil for making changes in her life to ensure her safety and the safety of Iris. Following clinical protocol, the clinician then conducted a risk assessment and reviewed with Zazil the safety plan devised in a previous session. She again offered Zazil the telephone numbers of bilingual domestic violence emergency shelters, which this time she accepted. Together, they thought of different ways of obtaining help and support when in a crisis occurred, including reaching out to the other women living in the same house.

Worried about Zazil's safety and the increased risk of miscarriage, the clinician asked if she had noticed any changes related to her pregnancy, which Zazil negated. The clinician then encouraged her to schedule an appointment with her midwife to check on her physical health and her baby's health, *"just to make sure everything was fine."* Zazil said that she had already called the clinic and was planning to see her midwife after her appointment with the clinician, and asked the clinician whether she could accompany her. Gently touching Zazil on the arm, the clinician praised her maternal protective behavior, and said, *"I'm so glad to hear that, and yes, I'd like to come with you to your appointment."*

Following the conclusion of this appointment, the clinician and Zazil walked together to the prenatal care clinic. Zazil seemed tense as she paced back and forth while they waited for the laboratory results. The clinician reassured Zazil that she had made the right decision about coming to get checked. Zazil's worried look dissipated when the midwife shared the good news that Iris and Zazil were both physically fine. During the appointment, the clinician provided support and clarification when Zazil seemed confused by the test results. The midwife seemed warmly engaged, perhaps seeing now how committed Zazil was to her pregnancy and the well-being of her baby. After meeting with the midwife, Zazil and the clinician met with the social worker to find out whether she could offer any further assistance to make sure Zazil followed through with additional safety recommendations and continued monitoring of the preeclampsia, which seemed to be under control at this stage of her pregnancy.

During the following session, Zazil reported that Pedro had come over to visit *"them"* at her aunt's house. She stated that he continued to be very remorseful about the previous week's incident and that he had not gone out drinking since then. Zazil reiterated that Pedro was aggressive toward her *"only when he drank too much."* She said that Pedro had called the domestic violence treatment program and scheduled his first group for the following week, and added that she had told Pedro that she was seeing a *"doctor who knew about what he did"* as an extra incentive to reinforce his attendance to the treatment program.

### Violence in the Present, Violence in the Past

During the next sessions, the clinician continued to monitor Zazil's risk of exposure to Pedro's violence. She also began discussing with Zazil her early exposure to intrafamilial violence. Zazil vividly recalled several incidents of violence by her father against her mother, and elaborated on how distressing this had been not only for her mother, but also for her and her siblings, who *"always"* tried defending their mother and were beaten by their father for trying to do so. Again, she said that this only happened when her father was drunk. The clinician acknowledged how difficult it must have been for young Zazil and her siblings to feel that they needed to defend their mother from their father, and talked with her about the negative effects on children of witnessing domestic violence. Zazil said she did not want to expose Iris to IPV or any other kind of abuse. During this session, Zazil disclosed the *"advice about marriage"* that her mother had given her. She remembered her mother telling her, *"Fight for your rights, even knowing what can happen to you . . . especially if you disrespect your husband and disagree with him. He will give it to you."* Zazil talked about how she thought that *"getting slapped, pushed, insulted"* was something normal that could happen in marital relationships, especially in those that had *"big problems"* like she was having with Pedro, referring to his drinking and their financial problems.

## Immigration, Grief, and Loss: "My Whole Life Is Changed; My Whole Life Is Lost"

A few weeks later, the clinician noticed drastic changes in Zazil's voice and facial cues that indicated a shift in her emotional and physical state compared to the previous week's session. Zazil seemed lethargic, was sighing more than usual, and the tone of her voice conveyed sadness and emotional pain. A brief open-ended check-in approach revealed that Zazil had an increase in her symptoms of depression. She specifically reported increased feelings of sadness, lack of sleep, anhedonia, excessive irritability, guilt, sudden bouts of crying, and emotional pain, which she had been *"unable to shake off for the past few days."* Zazil said, *"I don't know why I'm feeling like this . . . my relationship with Pedro is better now. He is no longer drinking and is now going to his groups* [domestic violence and AA] *regularly. We are moving back together next week; I'm happy about that. I'm working fewer hours so I can rest more. Iris is doing better inside of me."* Unable to discern what exactly was causing these changes in Zazil's mood, the clinician asked, *"What is then ailing your heart, your soul?"* Her eyes welling up with tears, Zazil said that indeed she felt bad, in pain, *"un dolor profundo en mi corazón* [a deep pain in my heart]." The clinician asked whether something had transpired this past week that perhaps had triggered the intense feelings of despair. After thinking for a few seconds, Zazil said, *"Yes, my father was sick,"* and said that her father had been taken to the hospital after falling ill. When the clinician asked Zazil how her father was doing, Zazil said that he was back at home and doing better, but added that she still felt extreme sadness and pain and could not understand why.

The clinician thought about the many losses that Zazil had experienced as the result of migration, including the loss of family, a well-established social support system, a familiar social environment, a set of traditions and social roles, self-identity, cultural heritage, and language. Holding this thought in mind, the clinician began contemplating whether being worried about the health of her father had triggered in Zazil a grief response or reaction as she realized that she could no longer be present for her father and her family. She was far away, removed from them and their reality. This realization, in turn, precipitated internal turmoil, an imbalance of the mind–body–soul, ultimately leading to a grief response. The clinician validated Zazil's feelings of sadness and pain when she heard the news of her father being ill, saying, *"I can only imagine the pain and sadness you must have felt when you realized how far away you are from your father, your mother, your sisters, your family . . . because they were going through a family crisis."* She added, *"You've also been going through a difficult time in your life, and I'm sure you needed them as well. You and your family needed each other to offer mutual support, to be there for one another."* Zazil listened quietly as tears rolled down her face. She then took a deep breath and continued crying, grieving. The clinician remained silent for a few minutes, allowing Zazil to express all her sorrow and pain, and then simply stated how difficult this was for her.

After a silence, Zazil continued to share how she experienced her many losses, her conflicted feelings, and the impact these losses had had on her life. The following narrative is a verbatim account of what she said, at times softly, at times between loud sobs.

*"I feel so bad for leaving my family to pursue my dream of a better life, but I also left them because I wanted to help them, send them money. I also feel very guilty that I cannot be there for them, especially now that they need me. I miss being with my family and wish I could be there with them right now, but I know I can no longer do that . . . We don't have much where we live, but I felt more comfortable and content. You know, sometimes I dream I wake up in my bed, in my house. I hear my grandma's voice early in the morning . . . then I wake up and I find myself here, in my reality. I also have this recurrent dream of finding a road here that can take me straight to my house . . . but it is just a dream. I feel even more frustrated and heartbroken to know that I have to stay here, especially now that I'm married, expecting a baby. With everything you hear on the news, I worry that my family might never meet Iris once she is born. That makes me feel very down. I only have my aunt and Pedro here . . .*

*"I also feel extreme guilt about living a better life, with modern life commodities, unlike my family who only have the bare minimum to survive, if that. I think about how different life is here compared to there. These thoughts come to my mind when I shop at the supermarket and see the abundance of food. If we want to, we could eat meat during the week, but back home you only have meat once a week, if that. I miss our food . . . , I also feel sad when I wash our clothes in the laundromat. You know we wash clothes by hand in the river and dry them under the sun. It's a lot of work but I missed doing*

*that . . . Pedro tells me that we should be happy with everything we have here compared to our families, but I am not. He sometimes gets homesick too. Maybe that's why he drinks.*

"*I want to go back home but I know my life is here now, and if I stay, I can financially support my family from here. They tell me the same thing, to stay here. I am so confused and guilty, hopeless at times . . . I feel sad, a deep pain in my heart. I sometimes feel like I'm no longer myself, that I have changed; my life has changed so much. My whole life is changed; my whole life is lost.*"

The clinician listened as Zazil spoke, and then said gently, "*You lost what your life used to be, Zazil. You are now grieving.*" Zazil continued crying, as she wiped her tears off her face. The clinician said to Iris, "*Nan [mother in K'iche' language] is very sad right now. She is telling me why she has so much pain in her heart. She misses her family, your family.*" Zazil wrapped her arms around her belly, around Iris, as she continued shedding tears of sadness, brokenhearted.

Throughout this time, the clinician showed compassionate support through gestures that conveyed interest and acceptance. She then said, "*You are feeling a lot of pain because of the many people and things you lost as a result of coming to the United States. You sacrificed so much to come here: your family, your friends, the healer, the partera, the community, all their support. You can no longer use your language, your mother tongue, to communicate with others. We talk in Spanish, and the world now speaks English. The customs are different here, even the way people interact with you is different. Also, you no longer can hear the sounds, sights, and smells of nature on the farm, or have the foods you enjoyed . . . so many things. Immigrants, like you, are separated from loved ones, people that are dear to them, that support them. These losses create intense pain and sorrow as the person tries to adapt to a new way of life. You are going through a normal process, the process of grieving these losses, as you adjust to living in this new and very different country, a different reality than what you were used to.*"

Zazil's affect intensity had diminished by now. She was now crying quietly, no longer sobbing. Her decreased emotional arousal showed in her body language. Her breathing seemed steady and slower, her shoulders were no longer tense, she was not grimacing as before, and she had a more relaxed gaze. This session showed the clinician that Zazil was able to tolerate a wider range of affect compared to previous sessions, when she used avoidance and isolation of affect to fend off intense pain.

Grieving these losses became a theme for the following two sessions. Zazil continued processing her intense feelings of disappointment and inadequacy, as she was confronted with a very challenging environment, particularly around receiving medical care. As she continued to process these losses, Zazil was able to regain emotional and physical equilibrium, corroborated by her increased ability to regulate her emotions when talking about her *aching heart*.

Zazil's experience of emotional dislocation is a common response to immigration, particularly in the context of trauma. The immigrant transitions from navigating a familiar sociocultural environment to being fully submerged into drastically different surroundings where even one's mother tongue is likely to be relegated to a secondary mode of communication. Although new opportunities present themselves, the immigrant must abandon what is familiar, known, and comforting. Through the process of acculturation, immigrants are exposed to a new culture, new customs and behaviors, a new system of beliefs and values, and often to a new language and even unaccustomed foods, altering their daily diet. During the adjustment process to the new cultural environment, the immigrant experiences profound loss and begins grieving personal and cultural losses. Some are tangible physical losses (e.g., separation from loved ones, language, personal possessions, support systems, and dietary habits), while others are intangible and symbolic losses, not necessarily evident to others (e.g., self-identity, cultural traditions, values, belief system, social role and status). Emigrating to a new country requires substantial adjustment and flexibility. If the acculturation demands exceed the immigrant's internal and external resources, especially social support systems, and if this process is compounded by trauma and/or discrimination experiences, the immigrant becomes emotionally overwhelmed and at risk of experiencing physical and mental health problems.

The experience of receiving empathic, meaning-making support as Zazil disclosed her many life adversities and their emotional impact had significant beneficial effects. Four months into the treatment, Zazil was more comfortable interacting with the clinician and better able to navigate different situations, including her prenatal care visits. She reported less difficulty communicating her thoughts and feelings to others and greater comfort in advocating for herself and her baby during her prenatal appointments.

### The Mother–Baby Relationship: "The Mother Hen and Her Brood of Chicks"

The target of treatment now became Zazil's capacity for reflective functioning to promote a secure attachment in her infant. This goal involved a dual focus on Zazil's understanding of herself and of her baby. Insight-oriented, trauma-informed interventions were vehicles for developing coherent trauma narratives and protective narratives to create sustaining meaning and greater emotional regulation in her day-to-day life. Culturally attuned psychoeducation provided concrete knowledge about the attachment needs of babies and the effects of IPV on attachment, maternal depression, and anxiety. Using nature metaphors and mindfulness exercises, the clinician elucidated for Zazil the importance of her role as a mother in providing sensitive, responsive, and consistent care to promote healthy development in her baby. She also used nature metaphors to describe symptoms of anxiety and *nervios*/depression, and taught Zazil mindfulness-based exercises, such as diaphragmatic breathing, visualization, and guided-imagery techniques for emotion regulation. Body-scan exercises were also included to encourage an awareness of body sensations and the feelings accompanying these bodily changes.

The clinician brought to one of these sessions pictures of a hen and her chickens to help Zazil access memories of growing up on a farm surrounded by nature and animals. She used the metaphor of "a mother hen and her brood of chicks" to illustrate that children need their parents to be a secure base for exploration and a haven of safety and comfort in times of distress. She also explained to Zazil how witnessing IPV can frighten the baby and disturb this biologically driven motivation to establish close relationships with primary caregivers for survival and protection. She said, "*I brought some pictures that may remind you of the time when you lived on a farm in your village. I remember when you told me that your grandmother raised chickens.*" Zazil smiled at the clinician and said, "*Those were the happiest days of my life.*" The clinician replied, "*I can see that. Those were really good times for you because you were with your grandmother.*" Pointing to one of the pictures of a hen and her chickens, she asked Zazil, "*Do you remember the mother hen and her chicks? Do you have memories of what happened after her chicks hatched?*" With a big smile, Zazil replied, "*They were so cute! They were always with their mother. They followed her everywhere she went.*" Also smiling, the clinician replied, "*You remember how cute they were . . . the picture brings back pleasant memories. Yes, chicks are always with their mother. Do you have memories of what the mother hen and her chicks did when they were roaming around the field?*" Zazil said with a smile, "*The hen used to find food for her chicks. She would cluck to call her chicks when she found a worm . . . I think she was teaching them what to eat. The chicks would also be playing near the mother hen, not too far away from her.*" The clinician said, "*Yes. She teaches them what to eat and lets them explore their world safely, not too far away from her. Do you remember what else she did?*" Zazil said, "*I remember how she would also call them out when it was bedtime and how they all went to sleep under her wings. It was so cute how her feathers would get so puffy, and the chicks would get inside to get warm and go to sleep.*" The clinician replied, "*You are right! The hen takes care of her chicks by making sure they have enough to eat and they sleep safely with her under wings."* Zazil seemed engaged and delighted to be talking about these joyful childhood memories.

The clinician continued the experiential exercise by asking Zazil, *"Do you remember what happened when mother hen sensed danger lurking nearby? For example, if a dog or another animal or a person came near her chicks?"* Zazil quickly replied, *"The hen would get sooo mad! She would spread out her wings and tail and would ruffle all her feathers; looking very mad, she would try to peck at the dog, or anybody else for that matter, and scare them away."* The clinician then said, *"So the hen not only took care of her chicks and sheltered them beneath her wings, but she also fiercely protected them, scaring away predators . . . those who could harm her defenseless chicks."* The clinician added, *"You know, Zazil, the mother hen reminds me of protective parents. The things she does for her chicks remind me of the things parents do for their children."* Zazil, with a look of interest, responded, *"I've never thought about that . . ."* The clinician continued, *"You see, like the mother hen, parents are supposed to do similar things in the lives of their children. Like the mother hen, parents are responsible for giving their children food, affection, and a safe place where to live so their children can grow healthy and develop."* Zazil smiled and said, *"Mother hens are very good to their chicks! Parents should be that way too."* The clinician said, *"Yes! However, there are times when parents are not able to give these important things to their children for a number of reasons. Can you think of those times?"* Zazil was quiet for a moment, and then said with a nervous smile, *"Hmmm when? I don't know when . . . I guess when parents are mean to their children."* The clinician replied, *"Yes, when they hurt their children, such as in the case of child abuse, but also when parents hurt one another, such as in the case of domestic violence."* Zazil seemed surprised and engaged, as she continued listening attentively to what the clinician was saying. The clinician continued explaining her point by adding, *"When there is violence between the parents—for example, one parent screams and yells at the other parent; one parent hits, slaps, and/or kicks the other parent; or both parents hit each other—children don't feel safe. They are watching their parents, whom they love very much, be very scary. They get confused and anxious because they cannot tell anymore whether it is safe to be with their parents, who are supposed to take care of them and protect them. It is hard to trust their parents. These children cannot develop a good relationship with their parents because they feel that their world is not safe. If children cannot feel safe and protected, they will have problems learning and their development gets affected."*

This intervention was transformational for Zazil's readiness to explore her experiences of physical abuse and witnessing domestic violence while growing up. She disclosed how scared she was of her father, especially when he got drunk and got into fights with her mother that often turned violent. She described how her mother was not able to

protect her from her father's harsh corporal punishment or from witnessing violence in the home. She said that now that she was becoming a mother, she wanted to make a conscious decision to be loving
and protective toward Iris, just like a mother hen. The clinician commented that for some reason Zazil's mother was not able to protect
her children in the ways that her own mother (Zazil's grandmother)
was protective of Zazil and her siblings, and added that now Zazil had
the opportunity to pass her grandmother's protective caregiving on to
her own child and the generations to come. Zazil seemed pleased and
empowered to hear this.

## Targeting Anxiety Symptoms: The Whirlpool Metaphor

During one session, Zazil recounted being "*bien nerviosa*" (very nervous) after waking up from a bad dream the night before. She dreamed
that something bad had happened to her mother, but could not remember any other detail of the dream. She could only feel the anguish of
knowing that something bad had occurred, and was not feeling well
when she woke up. The clinician asked her to describe what she meant
by "*not feeling well*." Zazil replied, "*When I woke up, I couldn't breathe;
my heart was beating very fast. When I got up, I began feeling a little dizzy,
so I lied back down on the bed. . . .*" The clinician asked, "*How would you
describe this feeling you were having?*" Zazil answered, "*I felt as if I was
being pulled into a hole and I couldn't get out . . . I couldn't shake those bad
feelings off. They stayed with me.*"

Searching for a helpful intervention, the clinician remembered
that in a previous session Zazil had talked about early childhood memories of fetching water from a river near her house. During that session, Zazil also described fondly how she used to go down to the river
to bathe while her grandmother washed clothes at the riverbank. She
had also narrated how dangerous the river was, especially in the rainy
season when the river swelled up, and some people were sucked into
a whirlpool and almost drowned. The clinician now resorted to this
whirlpool image as a metaphor to explore how Zazil felt after waking
up from her bad dream. She said, "*The way you are describing how you felt
after waking up from your bad dream reminds me of the time when you talked
about the whirlpools that formed in the river near your house on the farm,
especially when you said that you felt as if you were being pulled into a hole
and you couldn't get out. How long did these feelings last?*" Zazil replied,
"*I felt horrible! Yes, I felt as if I was being swallowed by a whirlpool and I
couldn't get out! It lasted for a few minutes until little by little I started to feel
better . . . I started to get out of the whirlpool.*"

The clinician asked Zazil whether she could describe what helped her "*feel better*." Zazil said that now that she thought about it, she did some of the things that she had learned in the previous sessions. For example, she took deep breaths, washed her face with cold water to slow down her heart rate, and visualized the greenery of nature surrounding her farming village. She also described how she felt the cold ground with her bare feet, touched her belly, and reminded herself that "*this was just a bad dream*." She then called her sister in Guatemala, who reassured her that her mother was well. She stated how much she missed seeing her mother. With relief in her face, Zazil said that this was the first time that she had been able to "*calm herself down relatively fast following a bad dream*."

The clinician praised Zazil's newly learned ability to manage her anxiety symptoms through emotion regulation and her skill in using the self-regulation techniques she learned in the sessions. She also highlighted the wisdom of checking whether her fears were real or imagined by calling her sister for concrete information. The next step in deepening Zazil's self-understanding was to tell her that dreams were a communication from parts of herself that needed to speak up. This insight-oriented approach led Zazil to connect her dream to a traumatic event involving her mother when she was a young child. The clinician then provided psychoeducation about the body's reaction to dreams and memories linked to traumatic events. Zazil was insightful as she was able to identify traumatic reminders as well as list her physical reactions triggered by her dream. These interventions illustrate the usefulness of integrating different therapeutic modalities—such as psychoeducation, affect-regulation strategies, and insight-oriented intervention—into a coherent intervention approach.

### Addressing Depressive Symptoms: The Storm Metaphor

In a subsequent session, Zazil talked about how difficult it had been for her to shake off her sadness during the week. When the clinician asked Zazil whether something specific had been bothering her lately, she said that she had been feeling homesick and elaborated on how much she missed her family, especially now that her due date was fast approaching. The clinician asked her to talk about the day when she started feeling sad. Zazil said, "*On Sunday, I woke up feeling sad. I had a dream that I was with my family back in the community. When I woke up, I realized that it was just a dream . . . my family is so far away. I am so far away from them. I cried and slept pretty much all day. The next day, I woke up thinking about my life and all the terrible things that have happened to me. I began feeling even more sad than the day before . . . I felt as if my sadness would never go away. I felt horrible . . . so down.*"

Relying on the usefulness of the whirlpool metaphor in a previous session, the clinician now searched for a different metaphor that could help with the depression symptoms. She said, *"You know, Zazil, the way you were describing how you felt last week reminded me of a storm. Do you remember what happens when a storm is approaching? Do you remember the storms on the farm?"* Zazil thought for a few seconds, nodded her head in agreement, and said, *"Yes, I do. It gets very windy, and the sky turns very dark. It gets filled with dark clouds, and everything is dark. I remember how the chickens would rush to go back to the coop to avoid getting wet. Even the animals go deep in the forest to find refuge. They know a storm is coming."* The clinician then asked Zazil, *"What happens when the storm arrives?"* Zazil replied, *"It starts raining very hard . . . the wind gets stronger . . . there are usually thunder and lightning . . . it can be scary at times because it gets so loud . . . I remember being scared as a child and my mother would always tell me it would pass. I felt better when she said that."* The clinician commented, *"Your mother knew how to help you feel better in the middle of the storm. No wonder you miss her so much."* Zazil smiled softly and sighed with longing, as she silently reflected on these memories reverberating in every one of her senses. Remembering her mother as a protector who could provide benevolent angel memories was a positive step in Zazil's ability to integrate positive aspects into her pervasively negative image of her.

The clinician continued elaborating on the metaphor by asking, *"Do you remember what happens when the storm passes?"* Zazil closed her eyes slightly as she took a deep breath and said, *"Everything is back to being calm, how it was before . . . well not everything . . . because everything is now wet from the heavy rain. It's easier to see now. It's hard to see when it rains hard. You can also hear again the buzz from the crickets. The air is so fresh, clean."* The clinician said, *"As I'm listening to you, it sounds like you went through a storm last week. Don't you think so?"* Zazil nodded her head, and said with an amused tone of voice, *"I guess I sort of did. It was a rough storm for sure, with thunder and lightning. I felt so sad then . . . I feel better from mis nervios* [my nerves] *today."* The clinician then asked Zazil, *"Was there something that helped you while you were going through your storm?"* Zazil said pensively, *"Well, I talked to my aunt on the telephone, and that made me feel a little better. She told me that my father is back to working on the farm and not to worry so much about him; my mother is also doing well. I also told Pedro about my sadness when he came home. It was hard to get going, but I forced myself to go to my prenatal class yesterday and came to see you today. So little by little, I started feeling better. Like today, I feel better than yesterday."*

The clinician reinforced all the things that Zazil had done during the week to improve her mood and decrease her depressive symptoms.

She also provided psychoeducation about the importance of regular physical activity, saying it releases brain chemicals (e.g., serotonin and endorphins) that promote positive changes in a person's mood. To give Zazil a sense of hope, she told her, *"During a storm, the sun is hidden behind the dark clouds, but it's still there. The sun appears once the storm passes, when the clouds disappear."* Zazil smiled at the clinician and continued listening. The clinician concluded by saying, *"Similar to the storm, one's sadness goes away . . . it dissipates, especially if one knows how to cope with and manage these strong and difficult feelings."* In this intervention, the clinician again presented nature as a source of beginnings or rebirths where calmness and cohesiveness occur in life.

## The First 4 Months Postpartum

### BABY IRIS ARRIVES

Zazil phoned the clinician to inform her that she had given birth to Iris, a healthy 7-pound, 11-ounce baby girl. She did not have birth complications as initially feared by her prenatal care team. She sounded joyful but also very tired due to a 19-hour labor. The clinician went to visit Zazil and meet baby Iris at the birth center later in the afternoon. By the time the clinician arrived in the room, Pedro had already left to go to work. Iris was sleeping placidly belly down on Zazil's chest. The clinician first congratulated Zazil on becoming a mother with a gentle pat on her shoulder, and as she got closer to them, whispered warmly, *"Welcome Iris!"* Knowing of Zazil's Catholic faith, she then joined her in thanking God, and also the spirits, her connection to her ancestors, for the blessing of a successful delivery and Iris's good health. Zazil, exhausted and sleep-deprived, told the clinician with relief on her face, *"I'm glad to finally have Iris with us."* The clinician touched her shoulder, and said with an affectionate smile, *"Me too."*

During this visit, Zazil was able to process briefly how different her delivery had been in the United States compared to the experiences of the women in her village—another migratory loss. This sense of loss was counterbalanced by her Mayan belief that motherhood is the culmination of a girl's passage to womanhood. Zazil was now a mother. Giving birth had transformed her into a woman. Although there had been no rituals marking her rite of passage to womanhood in this unfamiliar setting, Zazil still seemed very pleased for having accomplished this developmental milestone in her life.

During this visit, the clinician assessed the quality of Zazil's interactions with Iris now that the baby was physically present and real. She hypothesized that the combination of personal trauma and the sequelae of racism endured by Zazil could burden the bonding process with distorted mental representations of the baby if she experienced Iris as a flawed extension of her damaged self. While looking at Iris, the clinician noted aloud, "*Iris, you really like sleeping on your nan's* [mom's] *warm and cozy chest. You look so peaceful and comfortable. Like a little angel!*" Zazil nodded in agreement with a pleased smile.

The clinician then commented on "*Iris's beautiful, round baby cheeks and her abundant black hair.*" Zazil replied with a timid smile, "*You should see her when she is awake. She has my black eyes and I guess my hair too.*" With a warm smile, the clinician replied, "*Awww . . . she looks like you then.*" There was a subtle look of disappointment and a tone of irritation in Zazil's voice as she looked at Iris and said, "*She is bien morena* [very dark-skinned]." *Morena/o* is a term used in Latin American to refer to people with dark skin tones, including people of indigenous descent. Noticing Zazil's reaction, the clinician smiled warmly at both Zazil and Iris and said, "*Iris, you are such a precious morenita!*" In saying so, the clinician bypassed Zazil's disappointment by acknowledging that Iris was dark-skinned and celebrating this feature by using an endearing form of the descriptor (*morenita*) as an affectionate adjective that matched her joyful welcoming of the baby. There would be time later in treatment to explore the different emotional layers of Zazil's use of the word *morena*. The clinician understood that Zazil was simultaneously identifying with the oppressor and worrying about her daughter's future well-being in her negative perception of her daughter's skin color, which resulted from her experiences of discrimination and oppression as a woman of indigenous descent. This theme was too weighty to elucidate in this brief welcoming of the baby, and the therapist decided to look for other opportunities to address it.

During this visit, Zazil and the clinician discussed a break in treatment so Zazil could follow her cultural practice, which prescribed a postpartum rest period of inactivity. Zazil told the clinician that her aunt would be staying with her during this time of healing and respite. She also reported that Pedro continued not drinking, was attending his treatment programs, and would be taking time off from work to provide instrumental support (e.g., shopping and doing laundry) during this time of adjustment. The clinician and Zazil agreed to resume therapy when Zazil came to her follow-up appointment at 3 weeks postpartum and agreed to include Pedro in some of the future sessions. They also arranged to remain in contact by telephone. During these scheduled telephone calls, the clinician provided emotional support as well as advice on self-care and the challenges of caring for a newborn, which were particularly relevant for Zazil as a first-time mother. Zazil's mood remained stable throughout this period.

## Ambivalence Emerges: "Iris Is Awake All Night!"

The first postpartum session followed the usual greeting protocol, which now included both Zazil and the baby. After entering the room, Zazil placed Iris on the padded floor mat and sat next to her. The clinician commented that Iris was in a drowsy, sleepy state. Zazil answered that this was so because she had just finished nursing. Addressing Iris, the clinician said, *"Your nan* [mom] *knows you so well! You seemed content and sleepy because you just finished eating. You must be feeling pretty satisfied."*

The clinician then asked Zazil to tell her about the other things she had been noticing about Iris, mainly her likes and dislikes, during these past weeks. Smiling, but also showing a slight frustration on her face, Zazil said, *"What she really likes is to sleep all day and be awake all night! You naughty, spoiled little girl! Like last night, she was awake pretty much all night!"* The clinician said, *"Tell me more. It sounds like you and Iris had a rough night."* Zazil replied, *"Yes, we did have a rough night! If Iris doesn't sleep at night, I don't sleep at all! I don't mind it when we don't have appointments to go to, because I can also get some rest during the day, but when we have appointments, it's very hard for me to have energy to go out . . . I have to dress her, get her bag ready, and get myself ready. I don't know why she does not want to sleep at night."* Zazil added, *"Like right now, look, she is about to fall asleep again and here I am . . . I'm so exhausted! Sometimes I think I should keep her awake all day so she can sleep all night!"*

The clinician sympathized with Zazil's frustration, and asked her to describe how Iris was sleeping now compared to the previous weeks. Zazil said, *"Until recently, Iris used to wake up every 3 to 4 hours to breastfeed and then she would fall back asleep. I didn't mind that. But lately, she has been waking up and does not want to go back to sleep anymore! She is so stubborn!"* The clinician asked Zazil to describe what usually happened after she finished breastfeeding Iris. Zazil said, *"As soon as I hear Iris fussing, I turn on the light, pick her up, and breastfeed her. After she is done breastfeeding, I try to make her go back to sleep."* The clinician praised Zazil's caregiving, and then asked, *"How do you make her go back to sleep? Perhaps you are doing something different than before?"* Zazil responded, *"Now I turn on the light when I hear her fussing. While she is eating, I close my eyes until she is done. When she is done eating, I do different things to make her go back to sleep, such as talking to her, playing with her . . . I do everything that I can to make her go back to sleep, but she doesn't want to anymore! She starts crying if I stop talking to her. You know, come to think about it, I don't think I was doing all these things before."* The clinician said, *"Hmmm . . . so you are doing things differently. What did you do in the past?"* Zazil said, *"When she woke up, I would just feed her and then would go back to sleep.*" The clinician said, "*It sounds like Iris is now getting more stimulated at night . . . Do you think maybe she gets excited when she hears your voice, and sees the bright light . . . when you play with her? She might be getting confused about what she should do after she is done eating.*" Speaking to Iris, who continued to be in a relaxed state, the clinician said, "*Maybe it is confusing for you to know if you should fall back asleep or be awake with your nan* [mom] *who is looking at you, talking to you, playing with you?*" Zazil said, "*I never thought that doing those things could affect her sleep . . . I thought those things would help her go back to sleep faster.*" The clinician then suggested avoiding turning on the light or having a low-light lamp while feeding Iris at night and keeping her interactions with Iris to a minimum during these nighttime feedings. Zazil agreed to the plan, and said, "*I will try it and see what happens. I hope she doesn't cry all night!*" The clinician replied in a reassuring tone, "*She may cry a little until she gets used to it. She was able to do it before, so she showed you that she can do it. Let's see what happens.*"

During this session, the clinician also provided psychoeducation about the importance of night feedings for newborn infants. She explained, "*Iris cannot sleep through the night because newborns and young infants have very small stomachs and must wake up every few hours to eat.*" She empathized with Zazil and told her that as Iris got older, she would most likely be able to sleep through the night and establish a regular sleeping pattern. She also assessed Zazil's mood, and discussed how lack of sleep could affect her mood and her interactions with Iris and also with Pedro. The following week, Zazil arrived with a big smile on her face, and said, "*The plan worked! She cried a little the first few days, but now Iris is feeding every 4 hours and falling asleep after she eats! She is such a smart baby!*" Tactful psychoeducation had been sufficient to dispel Zazil's emerging negative attributions to Iris as a "*naughty, stubborn girl.*"

### Addressing Internalized Racism: "Iris Is Bien Morena"

Zazil and 3-month-old Iris arrived at the clinic for their dyadic therapy appointment after Iris's well-baby visit. Iris was a robust baby with abundant black hair adorning her tiny face. She slept throughout most of the session, but when she was awake her eyes were wide and curious, at times focusing intensely on her mother's tired but engaged face. Iris had a big appetite and protested quickly when hungry, a need that was diligently met by Zazil. Following customary greetings, Zazil placed the sleeping Iris on the padded floor mat and sat next to her with her legs crossed, directly across from the clinician. When the clinician asked how their well-baby visit had gone, Zazil initially reported an uneventful visit, saying that all had gone well with Iris's check-up. The clinician noticed that Zazil had a neutral expression but a flushed face, which made the clinician wonder whether she was having strong hidden emotions. When gently prompted for details about the visit, Zazil relayed in a matter-of-fact manner that Iris was growing steadily, had done well in her physical examination, and her vaccine schedule would start in a month. The clinician commented on what great news that all was. However, Zazil's body language continued to be constricted as she sat with her arms crossed, maintaining a somber demeanor.

The clinician sensed that Zazil was bothered by something. Remembering that Iris had a new pediatrician, she asked what the pediatrician was like during the visit. Doing an unusual amount of yawning, Zazil said that the pediatrician was "*all right,*" and that an interpreter had to be called in the middle of the appointment because of the doctor's rudimentary Spanish. The clinician wondered out loud, "*I wonder why they waited until the middle of the appointment to call an interpreter if the doctor didn't speak Spanish.*" Zazil yawned again, while excusing herself. When the clinician asked Zazil whether she was feeling tired today, she replied, "*Just a little tired.*" The clinician again speculated that Zazil's excessive yawning might be a combination of sleep deprivation and anxiety. She then considered whether something had happened during Zazil's interactions with the pediatrician and/or interpreter that provoked the feelings that her body language was manifesting. Following her intuition, the clinician said, "*I imagine it was difficult not to understand what the doctor was saying about Iris's health . . . and also the interruption in the middle of the check-up to bring the interpreter must have been stressful for you,*" and then, turning to Iris who was still placidly sleeping on the floor mat, added "*and for Iris, too.*" Zazil nodded in agreement but remained quiet.

The awkward silence reinforced the clinician's sense that something was amiss. She normalized Zazil's frustration over not being able to understand the pediatrician, the unexpected interruption in the middle of their appointment, and then having to wait for the interpreter for the check-up to resume. Zazil nodded as she turned to look at Iris, who was still sleeping, and murmured, "*It bothered me.*" The clinician said, "*It is hard to wait with a small baby like yours. It makes sense that you were bothered by this.*" The clinician then asked, "*For how long did you and Iris wait for the interpreter to arrive?*" Zazil said with irritation, "*We waited outside the doctor's office for 30 minutes until the interpreter arrived!*" She then described in detail what unfolded that had provoked such strong feelings in her. Once the interpreter arrived, the pediatrician asked Zazil to undress Iris for the physical exam. When Iris was undressed, the interpreter smiled at Iris, and said in a sarcastic and teasing tone of voice, "*Que morena eres!* [You are so dark!]." Zazil said that she felt so furious at the interpreter that she felt her blood boiling inside her and could not look at her anymore. She added that the interpreter was a light-skinned woman whom she had seen before at the clinic when she received her prenatal care. The clinician said, "*It sounds like her words made you very upset.*" Zazil nodded in agreement as her hands gripped her elbows, now showing clear anger on her face, and remarked in mortified tone of voice that she had been "*very offended by the interpreter's comment.*" The clinician replied, "*You are right. Calling somebody 'bien morena' can be offensive in Latino cultures, our cultures. It makes sense for you to be angry with the interpreter. What she said about Iris was offensive to you.*" She continued, "*I think you know how it feels when words like 'bien morena' are used offensively to describe a person . . . how it feels to be treated differently, many times badly, because of the color of your skin. What just happened I think reminded you of that . . . you felt these strong feelings in the past.*" Zazil was now looking down, her face flushed with anger. The clinician added, "*I remember when you told me about the way people looked at you and your mother when you sold fruit on the streets. I wonder if you felt similar feelings back then.*" As Zazil nodded in agreement, her eyes welled up with tears that soon began rolling down her face. The clinician stayed with Zazil's feelings, allowing her to reconnect safely with the feelings of anger at her cultural oppression.

The clinician then began to address the internalized aspect of this cultural oppression. In a nonjudgmental tone of voice and showing genuine compassion, she said, "*I was thinking . . . I remember what you told me when I first met Iris at the birth center . . . she was so little back then. She had just come into the world.*" Zazil, forcing a smile, said, "*I know . . . she has grown these past months.*" With displeasure on her face, Zazil added, "*I remember . . . I told you Iris is bien morena . . . To be honest with you, I wish Iris were más clarita* [lighter-skinned]." The clinician replied, "*I see . . .*" and, looking tenderly at the sleeping Iris, she added, "*and she is morenita . . . I wonder if you got angry at the interpreter, because she reminded you of that in a very insensitive way, without thinking how this could affect you because of your story, because of what you experienced growing up.*"

This profound moment was marked by seconds of deep silence. Zazil then said in a guilt-ridden voice, "*You know, I like light skin. I don't like my skin color. I actually hate it! I always despised the color of my skin . . .*" The clinician sat quietly, holding Zazil's self-loathing feelings, knowing that underneath this self-denigration lay immense pain. After a few minutes, the clinician said, "*I wonder if you learned this from your experiences growing up as an indigenous person in your society . . . in the town where you used to go with your mother to sell fruit, where they made fun of your traditional outfits, of how you talked, of your physical appearance."* Zazil seemed more engaged, and listened attentively as the clinician continued, *"Your interactions with others in your society taught you that being morena is not beautiful, it is in fact quite the opposite, ugly, and you believed it because that's the message you received from others starting when you were a young child. That was the message that your ancestors received as well."* Zazil answered, *"I never thought about that. I thought it was just a feeling that I always had. I just didn't like my skin color. I thought it was just my personal preference."* The clinician then asked Zazil, *"Let me ask you a question: who are the people who usually appear on TV and see in magazines also in this country?"* Thinking carefully, Zazil replied, *"They are usually light-skinned people, usually blond, with blue eyes . . . nothing like us."* The clinician agreed, *"Nothing like us. That's the message one receives, and then believes."*

Painful experiences of denigration and exclusion had clearly shaped Zazil's identity and sense of self, influencing her patterns of relating to herself and others. The clinician went on to reflect with her about the messages one receives from society that being light skinned is desirable and beautiful, when in fact *"that's just one truth that tends to become everybody's desired reality."* Ethnic and cultural groups devalued by the ruling majority internalize these dominant stereotypes and experience shame and the denial of their own identities.

Now calmer, Zazil described many instances when she and her mother were called derogatory names that referred to their skin color in the town plaza. The clinician said she could understand how negative ideas about dark skin color developed early on in Zazil's life, making her own dark skin something she hated. These exchanges enabled Zazil to continue making meaning of her past experiences as an indigenous woman, who had been discriminated against because of her skin color, belief system and values, language, traditions, music, clothing, and even food preferences. Zazil and the clinician had a lengthy discussion about how in Guatemala, indigenous people like her are still treated like second-class citizens. The clinician described the trauma Mayan people had endured throughout history, and how this history affected them for centuries and into the present. Through the processing of these early experiences and her people's collective trauma, Zazil was able to make a connection between her present states of cognitive and emotional disharmony and traumatic past experiences in the form of racial discrimination. The clinician and Zazil also discussed Zazil's worries about future discrimination toward Iris because, as Zazil put it, *"the darker and more indigenous the person is, the more likely she will be despised."*

Conversations about racism and racial/ethnic discrimination

became a recurrent and growth-promoting theme. In the course of treatment, the clinician spoke repeatedly about the fact that each race, culture, and language is rich and unique, and helped her to reflect on the joy and spiritual gifts that her own Mayan culture gave her. In helping Zazil treasure her cultural identity and reconnect with the spiritual legacy of her ancestors, she also taught her to find pride and value in herself.

### Dispelling Systemic Cultural Misconceptions: "That's How I Mother"

Iris was now 5 months old and thriving. During the previous 2 months, Zazil had been coming to therapy carrying Iris on her back using a baby blanket. The custom of mothers carrying their offspring on their backs with a richly colored woven cloth or shawl is prevalent in indigenous cultures across Latin America. To carry an infant on her back, the mother first places the swaddled infant on a woven cloth (a square cloth folded into a triangle) and then puts the baby on her back in order to tie the loose ends of the cloth into a secure knot across her chest. This baby-carrying method varies, depending on the age of the child and the environmental conditions. The clinician, who was very familiar with this caregiving practice, had seen its usefulness in promoting mother–baby bonding and maternal self-efficacy in her clinical practice. Others have also highlighted its adaptive usefulness for infants living in extreme weather conditions (Tronick, Thomas, & Daltbuit, 1994). Zazil stated that walking with Iris on her back was soothing for her child, who could feel the warmth of her mother's body and was soothed by the rocking when Zazil moved or walked. She added that carrying Iris on her back also allowed her to be more productive during the day, because she could finish her household chores when she was home alone. The clinician and Zazil had a session in which they discussed the importance of this baby-carrying mode as a means to reconnect with her cultural roots, a particularly important practice within the context of mothering in a foreign sociocultural environment.

One afternoon, the clinician received a voicemail message from the social worker stating that the pediatric team was concerned about Iris's safety, because Zazil had carried Iris to her appointment on her back *"using only a blanket."* The social worker reported that the pediatrician deemed this practice *"unsafe"* and was asking the clinician's assistance to address it because Zazil had left the clinic without scheduling Iris's follow-up appointment, and the pediatric team was worried that she would not return for her next well-baby visit.

Cultural clashes between immigrant patients and health care professionals due to linguistic barriers and cultural differences are all too common in the U.S. health care system, sometimes with devastating consequences (Fadiman, 1997). This telephone message reminded the clinician of the regrettable frequency of negative cultural attributions when service providers do not make an effort to learn about the cultural practices of the people they serve. She believed that mental health providers had an important role as cultural mediators who bridged the cultural gaps that interfere with the delivery of appropriate medical services, and decided to ask Zazil about this incident before speaking with the social worker or the rest of the pediatric team.

Following their usual greeting routine, the clinician asked Zazil how Iris's last well-baby visit had gone. Zazil said angrily, *"Not too good . . ."* and disclosed that the pediatrician told her not to carry Iris with a blanket on her back anymore because it was not safe. Visibly upset, Zazil declared, *"This was the first time I carried her on my back to that clinic! It is easier, more comfortable for me. That's the way I carry her."* The clinician said, *"I know that's the way you carry Iris. I'm very sorry to hear they said that to you. I can understand why you are so upset."* Zazil said tearfully, *"They made me feel like a bad mother. Iris is on my back. She is not going to fall out of the cargador [pouch] and get hurt."*

The clinician commented that she had not realized that Zazil only carried Iris on her back when she came to therapy. Zazil looked surprised, and said, *"I knew it was OK with you . . ."* Zazil said that she decided carry Iris on her back to the pediatric appointment that day because they were late, and it was easier to use the pouch than to carry Iris in a heavy car seat for the 10 blocks that she needed to walk to reach the hospital. The clinician confirmed the rightness of Zazil's decision, and said, *"I think the pediatrician is not familiar with your customs, and because of her unfamiliarity, she feared that Iris could slip out of the cargador and get hurt. She was worried about Iris. She doesn't know how well you tuck Iris inside the cargador, so she cannot slip out. She doesn't know that because she is not used to mothers carrying babies this way in this country. I wonder if it would help if you talk to them about it? So they learn from you. So when you or other mothers do it again, they won't panic anymore. If you would like, I can accompany you and Iris to your next visit."* Zazil thought about her offer for a moment and agreed to talk to the social worker about it. During this session, the clinician and Zazil also talked about using a bigger blanket because Iris was growing fast. Zazil said that she had already thought about doing this and that she had almost finished altering a pretty, colorful bedsheet that would serve as a bigger blanket. Indeed, for the following session Zazil carried Iris in this colorful bedsheet.

In the following session, the clinician and Zazil had a lengthy discussion about mothering behaviors that were valued in her culture and about the importance of keeping these childrearing traditions and practices. Zazil was worried that she could lose her identity as a mother if she was not allowed to carry Iris the way she was carried as an infant by her mother, saying, *"That's the way we carry our babies. I want to continue doing this."* The clinician answered, *"It is important to you because that connects you with your culture. You know, I just thought of something . . . Remember when you told me that your mother was strict with you about wearing your traditional trajes* [outfits] *when you went to the town plaza to sell fruit? I wonder whether she also felt very strongly about following her traditions and customs back then?"*

Zazil remained quiet as she pondered what the clinician had just said. Her eyes began filling with tears, as she was finally grasping what her mother really meant all those times she refused Zazil's request to not to wear their colorful dresses in the plaza. After a brief pause, she said, *"I guess I do feel like my mother. I want to follow my traditions. I used to get so angry at her for forcing me to do just that . . ."* To alleviate Zazil's sense of guilt, the clinician replied, *"You were so young back then . . . you did not understand what she was telling you, why she was doing that, why she was going against your wishes and not listening to you. You simply wanted to prevent you and your mother from experiencing the discrimination and mistreatment resulting from wearing your traditional clothes."* She then added, *"Now you want to be true to yourself, where you come from, your people. You probably learned that from your mother! I'm sure she will be very proud of you if you were to share what happened to you."*

Iris was now awake and gazing at Zazil. The clinician used this opportunity to include Iris by saying to her, *"Your nan* [mother] *knows how to keep you safe on her back, just like your grandma did."* Tears of pride and sadness rolled down Zazil's face as she said, *"I miss my mother so much . . . and my ati't* [grandma] *too."* The clinician took advantage of this port of entry to comment that Zazil was learning as a mother what her mother tried to teach her while she was growing up. Zazil said, *"I know she loves us and tried her best to be there for us when we were young. I remember she was always making so many sacrifices for us so we could eat . . . I just didn't like it when she forced me to go to the plaza with her because I was the oldest of her children, but I now understand why . . . I actually miss wearing my traditional trajes, which I didn't mind wearing in the community."* The clinician said, *"You felt safe there, among your people. It makes sense to feel comfortable there."*

Following this session, the clinician returned the pediatric social worker's phone call and described the cultural and personal meaning that carrying her baby on her back had for Zazil. She also provided psychoeducation about the importance of allowing mothers to follow safe mothering cultural practices. The clinician also informed the social worker that she would be accompanying Zazil and Iris to their next well-baby visit to provide support to the pediatric team. The social worker seemed relieved to hear this. Baby-carrying practices never again became an issue during treatment.

## The Last 2 Months of Treatment: The Dyad Becomes a Triad

During the latter part of treatment, Zazil's psychological growth enabled a shift in the therapeutic focus from the mother's traumatic experiences and mental health symptoms to developmentally relevant themes. In the context of this progress, Pedro's use of alcohol and propensity for domestic violence remained a pending issue. He had been sober for the past 7 months and continued participating in his weekly batterer treatment program and AA group. The time was right to invite him to join the sessions, and Zazil agreed. Pedro attended several sessions in which he talked candidly about the past violence in his relationship with Zazil, and committed himself to provide a safe family environment for his wife and daughter.

### FIRST TRIADIC SESSION

Zazil, Pedro, and Iris arrived 15 minutes early to their appointment. Pedro was carrying Iris, who was looking with great interest at her surroundings. The clinician first greeted Zazil, who readily introduced Pedro to the clinician. Once they settled in the office, the clinician acknowledged the extra effort Pedro had made to attend the session by taking time off from work, and thanked him for coming. Pedro smiled nervously and said that both Zazil and his group counselors had encouraged him to participate in some of Zazil's meetings. The clinician asked him what he had heard about the program that Zazil and Iris had been attending during these past months. Glancing at Zazil, Pedro replied uneasily, *"Zazil told me that this was a place for women who have problems with their husbands . . . she was told to come here because we were having many problems at that time. I couldn't control my temper. That was when I used to drink."*

This was a remarkably forthcoming statement. The clinician concurred with what Pedro had said, and added, *"When fathers learn to control 'their temper' by attending domestic violence treatment groups, their counselors encourage them to participate in some mother–baby sessions because fathers, like mothers, are very important in the lives of their children and the well-being of the entire family."* Pedro was listening attentively while glancing at Iris, who was now sleeping placidly on Zazil's back. Noticing this, the clinician told the parents, *"Your child depends on both of you, as her parents, for safety and security, so she can grow and develop. Look how placidly she is sleeping right now. She is sound asleep on your back, Zazil. She likes having the two of you here."* The clinician described the goal of the program as helping parents raise their young children safely and lovingly, so they can feel protected and learn about the world without fear. She concluded by saying that children raised in homes free of violence are more likely to develop into healthy adults.

Following this discussion, the clinician asked Pedro whether he could talk a little about the treatment program he had been attending. Pedro said that the groups, run by two male counselors, met once a week for 2 hours and that he had been attending consistently for the past 7 months. He added that this was his *"second time around"* in the program because he had dropped out of the first group over a year ago.

The clinician praised Pedro's consistent attendance, and asked him whether his experience in the groups this time was different from what he experienced the first time. Pedro replied, *"I initially hated the groups and felt like an angry bull who wanted to bellow in rage. Many of us in the groups felt that way. We did not understand why we were sent to these groups! I felt that I did not have a problem controlling my anger or my drinking. I didn't want to talk about my problems with anyone!"* The clinician said with empathy, *"You must have been very angry to be feeling like a bellowing bull!"* Pedro responded with feeling, *"Yes, I was! But you know, I now understand why I have to go to the groups. It was hard in the beginning to talk about my problems with the other men, but now I feel a little more comfortable."* The clinician said, *"It's hard sometimes to open up to others, especially when we are not used to talking about our problems with others."* Pedro replied, *"Yes, it was very difficult at first. But now when new group members start, they remind me of how much I changed. They act like bellowing bulls ready to gore when provoked. This is how I was in the past. This is because I grew up thinking that the man was the only one who had a say in the house, and that the woman was not supposed to question the authority of the man of the house, and if she did, she needed to be punished. In the group, we talked about how I learned this from my father who treated my mother that way."*

The clinician commented on how different Pedro's experience in the groups was this second time, saying that for one's behavior to change—such as stopping drinking or being violent—one needs to realize first that there is a problem, and Pedro had been able to do this by attending the groups. She then asked Pedro whether he felt comfortable describing how he learned about the behaviors that he now wanted to change. With sadness, Pedro described several incidents in which his inebriated father physically battered his mother in front of him and his siblings. Looking down at the floor and with a broken voice, Pedro stated that he felt very sorry for his mother and angry with his father for hurting his mother. He recalled a particular incident when he was 7 years old and he and his older brother tried to defend their mother, but had been severely beaten with a stick by their father, who became angry with them for interfering. The clinician reflected on how difficult it must have been for young Pedro to feel helpless and scared while witnessing these violent attacks against his own mother. Zazil listened quietly and attentively, as if only now realizing the similarities of their upbringings. When the clinician asked Zazil whether she had heard these stories from Pedro before, Zazil said sadly that she had not. Pedro said, *"I am ashamed of my story."* Zazil replied, *"The same thing happened to me."* There was a silence, and the clinician commented, *"Couples don't usually talk about the domestic violence that they saw as children, but they can get closer when they make the effort to talk about it because they can understand each other better."*

Pedro said that going to his groups had helped him understand that he had been acting like his father, whom he had hated as a child for his cruelty against his mother. He added that he felt ashamed and remorseful for hitting Zazil in the past, and that it took him some time to fully understand the consequences of his behavior. The clinician responded that children learn from their parents, and that boys grow up believing that they need to behave like their fathers if they want to grow up to be men, even if their fathers do hurtful things. She commented that both Pedro and Zazil grew up thinking that violence was a regular part of marriage, although it scared them so much while they were children, and now each of them was learning through their treatment that they did not need to frighten Iris the way they were frightened when they were little. She concluded by praising both Zazil and Pedro for their willingness to make changes in their relationship that allowed Iris to live in a safer family environment than what they had known.

There were two additional triadic sessions in which Zazil and Pedro talked with each other about aspects of their growing-up years that they had never told each other before. The clinician helped them practice ways of resolving without escalation some normative disagreements about Iris's care. Their growing intimacy as the result of these often tearful exchanges was touching to witness, as both parents were spurred by their love for their baby to change their expectations of themselves and each other and, in the process, learned to love each other more safely as well. Treatment ended when Iris was 6 months old. Zazil's depression, anxiety, and PTSD scores at the posttreatment assessment were not in the clinical range. By her report, Pedro remained sober, and there were no episodes of violence. Iris's development was on target, as assessed by the clinician's observations and a structured development test.

## Reflections on the Therapeutic Process

The treatment of Zazil and her family illustrates the use of P-CPP for the assessment and treatment of chronic and cumulative trauma beginning in childhood through exposure to family violence and ethnic persecution and oppression, and persisting into adulthood through IPV victimization and unresolved grief from immigration and historical trauma. Understanding Zazil's presentation through a biopsychosocial lens allowed the clinician to consider the intricate interactions between ecological, psychological, and biological determinants that gave rise to the complexity of Zazil's inner life and the unfolding of her social–emotional development. The inherent flexibility of P-CPP as a treatment model allowed the clinician to consider both the Western and indigenous Latino-specific paradigms to inform and guide the therapy process, fostering the formation and maintenance of a positive working alliance that ultimately led to a favorable outcome for Zazil and her family.

Several resonant themes emerged in each phase of the therapeutic process. Zazil's experiences of systemic racism and discrimination in her country of origin presented a significant challenge during the engagement process of the foundational phase. Her past interactions with other people in general and within social structures led to a legacy of distrust of mainstream institutions. Although the clinician did not belong to Zazil's Mayan cultural group nor have the same Guatemalan national origin, her commitment to learning about Zazil's culture and her awareness of how contextual factors impinged on her sense of self allowed her to address this potentially significant therapeutic hindrance early in the assessment process. The use of nonverbal communication in the therapeutic process played a crucial role in facilitating a strong alliance, countering the effects of racism and discrimination and preventing the premature termination of treatment.

The P-CPP core treatment phase highlighted the different dimensions of culturally informed interventions designed to promote safety, strengthen the mother–baby relationship, and prevent the intergenerational transmission of trauma. Through the harnessing of a strong therapeutic alliance, the clinician honed in on Zazil's cultural legacy to devise and implement relevant interventions that created a holding environment (Winnicott, 1960) where opportunities for repair could occur.

The clinician's acceptance of the cultural importance of family unity as a protective sphere against a dangerous world was crucial to the success of treatment. She aligned herself with Zazil's wish to preserve her marriage while upholding the necessity of safety for Zazil and her baby. Including Zazil's relationship with her husband as a therapeutic theme and inviting him to join the sessions were important components of treatment. As the closing phase neared, Pedro had developed a new capacity for self-reflection that led to positive changes in his behavior. His inclusion in the sessions expanded the depth and intimacy of the communications between husband and wife and consolidated the establishment of protective patterns of interaction that were also beneficial for the baby. In the joint meetings with Pedro, the clinician conveyed empathy for the origins of his violence in his own childhood experiences, while maintaining a clear focus on the destructive impact of domestic violence and on Pedro's capacity for change. This nonjudgmental ability to convey expectations for safe behavior served as a model for both Pedro and Zazil that the clinician hoped would extend to their growth as parents and protectors of their baby.

# Clinical Case 3.
# Treating Incest Pregnancy in a Young Adolescent

The sexual abuse of children is a widespread public health problem that festers in the secrecy enforced by perpetrators' threats and victims' fear and shame. The emotional burden carried by sexually abused children is particularly toxic in the case of incest, defined as sexual intercourse between close blood relatives or step relatives (Bernet & Freeman, 2000). Children who are sexually exploited by a family member must construct psychological mechanisms that reconcile inherently contradictory realities. They must maintain a modicum of trust in attachment figures who both fail to protect them and actively hurt them and create the illusion of safety in an unpredictable and frightening situation that by definition renders them helplessly at the mercy of their abuser.

Judith Herman (1992) wrote that the pathogenic relational environment of sexually abused children forces the development of extraordinary psychological capacities that are both creative and destructive. Their effort to cope with their plight fosters abnormal states of consciousness in which ordinary relations between body and mind, reality and imagination, and knowledge and memory no longer hold. These permeable states of consciousness engender psychological and physical symptoms that simultaneously conceal and reveal their origin in the abuse the child is experiencing. Vladimir Nabokov's novel *Lolita* (1955), which engendered controversy since it was first published more than 60 years ago, remains a masterpiece in part because of its exquisitely nuanced portrait of a young girl made into a sex object by her pathologically narcissistic stepfather. Lolita's despairing bedtime crying was the dark mirror of the tough daytime persona she adopted to cope with her lack of control over what he did to her body and to her life. Lolita has been routinely portrayed as a nymphet, a misperception that aligns with many readers' projections, and echoes the blame that many sexually abused girls endure in real life for "making it happen." The confusing mixture of acute pain, fear, shame, guilt, and precocious awakening of sexuality in the context of violation and bondage is an emotional burden that derails healthy development. Sensitive, supportive, and dauntless therapeutic work is necessary in an effort to prevent long-term distortions of personality structure.

This case illustrates the treatment of Anita, a 13-year-old bilingual Salvadoran girl, whose maternal uncle started sexually abusing her when she was 9 years old and who became pregnant at age 12 before learning how pregnancy happens. She grew up in a family environment in which the men were violent and/or absent. Anita's uncle subjected her to a pattern of sexual abuse that over the years moved from molestation to rape, along with intermittent rewards for complying and threats of hurting her and her mother if she disclosed the abuse. Anita's pregnancy was the event that brought an intergenerational family pattern of incest conducted in apparent secrecy into the open, leading to a family crisis of mutual blame, shame, and guilt.

The treatment of Anita focused on three distinct but interconnected conditions. First, Anita became pregnant well before she had the physical, emotional, and cognitive maturity to navigate safely the challenges of pregnancy and childbirth and cope with the responsibilities of motherhood. Second, the pregnancy resulted from sexual abuse by a close male relative who had assumed a paternal role, and who used a mixture of threats and material incentives to keep Anita under his control. Third, the family lived in such poverty that they often faced food insufficiency, unstable housing, and a lack of resources to meet the baby's needs. The co-occurrence of these three conditions necessitated the full range of P-CPP therapeutic strategies.

The overarching treatment goal was to promote Anita's capacity to empathize with herself as a prerequisite for healing and for becoming lovingly attuned to the needs of her baby. The core of the treatment involved a particular way of listening for, tolerating, and channeling regressive longings, fear, disappointment, and rage to redirect these feelings to their legitimate targets, and free the baby from becoming the representative of his mother's experiences of abuse and neglect. The clinician made use of psychoeducation and unstructured developmental guidance to help Anita learn about the pregnancy-related changes in her body, the process of labor and delivery, reproductive health and birth control, and the developmental and emotional needs of her baby. She used a trauma lens to understand and repair cognitive distortions and emotional dysregulation triggered by Anita's body sensations and by her negative attributions to the baby. She helped Anita learn and implement body-based strategies such as deep-breathing techniques to manage trauma reminders that provoked unmodulated anxiety. Insight-oriented interpretations enabled Anita to connect negative emotions in the present with their roots in experiences from the past. Coordination with service providers and community agencies for concrete assistance with problems of living helped stabilize the family's precarious economic situation and attain stable housing. All of these therapeutic strategies were deployed in the context of the clinician's empathic emotional support and reliable availability outside of the regularly scheduled sessions when needed and feasible.

# Referral and Presenting Problems

Anita had recently turned 13 years old when her mother brought her for a pediatric exam that revealed she was 32 weeks pregnant. By her mother's report, Anita was visiting her maternal family in their home country when she told her grandmother that she had *"worms moving in her stomach."* The mother reported that stomach parasites were a common condition in their tropical country, routinely treated at the local hospital. When the grandmother palpated Anita's stomach, she immediately noted that the child was pregnant and asked Anita about the circumstances of the pregnancy, but Anita did not believe her and said she did not know. The grandmother called Anita's mother to inform her of the pregnancy, and sent Anita back home for prenatal medical care. An exam at the pediatrician's office confirmed the pregnancy, including fetal movement and cardiac activity. The ultrasound exam revealed a normally developing fetus. Anita's mother expressed shock at the news of the pregnancy, but Anita seemed not to absorb the meaning of the information. She continued to insist that she had worms in her stomach, and was afraid that the worms were eating her insides.

Abortion was not an option because of the fetus's gestational age. When informed of this fact, Anita and her mother replied that abortion would not be an option even if it were legally feasible, because it was against the family's Roman Catholic religious beliefs. The pediatrician raised the possibility of adoption, but Anita immediately responded that the baby was innocent and should not be punished for the conditions of his birth. Anita's mother supported her, stating that Anita's decision to keep the baby was a generous, selfless act that contrasted with the selfishness of the as-yet unnamed perpetrator.

The pediatrician notified child protective services because of Anita's young age, and the child disclosed to the police that her maternal uncle, who was the brother of Anita's mother, had been having sex with her since she was 9 years old. This information prompted the uncle's arrest. Anita was referred to a midwife and to a public health nurse (PHN) who made home visits. The PHN became concerned about Anita's lack of interest in the fetus and referred her for P-CPP at 38 weeks gestation.

# Starting Treatment: The Foundational Phase

The first decision that the clinician (G. C.) needed to make even before meeting Anita was whether she should propose an individual session with the child or invite Anita's mother to join the session. This was an important decision, because Anita was a minor living with her mother, who would be presumably involved in every aspect of Anita's and the baby's life. The mother answered the phone when the clinician called to follow up on the PHN referral, and she readily responded that she and Anita had been waiting for the clinician's call and wanted to set up a meeting. This response suggested that Anita's mother, Luisa, saw herself as an integral participant in the services her daughter was receiving. Luisa's assumption was culturally appropriate in the context of traditional Latino family values, wherein a hierarchical relationship is typical, and parents have unchallenged authority over their children. Luisa's desire to be present suggested both a welcome emotional investment in her daughter and a potential hindrance if her presence inhibited Anita from expressing her own perception of her situation and asserting her own needs. One of the aims of the initial sessions would be to agree on the most useful treatment format, including the mother's role in treatment—a decision that would be influenced by the role allocation that developed between Anita and her mother for the care of the baby.

The clinician started the first session in an open-ended way, saying that the PHN told her that Anita was so young that she might find it helpful to talk with someone who understood what it was like to have a baby when one was still a child. Was there anything they wanted to tell the clinician? Anita's mother answered that her brother was the baby's father, that he was in jail, and that she was still in shock thinking that her brother abused her daughter and made her pregnant while she was still a child. Anita, who had been sitting quietly with averted eyes while the clinician and the mother spoke, said suddenly, and with much anger, *"You told me that he abused you and your sisters and your parents did not know. How could you not know that he was also abusing me and my sisters?"*

This exchange suggested that daughter and mother were both ready to acknowledge to each other and to the clinician the incestuous sexual abuse that resulted in Anita's pregnancy. It was a promising beginning that both of them could name and address the core aspect of this unspeakable transgression with the strong emotions of distress and anger that were appropriate to it. The exchange also highlighted a recurrent theme in child sexual abuse: the child's sense of betrayal that her mother relinquished her protective role as the attachment figure in not noticing what was happening and taking action to stop it. Understanding the reasons for Luisa's failure to protect and exploring ways to restore her capacity to do so would need to become one aspect of treatment given Anita's young age and her dependence on her mother both for herself and for her baby.

During this conversation, it emerged that the uncle had been living with Anita, her mother, and her two sisters and often spent time alone with Anita while the mother and the sisters worked. In response to Anita's urgent questioning of her not knowing, Luisa responded that she thought her brother had changed because "*he was now a grown man and would know better,*" and asked Anita, "*Why did you never tell me?*" Heatedly, Anita responded, "*Because he told me that you would never believe me!*" Anita's response was a classic illustration of the successful maneuvers of perpetrators of child sexual abuse, who routinely prey on the child's insecurities about the attachment figure to prevent disclosure of the abuse for fear of how the parent will respond.

The clinician intervened to move this exchange from mutual blame to greater understanding by speaking to Anita in a way that her mother could accept, saying, "*You are a child and he was making you do things that you did not understand. I would not be surprised if he was also threatening you and telling you that bad things would happen if you talked about what he did to you.*" Anita did not respond directly, but said, "*I was confused because he was very nice sometimes; he gave me things that I really liked.*" The clinician said, "*That is confusing for a child. What he did is not right, and he is the only one responsible for what he did to you even if you liked what he gave you.*" Anita said, "*He did the same thing to me and my sisters that he did to my mother and her sisters.*" Turning to her mother, she said again, "*How could you not know?*"

Anita's mother responded that she was working two jobs in order to support all of them and was exhausted when she got home. She added that her older daughter had three small children by three different men, all of whom were violent, and all of whom had left after each of the children were born, and she needed to care for her grandchildren after work. She then went on to say in a reflective tone, "*All the men in my life have been physically aggressive, including my father.*" The clinician asked if these men were also sexually abusive. Her immediate response was, "*Yes, all of them. My father was physically and verbally abusive, but not sexually abusive. But my brother abused all of my sisters, including me. Anita's father was the worst of all. He left us when she was only 4, and she missed him because he was nice to her, but he was really nasty to me, so I was glad when he left.*" This was important information, coming directly from Luisa rather than from Anita, about the physical and sexual abuse that was the family script and the particular role that Anita's father played in the child's inner life and in the complicated relationship dynamics between mother and daughter.

Luisa's economic dependence on her brother emerged as a complicating factor when she said that he came to live with them after Anita's father left, that he had helped pay for the rent, and that the family was in arrears now that he was in jail. Crying, she said that she was very angry with her brother, and did not want to see him anymore. It was clear that Luisa was overwhelmed by family and financial stresses and felt guilty and angry that her own sexual abuse was repeated with her daughters. The clinician extended support by saying, *"I can see that what happened to Anita is bringing painful memories and strong feelings that you were abused by your very own brother, and that he also abused your daughters and you did not know it. And to make things more complicated, you depended on him for rent."* Luisa agreed, crying. Seeking to make an empathic link between mother and daughter, the clinician turned to Anita, and said, *"Your uncle lied to your mother and he lied to you. He made both of you think that he was OK and that you needed him."* Anita responded, *"I feel guilty that he is in jail. He did awful things because he was using drugs. He was taking many drugs. He used to tell me not to talk to anybody about what was happening, because if I said something the worms would eat my organs and I would die, and my mother would not believe me."*

Worms had emerged as a recurrent theme for Anita with her grandmother, the pediatrician, the nurse, and now in the present session, and the clinician decided to explore the topic. She said, *"Anita, what he told you is so frightening. Tell me about the worms. The nurse told me that you still think that you have worms in your stomach."* Anita said, *"I remember that when I was about 9 years old, my uncle used to bring me candies, the ones I really liked a lot. Do you know them? They have the form of worms, and they are sweet and sour. I loved them! One day my uncle told me that he was going to make sure that those worms would not eat my organs . . ."* Anita started crying and stopped talking. The clinician said, *"I think maybe your memory is sweet and sour like the candies he gave you. On one hand, you were a little girl who really wanted to have the candies, the worms. I am wondering what happened after he gave you the worms?"*

Between sobs, Anita explained haltingly that her uncle put his *"worm"* inside her, and since that moment he started doing that regularly. The clinician explained that it was very confusing for a little girl to understand what was happening to her, that the *"worm"* he was putting inside of her is called a penis, and that a grown man's penis is too big for a little girl and hurts her. Crying, Anita said, *"I loved my uncle, I had fun with him, but he also did something bad to me and hurt me."* Anita was starting to sob uncontrollably, as if reliving her contradictory feelings toward her uncle, and the clinician guided her in using deep breathing techniques to help her regulate her emotions and come back to the present moment. Once she had calmed down, the clinician said, *"What your uncle told you is not true. You do not have worms in your stomach, and you will not die. You believed what your uncle said because you loved him, but he told you lies and he hurt you. You believed him when he said that your mom would not believe you if you told her what he was doing to you."* In making these statements, the clinician sought to support Anita's immature reality testing by describing the reality of her uncle exploiting her childish trust to satisfy his sexual impulses.

Anita's mother had been listening in silence as Anita and the clinician spoke. The clinician now tried to bring her into the circle of protection she was attempting to create for Anita and her unborn baby by saying, *"Your mom is bringing you here so that we can think together about how to help you feel safe, because she is very sorry that the same thing happened to you that happened to her."* The mother nodded silently, whispering, *"Of course I believe you. I never thought it would happen again."*

This first meeting set the frame for treatment. It revealed a remarkable willingness on the part of Anita and her mother to acknowledge Anita's sexual abuse by her uncle and to address the intense feelings it aroused. It also made clear that Anita was less mature and knowledgeable than a typical 13-year-old, as exemplified by her thinking of her uncle's penis as a worm, equating fetal movements with worms, and not knowing how babies are born. Although the interplay between her wishes, her fears, and unconscious equation of penis with worm was evident in how Anita thought of her unexpected and unwanted pregnancy, the clinician realized that it would be important to also ascertain Anita's cognitive and emotional capabilities to bond with and care for the baby.

At 38 weeks into the pregnancy, there was much concrete as well as psychological work to be done. The clinician conceptualized her preliminary treatment goals in terms of Anita learning about her body and about labor and delivery, giving self-forgiving meaning to the circumstances of her pregnancy, and transforming her perception of the fetus from the fantasy of a parasite harming her insides to a real baby-to-be that she could love and care for. Luisa's own experiences of sexual abuse by the same man who abused her daughter would need to be processed in a separate place, so that Anita's and the baby's needs could remain the focus of clinical attention. The immediate intervention modalities were psychoeducation, emotional support, and concrete assistance in addressing the family's difficult economic conditions. These interventions were consistently informed by the clinician's attunement to the psychodynamic themes in Anita's inner life and in her relationships with her mother, sisters, uncle, and absent father, who had abandoned the family when Anita was 4 years old, and whose loss might have contributed to Anita's longing for her uncle's love and approval as a surrogate father figure.

Mindful of the urgency of the immediate treatment goals, the clinician summarized this first session for Anita and her mother by commenting on the strong feelings that both of them were having and the importance of attending to each of their respective experiences. She asked Luisa whether she would be interested in speaking with a counselor of her own about what had happened to her and her family. Luisa responded that as she watched how the clinician and Anita spoke with each other, she realized that she also wanted someone with whom she could talk about her many worries and fears. She added that people from different agencies had been calling to offer services to the family, and that she and Anita were confused about the multiplicity of offers and did not know what to do. This is a common and paradoxical phenomenon. On one hand, there is a serious scarcity of services for underserved children and families. On the other hand, particularly dramatic clinical situations often elicit responses from multiple agencies, leading to uncoordinated, duplicative, and often mutually contradictory interventions. It is essential in these situations to form a systematic network of communication among providers that is based on shared goals, role allocation based on each service provider's expertise, and regular exchanges of information to maintain coordination and to respond to crises in a timely and effective manner.

The clinician offered to arrange a meeting the following week in which Anita and Luisa could meet the different potential service providers to clarify their roles and the services they were offering. She said, *"It is important for you to let us know what you need and wish for. Would you like me to schedule a meeting with them to gain a better understanding of who they are and what services they can offer?"* Anita and her mother paused for a couple of minutes, and then Anita spoke with considerable self-assertion, stating, *"Since I was a child, we've been moving from one place to another. We've been living with friends or in shelters. I want my baby to have a stable home. That is what I want to have, a place to live before my baby is born."* Anita's response provided some hope regarding her ability to keep in her mind the basic needs that her baby would have. The clinician validated her wishes and agreed to call a meeting with the service providers.

The content of this first session was wide ranging, illustrating the versatility of P-CPP to follow salient emotional themes, while also addressing the relevant safety needs and problems of living. Clinicians should endeavor to allot sufficient time in the first session to get to know the family and explore in some depth the different clinical priorities that will inform the foundational phase and treatment plan. Fifty-minute sessions are seldom sufficient for this purpose. The first session with Anita and her mother lasted 90 minutes, but it was time efficiently spent with an ambitious agenda.

Much had been accomplished. By the end of the session, a

promising clinical frame was emerging that comprised both psychological themes and a concrete intervention with problems of living. As the session progressed, Anita had revealed key aspects of her sexual abuse that elucidated the reality-based origins of her persistent focus on "*worms in the stomach*" and alleviated the clinician's worry about a thought disorder or intellectual delay. Anita had seemed to understand the clinician's sexual psychoeducation and the responsibility her uncle had for abusing and threatening her. Anita and her mother had moved from mutual recrimination for "mother not knowing, Anita not telling" to a beginning openness to each other's experience. Luisa had disclosed the broader family context of her own violent father and the violent men in her life. In particular, learning that Anita's father had been abusive to her but nice to Anita and that Anita grieved but Luisa was glad when he left would help to guide treatment, because it cast light into Anita's contradictory feelings of love, anger, fear, and longing toward her mother, father, and uncle as deeply troubled and pathogenic attachment figures. Luisa's request for a referral for individual counseling to address her own experience of personal and familial abuse offered hope that she could become more cognizant of the external and internal processes that created the current family crisis and more proactive in changing the family relational patterns. Finally but importantly, Anita had asked for specific help in preparing for her baby, who in the course of the session had moved in her mind from the perpetrator of stomach pains to a future being that needed the safe space she did not have either growing up or in the present.

These were impressive accomplishments for a single session. Anita's and Luisa's remarkable openness in speaking about their traumatic life events and feelings associated with them bode well for the possibility that treatment could help change their traumatic expectations, promote safer modes of relating to themselves and others, and place Anita's baby in a secure niche of relationships to interrupt this family's intergenerational cycle of physical and sexual violence.

### It Takes a Village: Partnering with Community Agencies to Address Multiple Needs

As agreed during the first session, the clinician invited all the service providers involved with the family to a meeting intended to clarify each provider's role and coordinate their goals. It was a tribute to the providers' commitment to the family that a meeting could be scheduled on such short notice. In addition to Anita, Luisa, and the P-CPP clinician, the meeting included Anita's school social worker, a school-based case manager, the PHN, and a clinician from a Department of Public Health

(DPH) program designed to help families become self-sufficient. This meeting allowed Anita and her mother to be active participants in planning how to address their needs. Long-standing food insufficiency and a lack of stable housing emerged as major problems during the meeting. A lack of material resources for the baby were another source of stress. The meeting participants agreed that the family would live in a shelter after the baby was born while the school-based social worker tried to secure housing, a goal achieved a few months after the baby's birth. The social worker and case manager also agreed to be in charge of securing basic goods for the baby until the family could become self-sufficient. The PHN took responsibility for providing concrete assistance with Anita's health and the care of the baby, including hands-on teaching of caregiving practices.

An important question that came up during the meeting was who would be the baby's primary caregiver: Anita or her mother? Luisa made an initial attempt to take on that role, arguing that this would allow Anita to continue her school attendance without interruption. Anita became vehement in responding that *she* was the mother and *she* would take care of the baby. She then added in a pointed tone, "*You can work.*" There was a silence and, in response to a question from the PHN, Luisa responded that she had stopped working several months ago because she was frustrated by the hard work and low wages of cleaning houses and felt that she did not have the energy to continue. This revelation raised the possibility that Luisa was having a clinical depression. The DPH clinician offered to provide individual psychotherapy for Luisa and to connect her with a job-training program.

This constructive meeting modeled for Luisa and Anita an approach to active and collaborative problem solving that led to immediate concrete improvements in the quality of their lives and fostered a strong working alliance among all the participants.

### Feedback Session, Clinical Formulation Triangle, and Offer of Treatment

The impending delivery date called for an abbreviated foundational phase so that the clinician could extend a timely offer of treatment, and the next clinical session took place 2 days after the providers' meeting. As agreed during the meeting, Anita came alone to her session with the clinician, who described how she understood what Anita needed and what treatment would look like.

The conceptual frame was that the baby's future healthy development was in jeopardy as the result of Anita's physical and psychological immaturity, the baby's conception as the result of rape and emotional betrayal, the fragmented family relationships, and extreme poverty. The fetal movements continued to be a traumatic trigger that reminded Anita of the repeated rapes she had experienced from her uncle. It is possible that, by attributing fetal movements to voracious worms rather than to the fetus, she was unconsciously protecting her baby from her rage. If so, this was a costly psychological strategy, because it resulted in Anita's dehumanized perception of the baby. This young girl had established an emotional distance from the fetus that interfered with the bonding process to the extent that she had expressed no love or excitement about the baby at any point since being informed that she was pregnant. A hopeful note was that Anita experienced a sense of duty toward the baby, as expressed in her refusal of adoption and her insistence that she, not her mother, would become the baby's primary caregiver.

This clinical formulation guided the clinician's feedback, which focused on the specific emotional themes that were most salient for Anita and used words that the young girl could understand. The clinician made an explicit connection between Anita's continued references to worms eating her organs and her uncle's sexual coercion, saying, "*I think it is hard for you to be pregnant, because the way your baby is moving inside of you is painful and reminds you of the worm-penis that your uncle put inside of you and that hurt you. You did not ask to be pregnant, and it is only natural that it is hard to imagine being a mom. If you agree, I can continue to meet with you now and after your baby is born to think and talk about these things and to help you prepare for the delivery.*"

Anita responded that she wanted to continue meeting and volunteered that she wanted to have a baby boy because "*bad things happen to girls and nobody can protect them.*" The clinician responded, "*Are you worried you will not be able to protect a baby girl, the way your mom could not protect you?*" Anita nodded in wordless agreement, and the clinician again sought to engender some intergenerational empathy by saying, "*And your grandma could not protect your mom. It's very sad that the women in your family did not know how to protect their daughters, and you were hurt so much.*" There was a painful silence, and the clinician added, "*It doesn't need to be that way. Women can learn to defend themselves and their daughters. Whether or not you have a baby boy, you and I can find ways that you can protect yourself and your baby.*"

The clinician then began to help prepare Anita for the concrete physical experience of labor and delivery, suggesting that because her due date was so near it was important to think about preparing for it. This conversation led to the co-creation of the birth plan, which incorporated Anita's needs and wishes, complied with hospital practice, was shared and approved by the OB/GYN team, and was given to the labor and delivery ward when Anita was admitted. Anita's main request was that her mother and the clinician accompany her during labor and delivery. She also said that she did not want an epidural, because some of her friends had told her it was very painful and because she was concerned about the effect of the epidural on the baby. This remark demonstrated a protective stance toward the baby and gave the clinician hope that Anita was making progress in adopting the maternal role.

After finalizing the birth plan, Anita informed the clinician that the following week she had an appointment for a sonogram, but her mother could not accompany her because she would be working. The clinician offered to attend with her, and Anita agreed gratefully. This session wrapped up the foundational phase of treatment and ushered the core treatment phase, with the understanding that emotional themes and practical interventions would be woven together to help Anita prepare to become a mother.

## Core Treatment

### The Sonogram Exam: From Being a Worm to Becoming a Baby

The ultrasound scan should not be considered a routine technical moment. It is an experience potentially loaded with emotional issues, because it serves as a bridge between the objective image of the fetus and the subjective fantasies of the mother. The ultrasound scan has been called "a revolution of representations" (Scacciati, 2015, p. 65) because it can elicit an important adjustment of the representations themselves and become a psychic organizer for parenting.

Anita and the clinician met 15 minutes before the sonogram appointment to prepare Anita for it, and in this brief interval she expressed anxiety about being hurt and a fear that the worms would be dangerous and scary. Her continued association of the fetus with worms in spite of repeated clarifications remained a clinical concern, and the clinician chose to provide reassurance that the procedure would not hurt and that it was very unlikely that she had worms.

When the sonogram scan started, Anita averted her eyes from the screen while the doctor described the baby's body and movements in a gentle, matter-of-fact tone. When he asked if Anita would like to know if the baby was a boy or a girl, she responded that she wanted to have a baby boy, as if the doctor could magically make that happen. The doctor asked how she was planning to name her daughter or her son, and she responded with only one option, "*Ethan*." The doctor then asked Anita if she would like to see Ethan. It was not until that moment that Anita turned her head toward the screen. She was silent for a couple of seconds, and then said in amazement, *"So it is not a worm! It is a real baby!"* The doctor described again the baby's head, arms, fingers, and legs. Anita exclaimed, *"I can't believe it! It is a real baby!"* The doctor mentioned that Ethan was moving a lot, and that he was growing and developing in a very good way. Anita asked him what was the sound she was hearing. The doctor said it was the baby's beating heart. Anita asked him, *"Are you sure this baby is mine? I thought he was a worm!"* The doctor encouraged Anita to look closely at Ethan's head, arms, and legs, saying that they were the head, arms, and legs of a baby. His repeated description of the baby's parts seemed to help Anita process the news that she really had a baby boy and not a worm inside of her. For Anita, this was the first real encounter with her real baby, with Ethan.

It is important to highlight the meaningful role that this empathic doctor played in creating a bond between Anita and Ethan while performing the sonogram. The clinician had met briefly with the doctor before the appointment to alert him to Anita's worries, and this preparation helped the doctor respond sensitively to Anita's reactions. The humanized description the doctor gave of Ethan and the vitality of his movements brought up strong emotions in Anita. In response, she now spoke directly to the baby, saying, *"I can hardly wait to have you in my arms. You are beautiful!"* This was the first time Anita had talked to the baby. The ultrasound appointment took place one week before delivery and was not only an emotional organizer for Anita, but also contributed to the strengthening of her relationship with Ethan and her perception of becoming a mother.

## Labor and Delivery

On the morning of the delivery, Anita's mother called the clinician from the hospital to let her know that Anita was having contractions. When the clinician arrived at the ward, Anita was anxious and afraid that she would not be able to cope with the pain. The clinician showed her how the contractions looked in the monitor and guided her in using during each contraction the deep breathing techniques she had learned less than 2 weeks before. Standing close to Anita, the clinician said, *"I want you to look at the monitor and see how the contraction begins. You will be able to see the peak of the contraction, and then you will see how the intensity of the contraction decreases. Make sure to focus on your breathing."* Anita responded, *"I don't know if I will be able to do it."* The clinician answered, *"Yes, you can do it. Remember with each contraction you are getting closer to being able to hold your baby in your arms."* The clinician asked Anita if she wanted her mother to help her, but when she looked at Luisa she found her sleeping on a chair. It was likely that Anita's labor was a traumatic trigger for Luisa that evoked the same emotional absence that allowed for her daughters' sexual abuse by her own abuser. The medical staff was remarkably understanding and thoughtful in allowing Luisa to remain asleep in the delivery room because her physical presence was important for Anita, who had come to expect the mother's emotional distance, but took comfort from knowing she was physically there.

The clinician left after the nurses explained that delivery was still hours away. When she returned several hours later, Anita appeared tired, sleepy, and dissociated. Luisa remained asleep. The clinician woke up Luisa and asked if she could hold Anita's hands and encourage her to practice the breathing and relaxation techniques. Luisa agreed, but a few minutes later said tearfully that she could not do it. The clinician invited her to step out of the room and guided her through the same breathing techniques she had taught Anita, but she was having difficulty staying in the moment and said that she was having memories of her own deliveries that were difficult to manage. The clinician validated her experience, and encouraged her to remind herself that those memories were in the past, that she was healthy and strong, and that her daughter was now going through her own delivery. Although she promised to try, Luisa remained a bystander during Anita's childbirth process.

The clinician could not be present during the childbirth owing to other commitments. The nurses later told her that during the phase of pushing Anita "*looked like she was not in the room; she looked very distant.*" It seemed evident that Anita had dissociated in order to cope with the experience of the delivery.

Ethan was born via a normal spontaneous vaginal delivery at 40 weeks gestational age without complications. His birthweight and length were within normal limits.

When the clinician visited Anita the day after delivery, Anita was in bed watching a movie, *Winnie the Pooh*. The baby was next to her, but Anita was absorbed in the movie and not holding or touching him. She looked like a very young child and showed no evidence of joy or excitement. Luisa was sleeping on a sofa, and her sister was talking on her cell phone. The clinician asked, "*Anita, how are you doing? I was here yesterday. I visited you because I wanted to know if I could support you in any way.*" Anita took her eyes from the screen, looked into the clinician's eyes, and said: "*Were you here? I don't remember anything. I just remember that there were moments when I thought I was in one of the corners of the ceiling, watching what was happening down here. I don't remember you were here. Can we see each other later? I am watching my favorite movie.*" This was an example of the developmental challenges Anita would face as a new young mother while continuing her adolescent development.

## Getting to Know Ethan and Addressing Negative
## Maternal Attributions

The PHN provided home visits after Ethan was born, helping Anita with postpartum self-care and with breastfeeding and other caregiving functions and providing developmental guidance and emotional support. The clinician had brief telephone conversations with Anita to maintain the therapeutic connection until Anita could resume treatment with Ethan. Joint sessions with Anita and Ethan started 3 weeks after the baby's birth.

During the first meeting, Anita reported that she was having a hard time breastfeeding. She said that her nipples were tender and painful and that the baby was biting her, adding "*He is doing that on purpose to make me feel pain.*" The clinician asked what made her think that the baby wanted to hurt her. She replied matter-of-factly, "*Because he is a man, and all of them do bad things to girls.*"

This was an important port of entry into Anita's negative attributions to her baby. The clinician guided her toward making a connection with the unconscious traumatic trigger she was responding to by asking, "*Are you remembering another time when your nipples were hurting you?*" Anita responded, "*My uncle used to play with my nipples and that was very painful.*" She said that she was just a little girl when he began to molest her. The clinician made an interpretation aimed at helping Anita differentiate between Ethan and his abusive father, saying, "*Maybe you worry that Ethan will be just like his father, hurting you on purpose. He is your uncle's son, and maybe it is hard to remember that he is also just a little baby who is hungry and learning to eat.*"

Anita seemed to soften, and the clinician followed up this intervention by taking a proactive protective stance and asking if Anita would like a nurse to check her nipples. Anita agreed, and they walked to the emergency room for a physical check that revealed a nipple infection. After receiving medical care, Anita commented, "*I told my mom, but she said that everything was probably OK.*" Not feeling protected by her mother remained an important theme for Anita, revisited often in the course of treatment.

The following session gave the clinician another opportunity to create a corrective attachment experience for Anita that she hoped would also protect Ethan. The baby began to cry soon after he and his mother arrived at the clinician's office, but Anita made no move to comfort him, as if she had not heard him. She remained instead focused on exploring the different toys that she found in the therapeutic playroom. In this interval of nonverbal communication, both mother and baby were making eloquent statements. The baby was showing his intense distress and his aloneness, as nobody seemed to hear him or moved to comfort him. He turned inward, unable to make eye contact or reach out as he cried, while flailing his arms and legs. Anita also turned inward, emotionally disconnected from her baby as she focused on her own developmental need to explore rather than to act as a precocious and unwilling caregiver.

The clinician sought to attune Anita to her baby's need for comfort by saying, "*Ethan is crying so hard. Anita, could we talk about what you think Ethan is feeling right now? What do you think he needs?*" Anita replied, "*I don't know. It seems that he is not feeling well, but I don't know exactly what it is going on with him.*" The clinician explained that babies cry when they need something, but cannot yet express that need in words, and added, "*I am wondering if he wants to be held, or he needs his diaper changed, or maybe he is hungry.*" Anita exclaimed: "*I completely forgot that it was his time to be fed!*" She picked up Ethan and offered him her breast. He promptly calmed down and fell asleep.

In the situation just described, the clinician provided an opening that Anita could use for problem solving about the reason for Ethan's distress and the appropriate action to address it. Offering feeling-based, unstructured developmental guidance allowed Anita to acquire a sense of agency in understanding Ethan's distress. This approach calls on clinicians to tolerate at times a baby's distress without intervening immediately in order to seek out the most effective therapeutic strategy to elicit enduring positive change. Immediate action might curtail long-term goals when the parent feels diminished by the clinician's greater knowledge and skill.

Moments like these give clinicians an opportunity for intervention as well as assessment. The clinician asked herself whether Anita "forgetting" that it was time to feed Ethan might be related to the sore nipples that she complained about in the previous session, and used the calm interval that followed Ethan's falling asleep after feeding to ask how her nipples were feeling. Anita responded, "*It was very hard when I was in so much pain, and it turned out that I had an infection. The doctor put me on antibiotics. My mother never believed me when I was telling her I was in pain. This is what happened to Ethan right now. I did not know what was going on with him, and I did not even try to find out.*" This intuitive understanding that Luisa not hearing her daughter's expression of need and Anita not hearing her baby's expression of need were parallel processes was truly impressive in such a young and traumatized adolescent. The clinician responded with empathic reassurance, "*You are just getting to know him and learning what he needs. You were able to respond to his needs immediately once you understood what he needed.*" Anita looked pleased and relieved. She was not used to receiving praise, and the clinician's supportive explanation helped to build her fragile self-esteem as a mother.

## Trauma Lives in the Body: Connecting Past and Present

Insights, no matter how deep, are not immediately transformational but need day-to-day implementation through practice. Despite her ability to equate not responding to Ethan's distress with her mother not responding to her own distress, Anita became very angry in another session, and yelled at Ethan when he latched on her breast. She was visibly dysregulated. Her tone of voice became loud and sharp, her body posture became stiff, and her facial expression revealed pain, anger, and frustration. The clinician chose to focus specifically on Anita's body experience. She commented, *"You seem so sore and upset. Could you describe how it was for you when Ethan was latching? What were you experiencing in your body?"* Anita said, *"It hurt me so much that I felt it in my whole body. I feel angry and I want him to stop hurting me!"*

Anita's nipples had healed from the infection, so physical pain was no longer a concrete factor in Anita's response. As the clinician asked Anita to tell her more about how she was feeling, Anita said that her feelings about the baby had changed suddenly, and that she wanted to push him away so that she was not close to him. She added that she did not know why these moments occurred most often when she fed Ethan. The clinician provided Anita with information about the body–mind connection, and explained that her body had stored the pain she felt during the abuse for so many years. Anita responded with much feeling, *"I hated it when my uncle played with my nipples and breast. I wanted to push him away and get away from him, but he didn't let me."* The clinician helped Anita to make the connection between these memories and body sensations she experienced when she offered the breast to her baby. Anita was overwhelmed with grief as she processed the realization that her baby latching to her breast reminded her of his father doing the same thing to her as a grown man.

The clinician guided Anita to practice deep breathing techniques as she helped her construct a coherent trauma narrative of the specific memories she had of her sexual abuse. The narrative moved back and forth between memories of the past abuse and her current experience with Ethan. The clinician used this alternation of past and present to guide Anita in differentiating between remembering her abuse and reliving it through her relationship with her baby. This process culminated in Anita saying, with much feeling, *"Ethan is just a baby. He doesn't want to hurt me. It is not his fault that his father is my uncle."* She then decided that she would stop breastfeeding because she wanted to enjoy the feeding moments with the baby without having to work at differentiating between the present moment and the intrusive somatic memories of her abuse. The clinician supported the decision to bottle-feed as a reasonable solution to Anita's persistent autonomic dysregulation to breastfeeding.

### Learning to Modulate Fear in Self and Baby

Ethan was 6 weeks old when Anita decided to start feeding him formula, a transition that he made without difficulty. The change in mood during the feedings was quick and positive, with Anita becoming very attentive to the baby's cues of hunger and satiety. This was the beginning of a more pleasurable feeding experience between mother and infant.

Several weeks later, Ethan had serious difficulties in breathing. Anita called the clinician to say she was going to miss her session because the baby was sick. She said, *"My baby is having trouble breathing, I can hear his chest, and he is not taking the formula. I am very worried and want to take him to urgent care."* The clinician offered to meet Anita at the hospital, and Anita agreed. The baby was admitted to the NICU and remained hospitalized for almost 1 week. This experience was a turning point in treatment. Anita began to feel more confident in her ability to identify Ethan's signals accurately and respond to them consistently. It was rewarding to observe that although Anita remained a young adolescent struggling with her own individual issues, as she felt heard and supported in treatment she was learning to relate empathically to her baby and to respond appropriately to alleviate his distress.

In spite of her increasing attunement to Ethan, Anita also continued to provide ample examples of the impact of her anxieties on her relationship with him. When Ethan was 4 months old, she asked the clinician to accompany her to a pediatric visit where both she and Ethan would receive vaccines because she had been *"afraid of needles"* since she was a young child and was worried that she could not be available for Ethan. The clinician agreed to join her for the appointment, seeing this as a valuable opportunity for therapeutic intervention with Anita's fear of body damage.

While in the waiting room, Anita was clearly anxious and said that she did not know what was going to happen. The clinician described the vaccination process and asked if she would like to receive the vaccines first, or if she would like Ethan to get them first. Offering this option gave Anita a sense of control and the ability to anticipate the process rather than be taken by surprise. This was a correction of her experience of having things done to her without her knowledge or consent. Anita recalled that as a child her mother used to scold her for being "*a crybaby,*" and again said she was terrified of needles. The clinician responded, "*It's understandable, you were a little girl and needed someone who could be with you during those scary moments. Today we are together to help you to go through this experience and to help Ethan. We are together, and we will be able to do it!*" Anita said, "*I want to get them first, but I want you to hold my hand.*"

The clinician agreed with her request, and the nurse explained that Anita needed two vaccines, and that it was important not to move during the procedure. Anita was pale, anxious, and tearful. During the first attempt, she moved, and the movement caused significant pain. She reported feeling dizzy. The clinician was holding Ethan in one arm while also holding Anita's hand. Ethan was looking at his mother intently with a sober expression, and the clinician said to him, "*Ethan, your Mom is scared about the vaccines she is about to get. I am here to help her and everything will be fine. I am holding her hand to support her. Everything will be fine.*" As the nurse got ready to try again, the clinician said, "*Anita, look at me. We are going to breathe together as you know how to do. I will be holding your arm, and you will not move your arm. Do you agree with this plan, or do you want something different?*" Again, providing some options was important for Anita to have some control. Anita said, "*No, I want you to hold my hand if you do not mind.*" The clinician agreed and asked her not to move her arm. Anita started deep breathing techniques while looking into the clinician's eyes, and the nurse was able to provide the vaccine without difficulty.

After it was over, Anita became tearful, and said with relief that it helped to have someone with her. She then said, "*Now it is your turn, Ethan. I am going to hold you, and we are going to look at each other while you get your vaccines. Everything will be fine. I am here for you.*" Anita held Ethan and covered part of his face with one hand so he would not see the needle. Anita kept looking at her baby, while breathing deeply. Ethan cried during the four vaccines, and it was evident that Anita was having a hard time looking at Ethan experience what she had just gone through. Once the procedure was over, Anita embraced Ethan and consoled him easily. She was able to soothe him, and Ethan cuddled on his mother's chest and appeared calmed. The clinician commented, "*You helped Ethan in a beautiful way. Although he was crying, you were available all the time and calmed him down easily. He knew that you were there for him. You were able to be with him in this difficult experience. Ethan learned that you are there for him.*" Anita said, "*I wish my mom could do that for me, but*

*I know she never had the support she needed.*" This statement showed that she continued to feel a longing for her mother's protection, but was moving from recrimination to a more empathic understanding of her mother's caregiving deficits.

P-CPP interventions aim at helping each partner in the child–parent(s) relationship move from a disorganizing to a self-organizing state to consciousness, and from that awareness to a supportive co-creation of collaborative states of consciousness. In the previous example, the clinician supported Anita in moving from a dysregulated state to a state of conscious self-organization to surmount stress, and then in reaching out to help her baby in co-creating reciprocity in their dyadic system that enabled Ethan to surmount his own stress.

In shepherding affect regulation, clinicians have their own emotional experiences. Sharing with a colleague what she felt during the session, the clinician realized that she had a strong countertransference reaction of internal disorganization when Ethan looked confused and anxious while his mother was crying. She understood that this countertransference response was an empathic resonance with Ethan's likely mental state of disorganized affect. Ethan had been looking intently at his mother, but after a few seconds he looked away and started making some inaudible noises. He was showing some signs of avoidance and withdrawal, arching away and making self-comforting body movements. However, when the clinician explained to him what was happening, Ethan became less dysregulated. The clinician commented to her colleague, "*As clinicians, we need to remember to ask—what does the baby see when he looks at his mother? The baby sees himself. Maybe Ethan was experiencing his mother's traumatic affect as his own. Maybe he was confused about what belonged to him and what belonged to his mother.*"

The scene at the pediatric clinic illustrates how the P-CPP clinician engages with moment-to-moment daily experiences through the creation of real and genuine relationships, which require that the clinician join in with the dyad and fully participate in creating a shared emotional experience. Ethan was not alone with his mother's traumatic experience. He experienced the clinician's presence, and he heard and saw how she was responding to his mother's experience.

During the treatment, the absence of Ethan's father was always present, and this absence enhanced the importance of the clinician's role as the third member of the essential psychological triad. Anita's mother was also in many ways an absence that was present. Anita needed to experience someone who could help her to manage her fear and anxiety so she could help her baby manage his own fear and anxiety.

*Identifying Ghosts in the Nursery:*
*From Feeding to Eating as a Joint Developmental Task*

Although the transition from breastfeeding to bottle feeding was easy, there were situations when the act of feeding became difficult for the dyad. Ethan was growing and becoming increasingly able to communicate his wishes about being hungry and/or wanting something specific to eat. When he was approximately 6 months old, Anita arrived to their appointment earlier than usual, saying that she was coming from school and she was hungry. The clinician offered an apple or a banana, and Anita chose the banana. Before eating it, she placed Ethan on her lap facing the clinician. Ethan was interested in what his mother was doing, and turned his body to look at her. The clinician commented, *"Ethan, it seems that you really want to look at your mom and see what she is doing."*

Anita peeled the banana and started eating it. Ethan moved his arms in the direction of the banana and smacked his lips. Anita did not respond to Ethan's attempts to communicate that he wanted to eat a piece of the banana. The clinician said to Ethan, *"It seems that you are trying to communicate what you want. You are trying very hard to look at your Mom."* Without saying anything, Anita moved the banana close to Ethan's lips, and as he stretched toward it, she took it away. She repeated this action several times. In spite of Ethan's frustration, Anita continued eating the banana and holding it within her son's visual field without offering a piece to him. Ethan got upset and cried. He tried to reach for the banana, and his mother moved it away from him without making an effort to console him. The clinician asked, *"I am wondering, what do you think Ethan is trying to communicate to us?"* Anita responded, *"He wants to eat the banana, but he needs to learn that he cannot have what he wants; he needs to learn how to wait. We did not always have food, and we learned to wait."*

The theme of being hungry had appeared in several conversations throughout the treatment. Anita had mentioned that there had been times when she did not have enough food, because her mother ate up the few food items that were in the house. Mindful that food insufficiency occurs often but seldom is discussed in the treatment of low-income children and families, the clinician kept in the office a basket with fruit, crackers, and cheese for clients, and Anita often started the session by asking if she could have a snack. The clinician now said, *"I am thinking how difficult it was for you as a child being hungry and not having food to eat. You were just a child, and you needed to eat in order to grow and develop."*

Anita explained that she was upset with her mother for not work-ing to bring food to the table. While she was describing to the clinician her experience as a young child, she offered the banana to Ethan and he had a bite of it. He smiled and looked at his mother. The clinician asked Anita if she had noticed what Ethan did after taking a bite of the banana. She said she did not, and the clinician highlighted the beauti-ful moment in which Ethan looked at his mom and smiled with satisfac-tion. Anita said, "*Sometimes I don't understand why I want him to feel what I felt as a little girl. It does not make sense, but that is what happens sometimes. I know what he wants, but I do not give it to him. I don't understand it.*" The clinician answered, "*We have been talking about your wishes for Ethan to learn several things, for example, to wait for what he wants. However, he is only 6 months old. We need to wait longer for him to learn to wait. Today, although you wanted him to learn a lesson, you did something different, you became aware of what he wanted, and you responded to his wishes. You did something different from what you experienced as a child.*" Anita responded, "*I don't want him to go through the same things I have gone through during my life. I want something different for him.*"

The clinician explained that Anita was doing something very dif-ferent: She was talking about her wishes, fears, and concerns. From that day on, Anita had a ritual at the beginning of each session. She would ask Ethan what he wanted to have for a snack; sometimes she allowed him to choose something from the basket and at other times, she chose what she wanted. For example, she chose crackers and cheese, but she did not offer them to Ethan. She said, "*You can choke, but I will give you a piece of a pear.*" The clinician commented in response that this was a beautiful way to protect Ethan from choking. This eating/nourishing ritual became an enjoyable beginning to each session.

Feeding situations are susceptible to escalating conflict that are difficult to avoid during the first year of life. The feeding exchange may trigger power struggles, misunderstandings, and conflicts often fueled by the parent's unresolved childhood conflicts. As in this case, exchanges around feeding can also provide the infant and parent the pleasure of creating a sense of reciprocity around nourishment when the parent is able to free the baby from the reenactment of the past in the present.

## Six-Month Assessment and Termination of Treatment

The 6-month assessment showed that Anita was not experiencing depressive or anxiety symptoms. The intense PTSD symptoms she had reported during the initial assessment had diminished significantly and were no longer of clinical concern, because she understood their origins and was able to manage them by using deep breathing techniques, by changing what she was thinking, or by making a conscious effort to trace them back to their origins in her real-life experiences. Ethan was growing and developing as expected.

Anita had enrolled in a school-based teenage pregnancy and parenting program when she found out that she was pregnant. She said she enjoyed school just enough that she wanted to graduate from high school and attend a community college. Ethan was enrolled at a child development center in that same school.

Anita had developed meaningful relationships with the service providers involved in caring for her and her infant. The PHN, who could provide home visiting services for 2 years, had become an important figure in her life, and Anita had an excellent relationship with the school social worker as well. The P-CPP clinician maintained regular communications with both of these providers to coordinate services. In addition, a regular Spanish-speaking pediatrician who provided primary care for both Anita and Ethan had been effective in helping Anita manage her fear of medical exams in general and needles in particular.

After the clinician shared with Anita the positive results of the 6-month assessment, Anita disclosed her wish to go back to her regular high school rather than remain in the teen pregnancy school program. She also said that in order to make the transfer, she would need to end therapy. The clinician listened carefully to Anita's coherent description of her plans, and concluded that the nonverbal message was significant and reasonable: Anita wanted to be a regular teenager.

## Closing Treatment: Planning for the Future

It was clear that being a young mother would pose difficult challenges that would take on different forms, depending on Anita's developmental stage and Ethan's development stage and individual characteristics. Toddlerhood, for example, was likely to bring up issues related to male aggression that could rekindle Anita's identification of Ethan with his father and the perpetrator of her sexual abuse. At the same time, the clinician believed that it was important to give Anita the freedom to decide that she no longer needed therapy and could rely on the support from other systems for the developmental guidance that she would need.

Reproductive health was an important topic during the closing phase. Along with her wanting to be a normal adolescent, Anita started talking about wanting to date—something that she had never done. She made a statement that was understandable but worried the clinician, saying, "*I want to know what it is like to have sex because I want to, not because I am forced.*" The clinician explored whether she was thinking of having sex with a specific person, and Anita confirmed that she and a boy in her class were becoming close, and he was asking her to have sex.

This disclosure triggered a strong countertransference response in the clinician, who believed that Anita was too young to engage in a sexual relationship, and who worried about Anita's romantic interests taking precedence over the care of her baby. The clinician channeled her responses into a therapeutic stance by helping Anita explore her feelings about this boy and imagine the specifics of what a sexual relationship with him would entail for herself and for Ethan. The clinician also asked Anita whether she was interested in becoming pregnant again, a possibility that terrified Anita and opened the door for a serious discussion of birth control. With Anita's permission, the clinician disclosed that Anita was considering becoming sexually active to the PHN, who engaged in psychoeducation about reproductive health and provided Anita with concrete access to birth control.

In the final session, Anita mentioned that she was planning to go to her home country for a visit because her grandmother wanted to meet Ethan. The clinician understood this trip as having a deep psychological meaning of repair, because the grandmother had discovered that Anita was pregnant and that she did not have worms. Anita was very excited about her trip. The clinician joined in the excitement, and extended the offer of ongoing support as she said, "*It will be wonderful for your grandmother to meet Ethan and for him to meet his great grandmother. You look very excited about your trip. I want you to know that you will have the doors of this office open if you need to come and talk.*" Anita replied, "*I know, it is not that we are going to disappear. We will be coming to visit you. I mean, because you will be here, right?*" Unlike the sudden disappearance of her father when she was 4 years old, this termination would offer Anita the opportunity to take the initiative in saying goodbye in a planned manner.

## Reflections on the Therapeutic Process

The treatment of Anita and her baby illustrates the importance of using a trauma frame to understand the symptoms of a sexually abused young girl and to interrupt the intergenerational transmission of traumatic reminders from mother to baby. The clinician blended different therapeutic modalities to identify traumatic triggers and to help the young mother understand how her somatic memories and affect dysregulation were influencing her perception of her baby and her interpretation of his signals of need. The treatment of Anita and her baby was guided by Bowlby's (1969) emphasis on the importance of reality as an organizer of psychic life. Anita needed to understand the language of her body as an expression of her pain, fear, and anger, and put her experiences of violation, neglect, and abandonment into words to create a coherent trauma narrative that the clinician witnessed and legitimized. Through this process Anita was enabled to read her baby's cues with empathy and love in spite of her young age and difficult circumstances.

As treatment ended, the clinician assured this young mother that she would remain available as a resource. This offer proved valuable: When Ethan was 1 year old, Anita returned for developmental help with his increasing autonomy strivings, which were clashing with her own. The clinician was pleased to see that Anita's emotional commitment to the baby was now unmistakable and largely free from contamination by traumatic reminders, providing hope that he would continue to hold a space of his own in Anita's psychic life.

# Clinical Case 4.  Treating the Traumatic Sequelae of Perinatal Loss during a New Pregnancy

*Perinatal loss,* a term that describes pregnancy loss through miscarriage, stillbirth, or early neonatal death, is a potentially traumatic event that can trigger clinical levels of long-lasting depression, anxiety, and complicated grief, depending on situational circumstances and individual vulnerabilities (Kersting et al., 2007). The common misconception that the parent–baby bond develops after birth often prevents the appropriate identification and treatment of clinically elevated parental responses following perinatal loss. Many parents report that their family and friends and the medical staff make efforts to console them for their loss by dismissing its importance and emphasizing that another pregnancy will soon help them forget and recover. These misguided attempts at support can be counterproductive when they make the parents feel isolated and criticized for the intensity of their grief response.

There is considerable debate about best medical practices following perinatal loss to help parents with their grief response. Many maternity units have protocols advising that parents should be encouraged to see and hold their dead infant after stillbirth. Having a funeral and keeping mementos of the baby are also common practices. There is no uniform endorsement of these recommendations. For example, a control-matched study found that women who saw their dead infant had higher levels of anxiety and PTSD than women who did not, while women who had not seen the dead infant had the lowest depression scores (Hughes, Turton, Hopper, & Evans, 2002). There are likely to be significant individual differences in parental preferences about the practices that they would find most helpful. Many of these preferences are linked to cultural and/or religious beliefs surrounding death and dying. Engaging the parents in a respectful dialogue about their wishes is likely to help them have a sense of agency following the shock of a perinatal death, although such a dialogue can often be difficult to establish in the rush of emotions and competing priorities that parents, family, and medical staff experience.

The loss of a pregnancy can involve feelings of grief, depression and anxiety symptoms, guilt and/or blame about causing the loss by doing something wrong (e.g., smoking, drinking, jogging, or having sex), and a sense in the woman that her body has failed and her femininity is undermined (Kersting & Wagner, 2012). Bessel van der Kolk's (2014) succinct naming of trauma-related somatic reactions as "the body keeps the score" is relevant to the vivid sensations associated with the process of miscarrying and with the contrast in the mother's somatic memory between feeling the fetus growing and feeling the fetal demise. These body sensations may carry into the next pregnancy as "trauma reminders" (Pynos, Steinberg, & Piacentini, 1999) that interfere with the mother's ability to claim and enjoy the pregnancy and with the prospect of life with the new baby.

This case illustrates the treatment of Ming and Lee, parents whose traumatic childhood experiences compounded their responses to their traumatic perinatal loss. Ming's heightened anxiety prevented her from enjoying and connecting with her developing fetus despite her deep wishes to do so. Treatment addressed the unfolding narrative of her traumatic experiences, focusing first on her perinatal loss and later on her childhood memories of family violence. The treatment focused on identifying Ming's immediate trauma triggers and helping her reconnect emotionally with her early attachment experiences of terror and lack of protection as she developed a new sense of herself as a mother. After the baby's birth, the father's own childhood traumatic experiences emerged in the form of unfounded fears for the baby's safety and overprotective behavior to keep her safe. Treatment fostered the mother and father's latent ability to give their baby the kind of safety, protection, and love that they did not experience in their own childhoods.

## Referral and Presenting Problems

Ming was a 34-year-old woman in the second trimester of pregnancy, who was referred by the perinatal clinic social worker because of unremitting anxiety about her pregnancy following two miscarriages, the most recent of which had occurred 2 years earlier.

Ming's first perinatal loss occurred very early in the pregnancy, when Ming and her husband, Lee, were still in China and recently married. The second perinatal loss occurred in the second trimester when the couple was already in the United States, and the miscarriage shattered their previously unconditional belief in the infallibility of the American medical system. While receiving treatment for this miscarriage, Ming learned that she had a uterine condition that interfered with blood supply to the fetus and caused the miscarriages. The current pregnancy was proceeding without medical complications, but the social worker reported that Ming was experiencing chronic stress and could not enjoy her pregnancy or establish an affective connection with the unborn baby in spite of medical reassurances that her condition was responding well to treatment, and that it was improbable that another perinatal loss would occur. She expressed trust in her medical team, but questioned how the advanced medical care she received did not prevent her last miscarriage and felt unable to fully accept her doctor's reassurances that another miscarriage was very unlikely now that her uterine condition had been diagnosed and was being treated.

Ming and her husband, Lee, had emigrated from China 5 years earlier and spoke English well. In China, Ming had a college degree in education. She spoke some English when she emigrated as an adult, and her ambition to regain her former professional status in the United States motivated her to achieve a high level of acculturation quickly. Her husband worked in a well-paid position, and they both agreed that they felt more at ease in the United States although they also missed many aspects of living in China. She told the social worker that she grew up in a high-conflict family in which her parents punished her harshly both physically and verbally, and in which she witnessed her father's recurrent violence against her mother. She said she felt grateful for living in the United States, where she experienced a sense of personal freedom that she had never experienced before. The perinatal loss shattered her trust in her new country, and she was grappling with anxiety that her medical condition was untreatable and that the reassurances of the medical care team stemmed from unrealistic optimism about their ability to help.

## Starting Treatment: The Foundational Phase

During the first session, the clinician (G. O. B.) greeted Ming by congratulating her about the pregnancy and by asking how she was feeling. Ming answered that she was feeling well, but did not elaborate and seemed guarded and ill at ease. The clinician tried to help Ming feel more comfortable by asking what the social worker had described to her about the referral. Ming responded that the social worker told her that she worried too much about the baby, and went on to speak with pressured speech about her constant worry of losing this baby as she had lost two other pregnancies. To help make the fetus more real, the clinician asked if she knew the sex of the baby and what she imagined the baby to be like. Ming said that she was expecting a baby girl, and described her as having an easy temperament and being kind, gentle, and smart. She described what she was doing to take care of the pregnancy and the baby, saying that she kept all her appointments, and adding, *"I'm taking care of me."* She then rubbed her belly and spoke to the fetus, saying, *"You are getting bigger and you are going to be OK; you are going to be born.*" As she completed this sentence, her voice broke down. It seemed as if she was reassuring herself, while talking to the unborn baby.

The clinician acted to confirm Ming's efforts at self-reassurance, asking what the due date was and whether they had a name for the baby. Ming's affect brightened when she answered that the baby's name was Lien, after her husband's much beloved grandmother who had died the year before the couple's emigration to the United States. The name choice was an affirmation of the parents' sense of belonging to their own cultural background and their comfort in honoring the continuity across their family's generations.

As she went on speaking about the pregnancy and her experience of the fetus, the narrative shifted without warning to Bao, the baby girl that she lost at the beginning of the second trimester 2 years earlier. The clinician thought to herself that the two fetuses seemed to have merged in Ming's mind. At first, Ming's speech moved back and forth between Bao and Lien as if both babies were the same. Soon Bao's memory took over her speech, and Ming sobbed profusely as she said, "*She was there, in front of me, she was dead.*" The clinician understood that Ming was reliving the tragic moment of Bao's death with the child's physical image clearly in her mind, and responded by saying, "*What a hard experience you had. This loss was very traumatic to you. I can see that Bao is still with you, that her loss is very present, it still hurts you a lot. Now I understand why you are so afraid of losing this pregnancy.*"

The clinician was deliberate in her use of the word *traumatic* to convey that she understood the enormous tragedy that this loss entailed for the mother. Ming continued to sob for a couple of minutes. As her crying subsided, she was quiet for a while, and then said, "*It helps me that you tell me this was traumatic. For some reason, I didn't see it that way until now.*" The clinician asked, "*How did you see it?*" Ming remained quiet, and then said, "*For me, it was just the loss of my baby, a painful experience in my life. I didn't think anything else.*" The clinician asked Ming how she saw it now. She answered, "*It feels that something was unlocked. I don't know how to explain it. It's like my feelings make more sense now.*"

The clinician explained that losing someone we love suddenly and unexpectedly is a traumatic event that stays in the body, and the body remembers how it felt every time there is a worry that something like that will happen again. The clinician added, "*When I asked you to talk about Lien, you started telling me what a kind, gentle, and smart baby she will be. After you said this, you started remembering all the things that you had hoped for Bao at this stage in your pregnancy with her. I can understand that your hopes for Lien are mixed up with the grief of losing Bao.*" Ming listened attentively, and her grief and tearfulness were transformed into genuine interest and a greater willingness to reflect on and answer the information-gathering questions that help set the frame for the foundational phase. Ming's open acceptance of the connection between the two fetuses seemed to warrant the risk that the clinician took when she made an insight-oriented interpretation linking the feelings connected with each of the two pregnancies. Ming clearly articulated that her grief now had more meaning to her because the clinician affirmed its validity, and her affect turned from initial guardedness to growing collaborative participation in the work of self-understanding and of preparing for Lien's birth.

As the session progressed, the clinician continued her efforts to make a space for Lien's separate existence in Ming's emotional space. She asked whether Lien recognized Ming's voice when she talked to her, and Ming responded, "*Lien is more connected to my husband than to me.*" "*What makes you think that?*" the clinician asked. Ming responded, "*Well, when my husband returns from his job and talks to her, Lien immediately starts moving. I hope that in time she connects also with me.*"

While listening, the clinician began to wonder to herself whether Ming felt undeserving of her baby's attention, preference, or love and whether she felt she was being punished for some wrongdoing. The clinician did not ask specific questions about these possibilities, because she sensed that it was too early in the development of the therapeutic relationship to probe into the maternal unconscious defensive structure. She felt a sense of achievement that Ming had responded well to the connection she had made between her conscious affective experiences by linking the fear of losing Lien to her grief for having lost Bao, and wanted to preserve the positive feeling that the mother expressed toward her following this new insight.

The clinician chose instead to provide a benevolent reframing of Ming's perception that Lien related more to her father, saying lightly, "*Do you think that Lien may be greeting her father after a long day away from him, but likes having you around all the time? It sounds to me as if she is saying 'hello' when he comes back from work, just as you do.*" Ming laughed and said, "*I never thought of it. Do you really think that is possible?*" The clinician responded, "*I really do. Fetuses respond to the things that happen around them, just like we do.*" Ming did not answer in words, but she smiled a little and her face softened in response, as if entertaining this possibility and enjoying the thought of it.

To reinforce these positive feelings, the clinician ended the session with a diaphragmatic breathing exercise as a body-based intervention to help Ming learn techniques that could help her regulate her anxiety and stress responses. The clinician introduced the invitation to practice these techniques as a way of helping her give Lien an experience of her mother's calm and relaxed body, so that she also could learn to relax even while in the womb, and mother and baby could enjoy together the shared experience of pregnancy.

As part of the invitation to the breathing exercise, the clinician asked the mother's permission to talk to Lien. With a soft smile, Ming agreed. The clinician turned her eyes to Lien (her mother's belly) and said, *"Lien, so many things have happened to your mommy. She really wants to welcome you, but she is very scared of losing you. She loves you so much, and she is coming to see me because she wants some help to be able to enjoy you and connect with you."* Ming smiled nervously and touched her belly. She again mentioned how guilty she felt after what happened to Bao. However, she was able to participate in the breathing exercise, and it soon became evident that the exercise had been a beneficial intervention because by the end of the session she was smiling, laughed easily, and had a relaxed posture.

Speaking to the fetus while indirectly talking also to Ming opened a space for Lien as an individual on her own right, uncontaminated by her association with her dead sister. Bringing the baby into the room as a participant helped Ming hold Lien in her mind as a living, sentient partner who could respond to her mother's moods just as she responded to her father's loving greeting on his return from work.

### Fear of Harming the Baby

The first session had supported Ming's ability to make meaning of her grief and to clarify her confusing of Lien with Bao. Ming's readiness to open herself to new insights allowed her to develop a therapeutic relationship with the clinician at a very fast pace.

Ming's trust in the therapeutic process led to new revelations in the second session of the foundational phase, when she talked about having intrusive thoughts about actions that could harm Lien. She described a specific situation of taking a very hot bath and then immediately having an intrusive thought that the hot water would harm the pregnancy. Her concern compelled her to get out of the bathtub and look online about the possible consequences of taking very hot baths during pregnancy. To her dismay, she found information that documented potential pregnancy harm in response to hot baths and immediately felt extremely sad and guilty. After a couple of minutes, her fear was so intense that she went back to the bathroom and took a long shower with lukewarm water to cool her body down. Only after taking the cooling shower and calling her doctor to report on what she had done and receive his reassurance, did she feel calmer again. The clinician empathized with her response and offered praise for her clear thinking and quick action in identifying a potential threat, informing herself about its potential accuracy, taking self-protective action, and seeking out expert opinion to ensure that she had left nothing undone. Ming responded with relief and gratitude to this benevolent reframing that highlighted her capacity to protect.

During the following session, Ming was able to make the link between her fear of harming Lien and her unresolved traumatic loss of Bao. As she started talking about Bao's loss, she said, *"I was alone,"* and started rubbing her belly. The clinician asked what she was feeling. *"My belly feels tense,"* answered Ming. The clinician invited Ming to do a brief relaxation exercise, after which Ming reported that her belly was no longer as tense as before and, without any prompting, continued talking about Bao. *"After I lost Bao, my mother told me that everything was fine, and that I would get pregnant again soon. She was not able to see how I was feeling!"* she said angrily. She continued, as tears began seeping down her face, *"The day before I lost Bao, I woke up very early with pain in my belly, but then the pain passed, and I thought that everything was fine and I went back to sleep. In the morning, I was getting ready to go to work. I went to the bathroom, and I was bleeding. I immediately went to the doctor, and was told that there was nothing more to do. And with the pregnancy in an advanced stage, it was necessary to deliver Bao."*

The clinician asked, *"Are you remembering when it happened?"* *"Yes, I was with my parents,"* Ming answered while gazing at the floor. *"They are retired, so they came from China to see me pregnant and to celebrate with us, because Bao would be their first grandchild. The plan was that they would come again for the delivery and stay for 6 months to help take care of the baby. I called my husband. He was on a road trip and drove all night to be able to meet me. I tried to wait for him, but I couldn't hold Bao inside of me. After the birth, the medical resident started to pass Bao to me, but then put her on the bed. Everything happened so fast! I saw her on the bed, but I couldn't reach out to hold her in my arms. I was terrified, I felt guilty. My parents were quiet, looking at us, but they did not do anything. Then somebody took Bao away, and I did not see her again."* Ming continued crying in a contained way, as she said that Bao was 18 weeks gestational age and was born dead.

After a pause, the clinician asked, *"I'm wondering if part of you feels that something you did caused her death."* Ming looked at the floor, and was silent for a while before replying, *"Yes, I felt guilty for a long time, and tried to explain to myself what I did that made it happen. Now I feel better."* The clinician continued, *"I'm wondering if there is still a little bit of fear in you of now harming Lien,"* and after a pause added, *"Do you remember what you told me the other day?"* Ming knew immediately what the clinician was referring to. *"Yes, I felt that when I took a hot bath, and I didn't know that could harm my baby."* The clinician pursued this theme, asking,

"*Tell me, how did you know?*" Ming said, "*I was tired, and I decided to take a hot bath, which relaxes me. I had a feeling that it was not OK. I was in the bathtub just for a little bit, but I couldn't bear the thought that it was wrong, so I got out of the tub and checked online. When I found out a hot bath could be harmful, I called my doctor immediately and took a warm shower to cool myself down. Only then did I feel calmer.*"

The clinician made a reassuring comment, saying "*Something inside you said that you did something that could harm your baby and something inside you warned you that you should protect her.*" "*Yes, it was like that,*" Ming confirmed. "*If you could have done something different with Bao, what would that be?*" the clinician asked. Ming thought for a while, and then said, "*I would have done more homework about how to take care of myself. I would have taken the first miscarriage more seriously. Maybe I could have done something else. Also, I would have hugged Bao after she was born. I wish my mother would have passed her to me.*"

The clinician brought her back to thinking about Lien, asking, "*Do you feel this way with Lien?*" "*No, with her I feel that I'm doing everything that is in my hands to protect her so that she can be born. I am making good decisions. I reduced my schedule at work when I had a little bleeding, even though the doctor said there was no need to rest. I went immediately to the hospital one day that I didn't feel Lien moving as usual, and I followed up with my doctor about my uterine problems,*" Ming responded. "*You are following your instincts and what the doctor tells you,*" the clinician added. "*Yes, now I know,*" she said.

Ming's narrative during this session included her processing of becoming a mother, her identification with her own mother, and her perception of her mother's emotionally removed stance and lack of help when Bao was born dead. Ming perceived her mother as insensitive for not giving Bao to her to hold and for commenting that Ming would become pregnant again soon. In parallel, she perceived herself as insensitive for not hugging or expressing emotion toward Bao when she saw the baby's body. The clinician hypothesized that Ming had responded with affective avoidance (a defense known in psychoanalysis as isolation of affect) as a way to manage an overwhelming traumatic event that made her feel angry in her position as a daughter but also guilty in her position as the grieving mother of a dead child. She also hypothesized that Ming's parents had responded with emotional withdrawal to the shock of their only daughter's miscarriage of their first grandchild, which turned their trip from China from a cause for celebration into a cause for mourning. It was a reflection of the emotional distance stemming from long-standing patterns of fear and anger that Ming and her parents could not come together for shared grieving, consolation, and support.

The clinician responded in the moment by offering compassion, saying that Ming had been completely unprepared for seeing Bao dead, and Ming's mother and father and the medical staff were completely unprepared to respond to Ming's needs, because they were themselves in shock. The doctors had told Ming that Bao could not survive, but she did not expect to see her daughter's body. Ming described multiple aspects of this scene repeatedly, including the sights, sounds, smells, and frantic movements of the medical staff surrounding her, along with the frozen response in her mother and herself in not being able to reach out to Bao and hold her.

Engaging in the details of this trauma narrative had a positive effect on Ming. At the end of the session, she reflected, *"I didn't know that I felt guilty, or that I am now afraid of harming Lien."* *"How is that for you?"* the clinician asked. *"I feel better now. I can talk about the things that happened to me without getting that upset and sharing how I felt. I can relax with your help. Breathing exercises really help me,"* she told the clinician.

## Maternal Behavior as a Reminder of Loss and Guilt

Ming arrived at the fourth session, smiling broadly. *"I finished my second trimester!"* she announced happily, and went on to say that now the baby could survive even if born prematurely. This relief was short-lived, because soon again she expressed the fear of losing Lien.

The clinician started exploring the origin of this persistent fear by asking Ming about her experiences while growing up. Ming responded, *"I normally prefer not to think of what happened to me. I normally don't remember the bad things in my past. I prefer to focus on the future."* As the clinician administered the structured questionnaire of adverse and traumatic responses, however, Ming was surprised at how raw and present the pain connected with her early traumatic experiences felt to her. She was also surprised to realize that she remembered events and details that she did not think she could remember. She talked about the physical, emotional and verbal abuse that she witnessed between her parents throughout her childhood; her father's unpredictable threats when he was angry about killing the entire family; and the bullying she experienced from her cousin.

These memories in turn brought her back to Bao, and she revisited the day Bao was born dead. She again sobbed, while saying, *"It was horrible. I felt guilty. It was my daughter, and I didn't react in any way. I was so in shock when my parents told me 'think that soon you will get pregnant again, try to forget.' How could I forget that?"* she said angrily. *"Can you imagine that?"* she continued. Her parents' repeated minimization of her experience and insistence that a future pregnancy would allow her to forget

Bao left a lasting impression, and she needed to describe these comments repeatedly as a way of processing them to gain increased understanding of why these experiences had affected her so deeply. Every time the clinician responded with empathy, using psychoeducation, emotional support, and body-based exercises to validate that Ming had the right to her emotions and to help her integrate intellectual understanding with efforts to change her sensory experience.

These intervention approaches were helpful in giving Ming a greater sense of meaning and control over her dysregulated affect. At the same time, an insight-oriented approach had a major transformative effect in diminishing Ming's intense guilt about Bao's death. The clinician asked, *"Could you tell me more about your guilt?"* Ming explained that she had felt very helpless, because even though the doctor told her that Bao was dead, she was not anticipating what it would be like to see her dead. She also believed that she didn't do enough to help Bao stay in utero. The clinician asked, *"Do you remember telling me how scared you are of doing things that can harm Lien? Did you feel that way before?"* Ming thought for a while, and then said, *"Yes, I thought many times that maybe I did something to provoke Bao's premature birth. I went over and over it in my mind for a long time looking for possibilities, and I think that it was a tea with roman chamomile that I had the day before her birth. Afterward, I read about the tea and learned that it is linked to premature birth."*

Ming again cried about the possibility that she did something that caused Bao's death. This topic became a recurrent theme during treatment. Ming was gradually able to link this persistent guilt to her chronic sense of internal badness in response to the relentless physical, verbal, and emotional abuse she had experienced as a child. She recalled her father and mother telling her, *"You are bad!"* whenever she did something they disapproved of, and her cousin mocking her for being *"ugly, slow, and awkward,"* wearing glasses, and not knowing how to dance. Her crying as she remembered these painful childhood scenes sounded like the crying of a despairing young child who had nobody to turn to for help and support.

A subtle cultural dimension also emerged in this psychological picture. In Ming's family's cultural traditions, food and drink had a special place, and her happiest memories were about the family cooking together, eating, and drinking tea as manifestations of being loved and cared for. Ming experienced as unbearably cruel the idea that drinking tea—something that gave her pleasure amid the fear of her family conflicts—could also be the source of her greatest grief. Ming interpreted this as a message that she deserved no pleasure, and would be punished for experiencing it. The clinician saw her role as providing

Ming with an unconditionally benevolent presence to support this vulnerable woman in understanding her self-blame as a reflection of her upbringing rather than as an objective truth, so that she could move from crippling guilt to greater self-acceptance.

### Feedback Session, Clinical Formulation Triangle, and Offer of Treatment

The feedback session allowed the clinician to speak with Ming about what they had learned together, to offer treatment, and to describe what the treatment would entail. The active role that the clinician had taken in providing insight-oriented interpretations, psychoeducation about trauma, and body-based regulation practices gave Ming a clear idea of what the tone of the treatment would be. These initial sessions illustrate the foundational phase as a time when clinicians perform a dual task: they gather systematic assessment information *and* test out how receptive the parent is to specific types of intervention in the range of P-CPP therapeutic modalities in order to maximize the effectiveness of the treatment.

At the beginning of the feedback session, the clinician asked Ming what she had learned from the previous sessions. Ming answered that she felt much better. Despite still experiencing fear, she was not as anxious as she was at the beginning of treatment. Through conversations with the clinician, Ming said, she had developed a better understanding of what was happening to her, and felt understood and supported while talking to the clinician. Ming's response made clear that she had established a solid therapeutic alliance with the clinician, and that an offer of treatment was appropriate given the remaining clinical needs.

The clinician recapitulated the work of the previous sessions, sketching for Ming the formulation triangle by linking her trauma history and the loss of Bao to her current fears about losing Lien. She presented treatment as an opportunity for Ming to gain a better understanding of herself in order to be more content and to give Lien the kind of loving caregiving she would have wanted to have while growing up and would have liked to give to Bao. Ming accepted the invitation to treatment readily and with gratitude.

It is important to note that the clinician explored racial and cultural topics with Ming from the beginning of treatment, including her experience of being pregnant in a foreign country with different practices and traditions from her own. The clinician pointed out that she was Latina and Ming was Chinese, and invited Ming to let her know if there were times when the clinician's assumptions and values were different from her own. Ming spoke thoughtfully about cultural matters. She said she felt happy to give birth to Lien in a place where there was advanced technology in case it was needed. She also commented on cultural differences. For example, she was constantly aware of her diet and adopted some customs that she learned from her family. She commented, *"In my country we are very careful with what we eat during pregnancy. The other day I asked my doctor if eating pineapple could be harmful, and she said no. Even though she reassured me that I was going to be fine, I didn't eat it, because I heard that eating pineapple could cause miscarriage. Also, women should not carry heavy things during pregnancy and after delivery. The period after the birth is a very special time when the woman is expected to rest and be taken care of."* She then asked, *"What are the customs in your country?"* The clinician answered that in her country there are also customs similar to those Ming mentioned, and described some specific examples of those cultural similarities. Ming smiled. She was pleased that the cultural similarities created an additional source of trust in the clinician.

## Core Treatment: Deepening the Work

Ming made the transition from the foundational phase to the core treatment phase with a good understanding of the roots of her fear of losing Lien and a greater ability to use breathing exercises to manage her anxiety when she had intrusive thoughts of losing Lien. Paradoxically, she also started to report recurrent difficulties with sleeping and nightmares that involved her parents. The ghosts of her past were emerging at this phase of treatment.

She arrived for the next four sessions with complaints about lack of sleep and intense, vivid, and scary nightmares, all of which involved parental figures. Every week she described horrific dreams that kept her uncomfortable during the rest of the week. Simultaneously, she reported having less anxiety about losing Lien. The clinician hypothesized that the fear of losing Lien was declining because the pregnancy was no longer considered high risk, and also because the therapeutic process was redirecting her anxiety to its original sources in the maltreatment she had experienced as a child. It was reassuring to witness that, in tandem with her intense emotional disequilibrium, Ming was able to maintain a positive motivation in preparing for Lien's arrival by washing baby clothes, preparing the baby's room, and getting newborn baby supplies. She reported that her husband was a loving partner in these "nesting" activities.

Ming described her father as abusive and her mother as depressed. Her childhood was filled with moments of chaos and panic, during which her father hit and hurt her mother and threatened to kill the entire family in moments of rage. These memories were now emerging in the form of dreams, including the following one: *"I dreamed that my father was hitting my mother, getting angrier and angrier, and my mother was screaming really hard and trying to run away, but he kept cornering her and hitting her harder. I tried to tell him to stop, but no words or sounds could come out of my mouth. I kept trying to speak but I couldn't. Then I saw myself as an adult and I woke up."* The clinician asked what Ming thought about that dream. *"I don't want to live that again,"* Ming replied. *"My father was very abusive toward my mother. I don't understand how she never left him. The way I see my father is without respect. I don't understand why he treated us that way."* The clinician commented that Ming did not want to repeat that experience with Lee and Lien. Ming answered that Lee was very different from her father, by saying, *"I was very careful in finding somebody that was not like my father. That is not the life that I want for Lien. Lee treats me with respect, and I'm grateful for that."* Ming added that she was proud of herself for feeling strong about this conviction, and finding a husband who would not treat her and their daughter the way her father treated her mother and herself.

Paradoxically, Ming's "angel" moments involved memories of her father being nurturing in the moments of safe connection they had together. She remembered lovingly a scene when she and her father were at the dining table at night and her father was helping her with homework, while the aroma of the dinner her mother was cooking wafted through the room. She had a vivid memory of her father's tenderness as he corrected her mistakes in a supportive manner. The clinician asked her whether the memory of moments like this with her father might have guided her in her search for a man like Lee. Ming teared up, saying that it made her so sad to know that her father had the capacity to be tender and supportive but displayed it so seldom. *"Life would have been so different if he had been able to be like that more often with my mother and me,"* she said. The clinician said that it sounded as if her father had given her just enough of his loving side to enable her to learn what she wanted and give her the tools to search for it and make it happen. This mutative clinical moment helped Ming gain some integration of her split paternal images into a more coherent image in which she could acknowledge and tolerate her ambivalence toward her father.

The nightmares continued, interspersed with memories of childhood that now became the core content of the sessions. *"I am very surprised,"* she said. *"I've never dreamt in this way in the past. I'm dreaming a lot, maybe because I have been talking about hard situations in my life. I normally don't like thinking about it."* She continued, *"I talk with my father but not that often, it still hurts me the way he didn't care for us. He barely spent money on us; sometimes my grandparents helped us, because we did not have enough to eat. Other times he would arrive and fight with my mother for any minimal reason, and he did not care if we were present or not."*

In quick succession, Ming then reported dreaming that she received a call from someone in China telling her that she should go back because her parents had a horrible accident. She woke up bathed in sweat and shaking with terror. While reflecting on the dream and with a very worried expression, she mentioned that she had talked with her mother a couple of days before the dream, and that her mother disclosed that her father had had yet another affair and his lover was now pregnant. Ming was shocked that her father would become the father of a child who would be born at approximately the same time as Lien. She expressed once again angry disbelief that her mother had never left him in spite of his lack of respect and care.

Ming then asked the clinician, *"Do you think that's the reason my mother and I never connected? She was always so preoccupied with my father's conflicts."* The clinician asked Ming what came to her mind as she thought about this question. *"It is possible,"* she replied. *"You and I have been talking about how the connection between mother and baby starts before the baby is born. My mom was probably struggling when she was pregnant with me. She is always struggling. Maybe I felt it when I was in her womb, and it continued all my life . . ."* Ming looked pensive and very sad as she realized that the distant and conflicted daughter–mother relationship stemmed from the depression and withdrawal her mother experienced in response to her traumatic life circumstances.

The following week Ming reported another dream. Her mother was lost in the forest with Ming looking at her from a distance. She got closer to her mother to convince her that she should go back home because it was getting dark. She took her mother by the hand, and they were able to find their way out of the forest and get home when it was already very dark. In the dream, Ming sensed that something bad was about to happen. Once she and her mother got out of the forest, they looked back and saw that a wildfire was consuming the forest. *"What do you think about my dream?"* Ming asked. *"It's such a powerful dream. What do you think it means?"* the clinician responded. Ming answered, *"After all the things that we have been talking about, now I realize that I have been through a lot. I feel that my dream shows how strong I am to get out of very hard things."*

The clinician supported this positive explanation, which emphasized the successful rescue motif of the dream. She also thought to herself that, among the dream's many layers of possible meaning, the act of rescuing herself and her mother (who perhaps in the dream was also a representation of herself as a future mother) might symbolize the psychological growth she was achieving in treatment. In the clinician's mind, the dream also depicted Ming's growing realization that her disorganizing anxiety had its roots not only in Bao's loss, but also in the explosive, potentially lethal violence she had experienced while growing up.

Memories of how Ming's mother treated her started emerging after this dream and brought to consciousness positive experiences that she had not remembered for many years, often associated with food and cooking. A positive identification with her mother became grounded in daily activities. She reported, *"My mom and I talk every other day now, she tells me stories about her pregnancy with me. She remembers it was an easy pregnancy, and she was happy that I was a girl. In the past she didn't talk to me about it."* The clinician was aware of the traditional preference for sons in Chinese culture and was relieved to see that Ming's mother had welcomed a baby girl. The clinician asked how this new way of talking with her mother was different for her. Ming replied, *"I feel closer to her. It's interesting because we were never close to each other. I like it, but it's definitively new."* The treatment was enabling her to take the emotional risk of creating a more integrated mental representation of her mother and their relationship. Treatment gave her the courage to talk to and connect with her mother in this new way.

### "Will I Be a Good Mother? Will Lien Be a Good Baby?"

The improvement in Ming's relationship with her mother ushered in new doubts about Lien. In a later session, Ming asked, *"Do you think that we can do something with Lien while I am still pregnant?"* "What do you mean, Ming?" the clinician asked. *"I noticed that when there are loud noises, she gets stressed out."* "How did you notice that?" the clinician asked. *"This week there were workers in my neighborhood fixing the street, and they used some loud machines that you can hear inside my house. My stomach got very tense and hard, and I had the feeling that Lien got all stressed out and scared."* "What did you do when this happened?" the clinician asked. Ming replied, *"I rubbed my belly and told her that everything is going to be OK."* "What a nice way of reassuring her. How do you want us to help her?" the clinician asked. Ming answered, *"I feel that she is going to be like that when she is born, get all stressed out. I fear that she is going to cry and cry, and I'm not going to be able to console her."*

This disclosure showed another facet of Ming's ambivalence toward becoming a mother. Her self-doubt about her capacity to be a good mother came to the fore now that her fear of being incapable of giving birth to a healthy living child was receding. The clinician facilitated reflection by asking, *"Is there a moment in your life when you felt like that? Like nobody was going to be able to console you?"* Ming's eyes filled with tears, and she cried while narrating the following story. *"Yes, I was around 11. We used to live in my grandparents' house. I don't even remember what got me that upset, maybe my cousin was bullying me. I remember being very upset and began sobbing loudly. I went to my room, hid in the closet, and stayed there crying inconsolably for what felt like hours. My parents started looking for me. I heard them calling my name, but I didn't want to come out of the closet. I didn't want to see them. I think that one of my little cousins found me, and together went to the living room where my parents were. My parents scolded me for hiding. I just stood there and listened to them until they were done. I then went back to my room and cried some more."*

The clinician linked the past with the present as she said, *"Your parents could not console you, and now you feel that maybe you are not going to be able to console your baby."* Ming cried with deep sadness, as she talked about her relationship with her mother and her need to be independent and strong. She described her mother as a cold woman, who never expressed love or allowed her to cuddle as a way of consoling her. *"My mother used to criticize me for being weak and crying for everything,"* she said. The clinician replied, *"That sounds very hard, not being able to trust and receive help from your mother when you were sad and scared. You were only a child, but you were not allowed to be afraid or to feel vulnerable."* Ming continued crying, as the clinician remained emotionally present but quiet, giving her room to feel her pain.

When the crying subsided, the clinician said, *"You had to make yourself be strong on many occasions when you felt alone and scared and needed help."* Ming started rubbing her belly, and the clinician asked, *"Is Lien OK?"* *"Yes, it's just that my belly gets a little hard,"* Ming answered. The clinician talked to Lien saying, *"Lien, your mom gets a little sad when she remembers things that made her cry when she was a little girl. She wants to listen to you and console you when you cry."* She then invited Ming to engage in a breathing exercise, which she readily accepted. As her belly softened and she felt more relaxed, Ming acquired greater trust that she was learning ways of soothing her baby effectively and she was not destined to repeat with her baby her childhood experience of unheeded cries.

### "Will My Husband also Die?"

Ming's memories of constant fights and her father's murderous rage were repeatedly associated with her parents' injunction that she needed to be independent from a very young age. Ming now started having intrusive thoughts that Lee would die and she would become a single mother. She said, "*I now have this fear of losing my husband to death. I don't know where it is coming from. I have always been very independent.*" The clinician helped her explore this new fear by using open-ended questions, and Ming realized that her apparent early independence was covering the need for connection and dependence on her parental figures that she had been denied. She suddenly said, "*I guess that I acted as if I didn't need anybody, but in reality I needed them. I guess I learned that from my parents, and now I behave the same way with Lee. I don't let him help me even if he wants to.*"

Ming's realization that she learned to be independent as a form of self-care in response to deprivation led to a conversation regarding the kinds of needs she would allow Lien to have and the ways she would like to respond to those needs. She recalled, "*I started working at a very young age. My aunt offered me a job and I took it. It was hard because I needed to commute to a different town every day and came back home very late. I took care of myself. I paid my expenses. My friends were surprised that I was able to do that and study.*" The clinician asked, "*How did your mother respond when you made those decisions?*" Ming responded, "*She didn't say anything. I was paying for myself, and she couldn't say anything. I rebelled and got angry when she tried to say anything to me.*"

The clinician made the connection with Lien by asking, "*How will it feel for you to have somebody dependent on you?*" Ming responded, "*I have been thinking about that. I would like to go back to work as soon as possible, but at the same time I want to be with Lien.*" The clinician spoke to the dual motivations that Ming was describing by saying, "*It sounds that part of you wants to continue to be independent and the other part wants to be responsive to your baby's needs.*" Ming nodded quietly.

This comment was an early manifestation of the conflicts many mothers experience between their role as mothers and their roles in the larger society, including their work activities. The clinician gave Ming space to experience the normative tug between her different motivations without any further interpretation, because she understood that the solutions to the many dilemmas she would encounter were part of the personal growth process that lay ahead.

### Preparing for Labor and Delivery: Concrete Plans and Processing Trauma

Ming was now 6 weeks before her due date, and the clinician used concrete assistance modalities to develop a birth plan. She introduced the idea of having a doula, a suggestion that Ming readily accepted.

The clinician and Ming also created the birth plan together, including the concrete topics routinely included in the plan. Most important, they had a conversation about the different medical questions that she needed to ask her doctor, including how to talk with her doctor if the need for urgent medical attention came up. This was very important to Ming, because her feelings of guilt for not doing "something in time to save Bao" continued to haunt her during moments of stress.

After giving Ming concrete assistance with the birth plan, the clinician started preparing her for the possibility of identifying traumatic reminders during labor that could bring her back to the trauma of losing Bao. Ming told the clinician that she had already thought about this possibility, and wanted to retell in every single detail what happened when she delivered Bao. The clinician felt internally divided about this wish for fear that Ming would lose her hard-earned ability to differentiate between remembering and reliving the trauma in the process of immersing herself again so fully in the trauma narrative. She was also respectful of Ming's conviction that this was what she needed to do, and agreed to this request.

During this new narrative of Bao's traumatic delivery as a stillborn, the clinician listened fully and with deep compassion but regulated affect to Ming's description. She went over every aspect of the experience in minute detail, including the room she was in, the people that were around her, including her parents, and the helplessness and horror that she felt when she realized that her baby had died. Her physical reactions in the retelling showed the permeable boundary between remembering and reexperiencing. Her face was red, she was sobbing uncontrollably at times, and she became nauseous. She was grieving fully by reliving systematically the events involving the death of her beloved Bao.

The clinician helped Ming use breathing to help her stay present in the room, but did not attempt to console her or intervene in any other way with her expression of grief. Afterward, Ming looked exhausted but relaxed. The clinician talked simultaneously to Lien and Ming, saying "*Lien, your mommy was crying for all the times that she didn't cry after losing your sister. Mommy is going to be OK, but she needed to cry, to mourn a big loss in her life.*" The clinician struggled internally with the idea of introducing Bao as Lien's sister, but decided that giving Bao a place in the family could facilitate a resolution of the grieving process that the mother was experiencing. Ming reacted well when the clinician used "sister" as a new way of referring to Bao while talking to Lien.

With Ming's consent, the clinician shared with the doula and the medical staff the story of Ming's miscarriage and possible trauma reminders, so that they could be prepared to respond supportively if Ming became dysregulated during the childbirth process. Possible trauma reminders included external triggers, such as the hospital room and the presence of doctors, medical personnel, medical technology, and the experience of first meeting Lien, while potential internal triggers included pain, contractions, and other body-based sensations inherent in the process of giving birth. The clinician also asked the medical staff to keep in mind Ming's fear of unexpected catastrophe and remembered to keep her informed of the procedures that they would employ. For example, if the delivery had to be induced, the medical staff could support Ming with brief explanations of what to expect during each stage of the process. Anticipating possible responses could give Ming a better sense of control and help her differentiate between the present delivery of Lien and the traumatic experience of delivering Bao.

## Inviting Ming's Husband to Join the Treatment

The clinician offered Ming the option of inviting her husband to join the sessions so they could talk about their shared fear that each of them would lose the other. Both parents had experienced the traumatic loss of Bao, and now it was important to offer support to Lee as an integral part of the family treatment.

During the first joint session, the parents quickly created an intimate shared emotional space, as the clinician encouraged them to describe what they needed from each other while waiting for Lien's birth. Lee cried openly when describing how he felt when he learned about the unfolding miscarriage while he was on a business trip and his frantic efforts to get back to town to be by her side. He said, "*It was terrible. I know that losing Bao is something that we will always remember. I kept imagining myself next to Ming while trying to be back in time for her delivery. I wish the doctors could have prepared us a little bit more for what was happening. It happened so fast that, by the time I got to the hospital, they had already taken Bao away and I could not see her. I never got to meet her or to hold her. We were so excited about her, and then we lost her.*"

Ming and the clinician were silent as Lee talked. He then added, "*Now I'm so happy about Lien but I'm also afraid. I am afraid to be too happy, but Ming's pregnancy is so different that I'm positive that Lien is going to be OK and I have plans for being a family.*" The clinician asked if he could tell her about these plans. He answered, "*My life is motivated by Lien, this is my first baby, and I feel so excited about doing things for her. I want to be there for her and be close to her. My grandfather was very present in my life as a child, and I want to be like that for Lien.*"

Ming and Lee then talked about their hopes as parents-to-be and the positive qualities that sustained them as a couple. They said that the family's cultural and religious beliefs gave them support and comfort at moments of stress. Their conviction that Bao was looking after her sister made them feel that they were all together as a family in one way or another. Lee joined two additional sessions, but now he focused on preparing for the concrete aspects of childbirth and baby care rather than on Bao. He said that he came from a loving family that belonged to one of China's many ethnic minority groups, but his parents were factory workers in a city far from their hometown and he lived during the week with his maternal grandparents, who were central figures in his life. The family got together during the weekends when his parents returned to the village along with many other parents in the same situation. He said his childhood had been *"effortful but good,"* guided by the expectation that he would exceed at school and get a good job that would help the entire family. His emigration to the United States was a sign of his success in his family's eyes but also a reason for sadness. Lee said briefly that he might not have considered emigration if his grandparents were alive, but his parents were supportive of his decision because they wanted what was best for him.

## Lien's Delivery and Birth Narrative

As part of preparing for Lien's birth, Ming and the clinician agreed that the doula would call the clinician to let her know about the delivery and the clinician would visit the mother and baby at the hospital. Ming wanted to honor the cultural custom of spending the first 30 days at home after the delivery, and planned to resume treatment after this period had elapsed. They agreed that the clinician would call weekly to check in, and that Ming could call the clinician if she had questions or concerns.

As planned, the doula informed the clinician that Lien had been born. Ming and the doula had established a close connection, and the doula was happy to report that Ming had a vaginal delivery with no complications and that both mother and baby were healthy. When the clinician visited Ming and Lien at the hospital, she found Lien peacefully asleep in her mother's arms.

Ming smiled and said with happiness and pride, *"Hi, this is Lien. She was born healthy and with no complications."* The clinician said, *"Welcome Lien, your mommy has been waiting for you! Look at you! You look so calm and comfortable in your mommy's arms."*

After asking routine questions about the baby's height and weight, the clinician asked Ming how she was feeling. Ming showed a deep sense of calm, and said she felt very happy. She described the labor and delivery process in great detail. *"The pain started 2 days ago. I was in contact with my doula, and she helped me understand what was happening with my body. First, she asked me to pay attention to the frequency of the pain. I was doing OK with the pain, and then suddenly the pain increased. Lee and I decided to go to the hospital, but when we got there they told us to go back home, and I was feeling very uncomfortable. We waited a few hours before they admitted me to the hospital. My doula arrived directly at the hospital. It was great to have her help, because she knew so much and was so supportive. Lee was also there with me. I tried to stay focused on the pain and to keep breathing. After a while, I asked for an epidural. After a couple of hours, Lien was born. It was easy! I'm so fortunate! Lee was nervous because he does not do well when he sees blood, but he could still support me."*

The clinician congratulated her on such an uncomplicated and easy delivery and on her healthy and beautiful baby, and chose not to pursue Ming's comment about Lee at this moment of celebration in greeting the baby. Ming responded, *"Seeing Lien was the most beautiful experience in my life. I didn't want to separate from her, not even a minute. She is beautiful,"* she added with tears of happiness. *"She has been here with us all the time. My husband doesn't want to separate from her either. Our family is complete!"* she added.

Ming's statement that her family was complete was particularly noteworthy, because it implied that she was not experiencing the absence of Bao as a form of incompleteness. She did not mention Bao, and she did not compare the two deliveries. The clinician interpreted this fact as a positive sign, because it suggested that Lien had been given a space of her own that she could inhabit fully, without having to share it with her sister in her mother's psyche.

As agreed, the clinician and Ming had weekly telephone conversations that lasted between 15 and 30 minutes and were devoted to checking on the baby, the mother, and family well-being. These calls maintained the continuity of treatment in the weeks after the delivery. Ming described the adaptations they were making as a family, and was thrilled in particular by Lee's devotion and skills as a father. The mother also felt supported by the visits of a public health nurse who gave her practical hands-on information and made her feel that there was an expert keeping an eye on Lien's healthy development.

### Lien Joins the Treatment

Ming returned to treatment when Lien was 6 weeks old. The baby's presence during the sessions allowed the clinician to witness Ming's solicitous caregiving and her growing knowledge of her baby. She quickly learned to understand what her different cries could mean, such as when she was hungry, tired, or simply needed her mother's body close to her.

During the first six sessions after resuming treatment, Ming raised topics that mainly involved the baby's care, such as patterns of feeding, sleeping, crying, and soothing. Ming was a very kind, loving, and attuned mother. In one session, as the clinician commented on how well the mother and baby responded to each other, Ming made clear that she was consciously differentiating herself from her mother. She said, *"The other day when I was talking with my mom on the phone, Lien started crying, and I didn't know what she wanted. My mother told me to let her cry. I felt so overwhelmed that I ended the call."* The clinician asked what made her feel overwhelmed, and Ming responded, *"I remember the many times I cried alone in my room. If I was sad, upset, or angry; nobody was with me. I would fall asleep while crying, even during the day. Then I would leave my room as if nothing had happened, and nobody paid any attention to me. I don't want that for my baby."*

During a session a couple of months later, Ming expressed some concern about Lee's anxiety about Lien's well-being. *"Lee is a very involved and loving father, but since Lien was born he has just been so anxious and worried about her. At times, I feel he is overprotective of her, and she is not even 4 months old."* The clinician asked what her thoughts were about Lee's anxiety, and Ming responded, *"At first I was OK with it, but I feel that now it is a little too much. He wakes her up when she is not even crying. I talked to him and explained to him that she is OK and we should let her rest, but he wants to make sure that she is fine and held all the time."* As the conversation continued, Ming said, *"I think that he is scared that something might happen to her. He told me that after delivery scary memories came to his mind. I'm grateful he trusts me that much to tell me."* The clinician commented, *"I remember you told me that he does not do well with blood and got nervous during the delivery. Do you think maybe something got triggered in him after seeing blood when you were giving birth, and now he constantly worries?"* Ming said, *"Yes, he is more afraid that something will happen to her now than during the pregnancy."* The clinician now included Lien in the conversation, and said, *"Your mommy is telling me that daddy cares a lot about you, but mommy doesn't want him to be worried all the time. You are OK, mommy is OK, and mommy wants daddy to relax and enjoy you now that you are all together, complete."* The baby's ready smile in response to the clinician brought a moment of shared joy. The clinician then ushered an invitation for Lee to join treatment again if this was something that he and Ming thought would be helpful to them.

## The Father's Story

At the next session, Ming told the clinician that she asked Lee to join the sessions, and he quickly accepted because he felt burdened by his intense fear of losing Lien. During a session involving Lee, Ming, and the baby, the clinician asked Lee when he noticed that his fears intensified. Lee said that he felt extremely vulnerable during the delivery. He had been very excited about welcoming Lien. Their doula had told them while talking about the birth plan that sometimes fathers cut the umbilical cord, and he liked the idea of being an active participant in the delivery besides giving support to Ming. They agreed with the doctor that he would cut Lien's umbilical cord at birth, and they added that to their birth plan, feeling excited that he was going to be involved in the baby's birth. Then he became dizzy when he noticed the amount of blood during the delivery. When the doctor asked Lee to cut the umbilical cord according to the birth plan, he was not able to do it. At the time, the doctor simply took over, and nothing more was said about what happened, but the moment lingered in Lee's mind as a source of shame and regret.

The clinician responded to Lee's narrative by asking how he understood his reactions in the delivery room. He answered that when he was 8 years old, his mother had a difficult home delivery. He remembered his mother's screams and the blood that surrounded her before the midwife sent him to play outside, but he stayed close to the house and continued to hear her crying and screaming for a long time. Lee's hands were shaking, and his voice was hoarse as he remembered this scene. Ming seemed very impacted by Lee's experiences, making grimaces and showing tension in her neck and shoulders. Lien began to cry in response to her parents' affect. As Ming rocked Lien gently to calm her down, the clinician said to the baby, "*Your daddy is telling us that he has a lot of sad feelings, and you and your mommy are also sad for him.*" Turning to Lee, the clinician said that he was talking about a very important part of his life that shaped how he felt now about becoming a father. Lee agreed, adding that his mother had delivered twins at the time, but only one of the twins had survived. Ming startled when she heard this information, which Lee had not told her before. The clinician understood at that moment the likely connection between the perinatal loss experienced by Lee's parents, and Lee's current fears about Lien's health and well-being as reported by Ming.

It seemed that talking about these powerful memories during the triadic session was dysregulating not only to Lee, but also for Ming and Lien. The clinician used this understanding to offer Lee the opportunity to meet individually with him. To model pacing and modulation in the recovery and sharing of traumatic memories, she said, "*I want to hear all the important things that you are describing, and at the same time, I am seeing how much Ming and Lien are also affected because you are so important to them. You and I met only a couple of times, and I am wondering if it might be helpful for you and I to meet separately to think more about how this experience is continuing to affect you."* Lee and Ming agreed that this was a good idea. Lee and the clinician scheduled an individual session for the following week.

Lee opened his individual session by saying that he realized he worried excessively about Lien's safety and well-being, and his memory of his mother's delivery made him realize that the two experiences were connected. He again talked about his inability to cut the umbilical cord, explaining that he became dizzy and disoriented when he saw Ming's blood. He seemed disappointed and ashamed for his perceived failure. The clinician empathized with his regret that he was not able to accomplish something that he really wanted to do as a ritual during the delivery of his daughter. She then asked, *"You previously mentioned how difficult it was for you to be present during your mother's delivery when you were only 8 years old, and that many images came to your mind during Ming's delivery. Can you tell me more?"*

Lee became very serious. He said he remembered thinking that his mother was going to die when he heard her screams. When the midwife told him to go outside, he was so scared that he did not know what to do. *"My grandfather was arriving at his home next door and saw me there, waiting outside the house by myself. He told me to go home with him. I felt so much better to be with him. I stayed the night at my grandfather's house. The next morning I ran to my house looking for my mother. My mother was sleeping. The midwife was cleaning up the room, and there were many bloody sheets on the floor. I asked for my baby brothers, and my father told me that one of them had died. I remember feeling guilty as if it was my fault."*

Lee's body seemed stiff, and he paused frequently as he spoke, at times having difficulty saying what he wished to convey. The clinician empathized with him, saying it was a frightening story. Lee agreed, adding that his father did not explain anything else, and the family never spoke about the twin baby's death.

Lee then proceeded to tell another frightening story, as if he needed to unburden himself of the unspoken traumas of his childhood. When he was around 10 years old, he went to town with his grandfather to buy groceries at the farmers' market. They both enjoyed doing this errand together because his grandfather taught him about the different fruits and vegetables, including what grew in what season and how to buy the best and least expensive produce from vendors that they knew and trusted. They were buying groceries when a drunk driver ran his truck into the farmers' market. His grandfather pushed him out of the way to protect him from the truck, and then he heard people screaming and chaos. Lee ran to his grandfather, who was lying on the ground and who asked Lee if he was all right. Lee was not hurt, but the truck had hit his grandfather and other people who had been shopping. Lee saw a dead person and a lot of blood on the sidewalk. Later on, the police arrived and carried away the deceased person in their vehicle. His grandfather was taken to the hospital, where he died a week after the incident. Lee cried intensely while describing this story. He remembered how painful it was for him to lose his grandfather. "*I normally don't talk about this,*" he said. This was close to the end of the session, and the clinician guided Lee through a breathing exercise to help him leave the session in a more regulated state. They agreed that Lee would return the following week for another individual session. The clinician called Ming on the telephone to make sure she would be fine with Lee having another individual session the following week. The clinician was glad to hear that Ming supported this plan, and invited her to reach out to her by telephone if she wished to talk about Lien and/or herself during the week.

During the following individual session with Lee, he told the clinician that he had never spoken about his memories in detail and that he found it painful but relieving to give words to the images that he had carried since he was a young child. He said that Ming knew about the death of his grandfather, but he had never told her in detail about his feelings about his mother's delivery of the twins and his grandfather's death. He added, "*It is good that she was not here to hear what I said.*" The clinician then asked, "*I have been thinking about all the things you told me, and I have been wondering. Do you think the blood in Lien's delivery brought you back to those moments? Blood seemed to be a reminder of the traumatic experiences that you had. In both of them, you lost a family member. You thought that you were going to lose your mother.*" Lee became tearful but remained calm as he completed the clinician's thought by saying, "*I thought something could happen to Ming and Lien as well.*" During this session, Lee explored the connections between his past and his present and gained a new understanding of his protective fear, and his efforts to make sure Lien was safe allowed him to understand his present fears about Lien. A third individual session with Lee served to consolidate the insights he had acquired during the earlier sessions and help him anticipate and practice ways of reassuring himself, instead of waking Lien up to make sure she was all right.

### Re-Creating the Triad

Ming, Lee, and Lien arrived together as agreed to the following session. Lee said that since his individual meetings with the clinician he had talked more with Ming about his past experiences of loss. Ming added, "*I am very moved by what he told me. I knew about what happened to his grandfather, but I never knew about his twin brother and I never thought that Lien's birth would bring these memories back."* The clinician commented, *"The two of you had so much pain in losing loved ones, and now it makes sense that you are afraid it can happen again."* There was some talk about what would be the most useful format for the sessions in the future, which led to an agreement that the parents could decide on an ongoing basis what would work best for them in any particular week. This flexibility was a way of affirming the clinician's trust in the parents' capacity to make the right decisions for themselves and their baby. It gave them the autonomy to navigate solutions to the question of how to balance their individual needs with their needs as a couple learning to co-parent their first child.

## Negative Maternal Transference Emerges

Ming arrived alone with Lien to the following session. She seemed distant and formal, in contrast to her previous demeanor. Although there had been brief telephone contacts between Ming and the clinician during the 3 weeks spanning Lee's individual sessions, she now seem guarded and detached.

With Ming's history of detachment and anger at her mother in mind, the clinician asked her if the weeks of not having her regular sessions brought up some feelings for her even though she had agreed to the arrangement. Ming seemed surprised by the question, and asked, *"How do you know that I had feelings about that?"* The clinician replied that it would be understandable to have feelings about it. Ming said, with tears in her eyes, *"I don't know why I feel like that if I know that Lee needed you and that it is important that he gets support with his relationship with Lien."*

It was very difficult for Ming to talk about needing the clinician and feeling jealous that the clinician had turned her attention to Lee. Lien had been looking at her mother with an interested expression as Ming spoke, and she became fussy when Ming started crying. The clinician turned to Lien and said, *"Your mommy is feeling sad. Are you feeling a little sad too?"* She asked Ming if this was the first time that Lien saw her crying, and Ming assented. The clinician continued, *"It's different for you to see mommy crying, but she is going to be OK. Mommy is very important to you, and you are not used to seeing her cry."* As Ming started echoing the clinician's words in speaking to Lien, the baby returned to a state of interested calm.

During the following 2 months, Lee attended sessions sporadically and reported that his fears related to Lien had decreased considerably. He now could guide himself out of overprotective actions by identifying the internal states that he was experiencing. Ming confirmed Lee's accounts, stating that she no longer found him hovering over the baby. During the triadic sessions, he was attuned to the baby's signals and mostly responsive to the baby's bids for autonomy and closeness.

### The Father–Baby Relationship

Lee's reflexive wish to protect Lien from any distress continued to emerge from time to time. During one triadic session, Lien was on the floor playing with toys while the parents and the clinician were talking. Lien started to turn over from back to front, and Ming reported that Lien has been practicing this at home and she felt excited to see it happening. While Lien was trying to do the turn during this session, Lee returned her to her back. Lien tried to turn over again, and again Lee put her on her back. Ming watched in silent disapproval but did not intervene. This happened two more times before Lien started crying in frustration for not being able to practice her new achievement.

The clinician wondered with Lee what it was like for him to see Lien trying to turn to be on her belly. Lee said, "*I fear that she is going to hurt herself. She is still so little.*" Lien tried again while her father was talking. The clinician said, "*Lien, your daddy is telling me how much he loves you that he doesn't want you to get hurt, but you are so ready to practice something new. You are so proud of yourself that you want to show your mommy and your daddy that you can do it.*" Lien tried again, and this time was able to turn over from back to front while both parents applauded her. Lien smiled while lifting her neck. Lee said in a surprised tone of voice, "*I never thought about what it was like for her to do these kinds of things. I guess I was just thinking about me.*"

Other themes emerged in different ways in Lien's relationship with her mother and father. For example, when Lien was ready to start solid food, Ming experienced a period of increased anxiety, because she was fearful of giving Lien something to eat that could cause her to choke. This anxiety decreased and became more reality based with some exploration of the links between the mother's past experiences of danger and Lien's moving into new areas of development.

## The Closing Phase of Treatment

When Lien was about to turn 6 months old, the clinician reminded the parents of the original agreement that treatment would last until about this time unless there were difficulties in their relationships with the baby or with the baby's development. The clinician then started the posttreatment evaluation to assess how the parents perceived themselves and how Lien was developing.

The evaluation measures confirmed the clinician's observations. Ming's anxiety and PTSD symptoms were no longer clinically significant, although her anxiety score remained subclinically elevated. Lien met all the developmental expectations for her age. Lee had not filled out assessment forms at any of the treatment phases, but it was clear that he was feeling comfortable with himself and his functioning as a father. The family was doing well, individually and in relationship with one another. There was no clinical reason to continue treatment.

In spite of this positive overall picture, the termination of treatment brought up a reemergence of the previous themes of loss, and coming to the final sessions was difficult for both Ming and Lee despite the clinician's efforts to prepare them ahead of time for the end of treatment by pacing the termination over the course of seven sessions. This was an agreement reached with the parents as a corrective experience in response to their history of sudden traumatic losses. The clinician and the parents had extended conversations about all the things that were going well for them and Lien. These preparations alleviated but did not eliminate the intensity of the difficult feelings associated with saying good-bye to the clinician.

Ming missed some appointments without notice for the first time in the course of treatment. The clinician helped her link these absences to her fear of pain about saying good-bye to the clinician. Ming also reported a dream in which she was delivering a baby, but did not know what happened to the baby and woke up in a state of great agitation. She understood this dream as a statement that, as much as she had made progress in modulating her grief over Bao's death, the feelings might reemerge as an integral part of her inner life when she encountered reminders of losing people who were important to her.

Lee was more forthright in his expression of anger at the termination of treatment. He said, *"I didn't have the opportunity to say good-bye to my grandfather. The day that he died was the only day that I didn't go to visit him. I remember feeling guilty and mad that something like that happened to him. I felt mad at my father for asking us to go shopping, I was mad at the drunk driver, at the police, at my grandfather, at myself . . ."* The clinician said gently, *"And maybe also at me?"* *"At you too,"* admitted Lee, adding humorously, *"You became too important to us."* The clinician thanked him, and said that she would miss them too. Therapy, she added, was a little like parenting in terms of thinking about when it was the right time to let go. There is a time when people are ready to be on their own, but the feelings of closeness remain.

The extended termination process gave the parents the opportunity to revisit their unresolved experiences of loss and differentiate them from the realistic regret of bringing to an end a therapeutic connection that was very meaningful to them. The clinician spoke about how the opportunity to talk about how a planned and thoughtful "good-bye" could begin to heal the previous "good-byes" that were painful, horrifying, and unpredictable.

In one of these sessions, Ming said, *"Lee and I were talking about what you said about how difficult it is for us to say good-bye, because of our previous good-byes. We know that it is difficult, but we want Lien to learn that sometimes you have to say good-bye to people that are important to you."* It was touching to see the couple's identification with the clinician and their efforts to cope with their own feelings about saying good-bye by converting the termination of treatment into a valuable lesson for their baby daughter. It was perhaps a sublimation of their lingering anger at the clinician for not being able to be the unconditionally available parent figure that a part of them still longed for.

Lee was not able to attend the last session, and the clinician asked herself whether having an actual good-bye was perhaps too difficult for Lee owing to his experience of losing his grandfather. Lee was able to call the clinician to express his thanks and say good-bye through the safe nonvisual medium of the telephone.

Ming and Lien arrived on time to the last session and spent time on the floor playing with age-appropriate toys. The clinician acknowledged that this was the last session. Ming cried as she expressed her gratitude for all the support that the clinician had provided. The clinician accepted her gratitude, acknowledged the hard work she had done during treatment, and said that she would always remember Ming, Lee, and Lien with very special feelings. The clinician included Lien as she spoke, saying, *"We are sad because today we are saying bye-bye. The two of you are doing so well together that you don't need to come see me anymore. Your mommy and your daddy have been so brave in wanting you to learn how important it is to say good-bye in a planned way."*

The clinician then asked Ming what she wanted to do during this last session. Ming said she wanted to read a book. The clinician had talked about the importance and benefits of reading books to babies in previous sessions, and encouraged Ming to read baby books to Lien. For their last session, the clinician suggested reading *The Invisible String* (Karst & Stevenson, 2000), a book that describes how feelings of love endure in the face of physical absence. Pleasurable mutuality could be seen in the mother–baby dyad as 8-month-old Lien sat on her mother's lap while she tenderly read the book to her. The clinician listened quietly, while noticing Ming's confidence and comfort as Lien's mother. She felt reassured that the loving attunement between mother and baby validated her decision to bring the treatment to a close.

# Reflections on the Therapeutic Process

The treatment of Ming, Lien, and Lee illustrates the importance of using a trauma framework to understand the dual emotional impact of perinatal traumatic loss and the parents' childhood traumatic memories on the parents' experience of a new pregnancy. This clinical example also shows the usefulness of a close collaboration between perinatal mental health services and primary care, both to facilitate the referral to treatment of families in need of mental health treatment and to create integrate models of care when medical issues and mental health issues overlap.

While pregnant with Lien, Ming's unresolved grief for Bao demonstrated the difficulty of disinvesting emotionally from the deceased baby (Gaudet Séjourné, Camborieux, Rogers, & Chabrol, 2010). This inability to disinvest entails a decrement in perinatal attachment to the new fetus (Armstrong & Hutti, 1998). During the different treatment phases, Ming was able to process the traumatic loss of Bao and become reconciled with her loss. The resolution of her grief allowed Ming to invest her emotions in connecting with and preparing for Lien's birth. Lee's participation in the treatment was guided by clinical needs. The intensity of Ming's anxiety during the initial months of treatment called for a sustained focus on bringing some closure to her traumatic memories of her miscarriage, which Lee did not witness because he was on a business trip. The clinician was flexibly attuned to the parents' messages of when they needed to address their experiences individually and when they wanted to be together to create a shared approach to the pregnancy and their baby. This flexibility of response to clinical need and parental wishes is one of the hallmarks of P-CPP.

The intensity and severity of the symptoms experienced by Ming and Lee called for the versatile deployment of multiple intervention modalities in coordination with one another. Psychoeducation and unstructured developmental guidance helped the parents use their intellect in creating an understanding of their emotional states. Body-based exercises helped them to use active, immediate tools to modulate emotional dysregulation. Insight-oriented interpretation had the long-lasting effect of giving existential meaning to key aspects of their inner world by linking present experiences to their childhood traumatic memories and to benevolent memories to create more nuanced representations of their attachment figures and themselves.

The crucial contribution of baby Lien to her parent's therapeutic progress cannot be understated. Her uneventful birth provided a much-needed corrective experience to the parents' anticipatory anxiety of a repetition of Bao's traumatic delivery. Lien's easy temperament made the parents feel effective as they delighted in her regular biological rhythms, easy adjustment to transitions, quick responsive-ness to their soothing interventions, and predominantly positive affect. As Selma Fraiberg (1980) observed, working with babies is "a little like having God on your side." The clinician harnessed this celestial help by joining the parents' celebration of the baby, and in this process helping them to celebrate themselves.

# Section IV

# Common Obstacles
# to Attuned Caregiving

This section provides brief clinical illustrations that target frequent parental experiences that become obstacles to bonding with the baby. The purpose of this section is to enlarge the scope of the extended case presentations described in Section III by including additional topics that emerge during the perinatal period. One theme—infant crying—occupies the normative stress part of the range from developmentally expectable stress to traumatic stress. The impact of prematurity is included as a frequent challenge to the infant–parent relationship in the perinatal period. One theme involves immigration-related family separation, with the challenge of creating a semblance of family integration when an international border that they cannot cross legally separates the mother from her older children. Other themes involve the reemergence during pregnancy of specific childhood traumas, including foster care placement, separation from a parent, growing up witnessing domestic violence, childhood incest, and the death of the mother's mother during childbirth. Some of the specific events resemble those of the clinical cases in Section III, but these brief vignettes have the purpose of illustrating the enormous individuality of responses to traumatic experiences. The illustrations also expand on the clinical versatility that is called for to help parents integrate their experiences of fear, anger, and sorrow into an overarching commitment to parenthood that puts their baby at the core of their emotional life. For the sake of conciseness, each vignette includes basic contextual information and the facts that are immediately relevant to the clinical intervention.

# Vignette 1. Infant Crying as a Trauma Reminder

A baby's cry is a universal, adaptive behavior and the baby's most effective form of communication during the preverbal developmental stage. Infants have at least six types of cries, and each type communicates something different: pain, hunger, fatigue, boredom, discomfort, or the need to let off steam at the end of a stressful day (Brazelton, 2006). Crying is most often the first indication of life outside the mother's body, and for many parents it presents the first challenge they face after the baby is born. Parents are immediately thrust into the challenge of learning about the meaning of the baby's cry and figuring out how to console the baby on one hand, while at the same time they register for the first time the affective response that their baby's cry evokes in them. Infant crying can become a dysregulating factor in the parent–infant relationship when it triggers unbearable memories and feelings that the parent has suppressed, denied, or converted into defensive strategies for the management of affect. The affective mismatch between parent and infant in these situations can disrupt parental attunement to the baby and decrease affect synchronization and co-regulation in the dyad (Stern, 1985).

Fraiberg and colleagues (Fraiberg, Adelson, & Shapiro, 1975) hypothesized that a mother cannot hear or respond empathically to her baby's crying when her own crying was not heard or responded to in childhood. This vignette illustrates the value of learning about the specific meaning that the baby's cry has for a mother or a father when the baby has dysregulated bouts of crying. Affective synchronization between parent and infant can occur quickly when the parent becomes aware of internal obstacles that interfere with their prompt responsiveness.

It is important to keep in mind that colic in the first months of life is a real phenomenon, and that some infants experience intense physiological distress that is not quickly responsive to even skillful and solicitous parental ministrations. Even in these cases, however, the interpretation that the parent gives to the crying can change the quality of the emotional experience for the parent and the baby. The parent's ability to tolerate the baby's distress and remain present and attentive becomes a protective factor for babies prone to physiological dysregulation.

## Maternal Depression as a Harbinger
## of Unheard Infant Crying

An, a 25-year-old Vietnamese American woman, started treatment due to severe depression when she was 30 weeks pregnant with her first baby. Her pregnancy was unplanned and unwanted by the baby's father, who asked her to have an abortion. An decided to have the baby, but found herself abandoned by the baby's father and quite unsupported by her own mother and father. Her difficult present circumstances were exacerbated by the impact of her childhood adversities and traumatic stressors, which included her father's alcohol abuse, domestic violence, physical abuse of An and her siblings, and verbal abuse in the form of insults and threats by both parents. The father regularly threw the family out of the house during drunken rages, at times in the middle of the night.

There were also positive memories. An mentioned her maternal aunt as a reliable figure, who made her feel safe and protected. She also derived a strong feeling of comfort from nature. She remembered a special hill that her mother and siblings would escape to when her drunken father threatened them. She described in vivid detail the plants, the smell of the trees, and the stars in the sky when they went there at night. The emotional availability of protective factors served An well in enabling her to make a strong connection with the clinician (G. O. B.) and to use the treatment to become gradually more confident of her capacity to become a good mother to her baby in spite of her depression.

### *"I Fell Off of a Ladder, and My Mom Did Not Care"*

One memory stood out among the many stories that An told the clinician during her pregnancy, as described in the following account. *"I was around 7 years old. My cousins and I used to play outside the house. We lived next to each other. The neighbor, two houses down, had aggressive dogs that sometimes bit people. We ran every time we passed in front of that house, because the dogs would bark loudly and we were afraid they would bite us. One day the dogs chased us, and to get away we quickly climbed up the ladder on the side of our house to reach the rooftop. We stayed there for a while until my mother came outside looking for us. She got mad when she saw us on the rooftop, and yelled, 'Get down now!' My cousins came down, but I was scared. My mother kept yelling at me to get down. When I finally decided to climb down, I was so nervous that I slipped and fell on the ground and hurt my foot.*

*I remember I was crying because I was in so much pain. My mother was very angry and said, 'That's what you deserve for not obeying me, now deal with the consequences!' My foot was hurting a lot and I couldn't move it. One of my cousins tried to help me get up, but my mother told him to stop and to go back inside the house. She said to me, 'You get up on your own so you learn your lesson.' I stayed there for a while trying to stand up, but I couldn't. It was getting dark, and the animal sounds from the woods frightened me. I felt so scared and all alone. Finally my grandpa arrived home and carried me in his arms inside the house. I remember I couldn't walk and stayed in bed for a long time. I don't remember for how long, but then a doctor came to the neighborhood to treat the neighbors' cows and my grandpa asked him to treat my injured foot. I remember my mom was very angry because the doctor charged a lot of money."*

This dramatic story served as a warning in the clinician's mind for the challenges that An was likely to encounter in becoming attuned to her baby's signals of need. An remembered the fear she felt during this experience, but she did not seem to hold her mother accountable for the danger she was in. The clinician sensed that An felt an implicit identification with her mother's anger for having to spend scarce resources on An's injured foot. This is a graphic example of young children holding themselves as the culprits when their parents are abusive with them. This childhood response is often the first developmental stage in the process of forming a projective identification, where the child takes on herself the feelings projected on her by an abusive parent. It remained to be seen whether An would be vulnerable to the second element of projective identification, blaming her baby for the feelings that his expression of need triggered in her.

## *"My Baby Doesn't Stop Crying"*

The first weeks of little Tuan's life were uneventful, but when he was about 2 months old, An started complaining that Tuan cried for as long as an hour at a time, particularly in the mornings and at night. The pediatrician and the public health nurse who provided home visits did not find a medical reason for the crying and attributed it to colic. During one session, An described her concern about the neighbors' complaints and her concern that the manager of her apartment building would not renew her lease. The clinician asked An how it felt when Tuan cried. She responded that it was hard, especially because he cried in the mornings when it was time to go to work and in the evenings when she was tired from the workday and facing a long night alone with him. The clinician wondered aloud whether Tuan might be having a hard time with the transitions at the beginning and the end of his day. An ignored this comment and mentioned that the public health nurse recommended that she go to another room in order not to hear the crying, but this only made Tuan cry more. The clinician turned to the baby and said, "*Tuan, your mom is telling me that sometimes you cry, and she doesn't know what you need. She tries everything, and it is hard for her and for you because she doesn't know how to help you.*" An took a toy and moved it in front of Tuan's face, saying, "*Yes, yes, yes, you cry a lot . . . ,*" as if confirming what the clinician had said. Tuan smiled and the mother smiled back, but she then pulled back and remained quiet. The clinician asked her again how it felt when Tuan cried, and An's face contorted suddenly in an angry expression that the clinician had never seen and that went away instantaneously. She then went back to her usual neutral affect and said that she was tired.

The clinician then took a chance and commented that she had just seen an expression in An's face that she had not seen before, as if she was angry with Tuan for crying. An looked at the clinician with a puzzled expression, and the clinician held An's gaze with an interested, accepting facial expression. While they looked at each other, the clinician thought that An's response reminded her of the duality in projective identification, in which a person holds polarized perspectives in an interaction, such as being simultaneously a victim and a victimizer. After a brief silence, the clinician said, "*We talked about Tuan crying and your frustration. Does anything come to your mind when he cries? Or right now?*" An was silent for a while, clearly struggling to regulate her emotions. She then said in a chocked voice, "*I remember crying many times, and my mother just being impatient or angry about my crying. She never asked me what happened to me. She just scolded me for crying.*" She then returned to the memory of her fall from the ladder and her mother's punishing response, saying she wished her mother had been more patient and more interested in her feelings and in what made her cry. The longing for a protective maternal response to her childhood fears was touchingly apparent in this response. The clinician understood this exchange as an expression of An's readiness to explore the possible connections between her past experiences as a child and her present experiences as a mother.

The ensuing conversation confirmed the clinician's impressions that An's interactions with Tuan when she was alone at home with him paralleled her own interactions with her mother when she was a child. She disclosed with deep shame that she sometimes yelled at Tuan to shut up or went to the bathroom and closed the door in order not to hear his cries. "*I do not want to be like that with him,*" she said. The clinician asked, "*If you could say what you wish your mother had said, what would it be?*" An answered, "*I wish she could have said, 'I am sorry you are crying. Are you OK? What happened to you?' She was just not interested in me.*" The clinician asked her, "*Do you think Tuan also wishes, in his own baby way, that you would say that to him?*" There was a profound silence following the clinician's question.

Tuan was kicking and babbling, while looking at his mother during this exchange. The clinician turned to him and said, "*It seems to me that your mommy wants to learn to be patient with you when you cry. She wants you to feel that she can support you and understand what you need.*" An looked at the clinician and nodded while smiling.

It was time to end the session. An gently told her baby that it was time to go. She took him in her arms and put him in the baby carrier. The clinician asked her how she was feeling as she was leaving the session. An answered, "*Better. Thank you.*"

This session was the last time that An reported Tuan's long, inconsolable crying. During subsequent sessions, the clinician asked if Tuan was still crying for long periods, and An consistently responded that this was not happening anymore. The clinician asked An what she thought had happened, and An said, "*After the time that we talked about it, I felt something change.*" "*What do you think changed?*" the clinician asked. "*I feel less stress when he cries, and I'm able to think about what he wants and how to respond to him. It is interesting that he does not cry that long anymore,*" An said. "*It sounds like you are more patient with him. Do you think maybe he learned that he can tell you how he is feeling and you understand what he needs?*" the clinician said. An nodded with a bright look, while turning to gaze at Tuan. "*Your mom feels very good that she can understand what you need and help you feel better, Tuan,*" said the clinician. An moved closer to Tuan and touched her nose with his.

This relatively straightforward conversation about crying enhanced An's reflective functioning, giving her the opportunity to understand her baby's crying by connecting with her own crying as a child. The first step was to help An turn inward to understand what Tuan's cry evoked in her. She was then able to make a conscious connection between her feelings about Tuan's cries and her painful childhood experiences with her own mother. Reaching this level of awareness led to a noticeable shift in her feelings toward Tuan that allowed her to respond to his needs in a loving and soothing manner, paving the way for positive experiences of co-regulation that hold the promise of becoming imprinted in Tuan's future self-regulation.

# Vignette 2. Prematurity

Preterm birth has become a public health issue in industrialized countries, with approximately 1 in 10 infants born before 37 weeks of gestation in the United States (Hamilton, Martin, Osterman, Curtin, & Mathews, 2015). Rapid advances in neonatal care have led to increased survival rates for infants born preterm, a benefit that should not obscure the importance of addressing two intertwined areas of risk: the risks to the baby's life, health, and developmental course and the mother's and father's immediate and long-terms emotional responses to these risks.

The etiology and epidemiology of prematurity are beyond the scope of this book, but perinatal clinicians need to learn about the many facets of this phenomenon. Reviews of current research on this topic serve as excellent introductions (e.g., Shah, Browne, & Poehlmann-Tynan, 2019).

Prematurity puts the infant's life and developmental course at risk. Mortality increases in proportion to the decrease in gestational age and is highest in babies born at less than 32 weeks gestational age (Simmons, Rubens, Darmstadt, & Gravett, 2010). Babies born prematurely are also at increased risk for health problems and neurodevelopmental disabilities; prematurity also entails less optimal self-reported quality of life for children and parents (Natalucci et al., 2017). Mothers and fathers experience intense psychological distress in response to fears for the baby's survival and well-being, violated expectations about a healthy baby, disrupted caregiving when the vulnerable infant requires a stay in the NICU that interferes with physical contact and normative routines, and intrusive medical interventions (Davis, Edwards, Mohay, & Wollin, 2003). This distress is compounded when the childbirth process endangered the mother's life and health.

The P-CPP model includes the perinatal clinician's physical presence in the NICU when appropriate to gain a firsthand understanding of the baby's condition, the quality of the interactions between the parents and the medical team, and the parents' response to the baby. Mental health consultation with the medical team and mediating between the parents and the medical staff can decrease mutual negative attributions that prevent constructive collaboration on behalf of the baby.

Clinicians who are not based in a hospital are also able to work effectively to support the parent–infant relationship using a variety of therapeutic strategies. Therapeutic intervention with parents of preterm babies must attend to the many facets of the clinical situation. Concrete assistance and crisis intervention are often the most immediate intervention modalities, along with emotional support to give the parents a safe place to process their reactions. Developmental guidance and psychoeducation about the specific features of the baby's condition help the parents understand the needs of the baby and learn caregiving practices that are adapted to the baby's individual characteristics. Insight-oriented framing of traumatic triggers is used when the specific stressful and traumatic aspects of the experience evokes maladaptive responses to the baby.

The following vignette illustrates how the clinician (G. C.) addressed feeding difficulties with a premature infant in the context of a therapeutic relationship that began late in the third trimester of pregnancy and spanned the transition from the NICU to the home.

## Guilt, Grief, and Fear as Sequelae of Premature Delivery

Alice, a 32-year-old European American woman, started treatment when referred by her OB/GYN physician because she was not gaining weight as expected. In the two P-CPP sessions before she delivered, she reported profound feelings of anger and sadness following the breakup of her relationship with the baby's father, who left the home abruptly when he found out that she was pregnant 6 months after they married following a 1-year relationship. The clinician's interventions in the two prebirth sessions focused on emotional support to help Alice process her anger and grief and to start differentiating between her anger at her husband and her feelings about the baby. She disclosed in this process that once she married her husband she thought they were both ready to have a child and stopped using birth control. She had assumed that her husband's not inquiring about birth control meant that he was open to a pregnancy, although they had not talked explicitly about it. She was shocked and dismayed when he responded angrily to the news of her pregnancy, and left her after she refused to have an abortion. This was Alice's first pregnancy. She did not have family in the area where she lived and felt isolated from her friends, who, she reported, were primarily interested in a casual lifestyle of partying and not interested in babies. It was clear from these initial interactions that pregnancy and motherhood represented a major life change for Alice with far-ranging psychological implications.

Alice delivered baby Hope at 27 weeks gestational age and a birthweight of less than 3 pounds. The baby was rushed for breathing support to the NICU, where she stayed for 13 weeks. Alice was discharged after 2 nights at the birth center, where she met with the clinician the day after giving birth and spoke about her guilt and grief for the premature delivery, attributing it to her failure to eat properly and gain adequate weight. The clinician expressed understanding and support, primarily letting Alice speak about the shock of the unexpected delivery, her fears for baby Hope, and her sense of foreboding in facing the challenge of raising a baby on her own. She did not articulate her self-doubt about her early decision to keep the pregnancy, but the clinician could sense this ambivalence clearly expressed in her body language, tone of voice, and content of her speech. The clinician chose not to follow up on these hints of ambivalence in order not to risk the premature mobilization of her defenses. The immediate priority was to support and reassure Alice as the foundational steps toward a therapeutic alliance that could promote the mother–baby relationship. There would be time to help Alice become conscious of her ambivalence and integrate it when it became a more salient clinical issue.

During the clinician's visit to the hospital, she and Alice agreed that they would meet regularly at the NICU as the setting for the treatment. However, Alice did not show up for the first appointment. The NICU nurses told the clinician that she had not come to visit the baby since the time she was discharged, and the clinician telephoned Alice at home to follow up on her not coming to the appointment. After asking about her overall well-being, the clinician asked Alice whether perhaps it was difficult to come and see Hope and the other babies in the unit. Alicia responded, *"Yes, it is very difficult to see how they are struggling to survive. It is so painful to watch the pain they are suffering with everything the doctors and nurses are doing to them."* The clinician responded, *"Yes, some of the interventions are very hard, and the doctors and nurses also wish they did not have to do them. They do all these procedures to help the baby mature in the outside world."* Alice was silent. The clinician offered to meet her at the NICU to explain the purpose of each procedure, adding that babies are better able to tolerate pain when there is a familiar and supportive person by their side. This explanation seemed to have some of the desired effect. Alice started visiting Hope, although not as often as the clinician and the medical team would have wished. She often seemed awkward and tense with the baby, but there were also moments of deep tenderness and interest in Hope's experience.

The clinician offered therapeutic support and psychoeducation either by phone or at the NICU during the 13 weeks of Hope's hospitalization. The physical barriers that prevented Alice from close contact with Hope were alienating to her, and she responded by feeling emotionally distant from her baby. One of these sessions offers a glimpse of her frame of mind and the resulting clinical intervention. Alice arrived at the NICU looked tired and irritable, and her first words to the clinician were, *"Coming to the NICU is very difficult. I cannot hold Hope in my arms because she is hooked up to so many devices. It is hard to watch how easily the nurses take care of her. I feel inadequate as a mother."*

The clinician validated Alice's emotional response, and commented that the nurses were at ease during the ministrations because it was their job and they had been doing it for years with many dozens of babies. She added, *"Alice, for you there is only one baby. For you, Hope is not a patient, she is your little daughter that you want so much to protect. It makes sense that you feel you are not as competent as the nurses are. For you, it is not a job, it is your life."* Alice responded, *"Yes, but I am afraid that Hope will be more connected to some of the nurses rather than to me."* The clinician acknowledged this possibility and gave it a benevolent interpretation, saying that indeed babies become connected to the people they know best, and that it was actually helpful for Hope to feel connected with the nurses who treated her, because this familiarity helped her feel more comfortable during the procedures she had to undergo. She added that babies can connect with several loving caregivers, and that Hope would connect more deeply with Alice as she spent more time with her.

Alice then said, *"I am very worried about her brain development. I don't know how being premature will affect her."* The clinician responded, *"Alice's brain needs human connection to grow because we humans are very social creatures. We need to be in a relationship with others to learn about the world, even when we are babies. Hope is very sensitive to what is happening to her. You can use your voice and your touch to give her a feeling of love and goodness to counter all the painful procedures that she cannot escape. You can talk or sing to her, and you can touch her gently to give her pleasure. That will help her connect with you, and it will also help you connect with her until the time when you are able to pick her up and hold her."* The clinician joined action to words as she provided this kind of developmental guidance, guiding Alice to approach the baby and talk or sing to her, while touching her gently. These interventions encouraged the beginnings of a tentative bond, as the clinician helped Alice notice that Hope seemed to relax and listen in response.

### Addressing the Baby's Failure to Gain Weight

The setting of the treatment changed to the clinician's office after Hope went home. During the first postdischarge session, Alicia came to the office looking tired, tearful, and irritable. She mentioned that the pediatrician said during the most recent pediatric visit that Hope was not gaining weight as expected, and that he would need to hospitalize her for nasogastric tube feedings if she stayed at the same weight for much longer. The clinician asked Alice, *"How was it for you to hear that information?"* Alice responded tearfully, *"I am afraid that she will die. I read on the Internet that babies as premature as Hope are at risk of dying."* The clinician validated her fears and sat quietly with Alice as she sobbed with deep anguish.

Hope became restless in her mother's arms and soon began to cry, perhaps in response to the tension in Alice's body. Alice promptly stopped her own sobbing and offered her the breast, but Hope struggled to latch on to her nipple and, after a few failed attempts, turned her head away from the breast. Alice forcefully shoved her breast into Hope's mouth, and the baby started to gag. This scene of maternal misattunement to the baby made the clinician focus on the specific details of what transpired between Alice and Hope during feedings. The clinician asked, *"When was the last time you breastfed Alice?"* She responded: *"Just before we came in. I fed her in the waiting area. I think that she is missing the nurses. I am sure she prefers to be fed by the nurses."* The earlier theme of maternal inadequacy and Hope's perceived preference for the nurses was surfacing again in this exchange.

The clinician made use of the mother–infant exchanges that she had observed earlier in the session to guide her response to Alice's perception of her daughter's rejection. She had observed a clear mutuality between mother and infant in social exchanges, in response, for example, to smiles, gazes, and signals of distress. Hope followed her mother with her gaze as she moved and made anticipatory body movements to collaborate when Alice picked her up. It seemed from these observations that feeding was particularly charged with negative attributions for Alice, and the clinician thought of the parallel between the baby's failure to gain weight and Alice's own difficulty eating and gaining weight during her pregnancy—a factor that Alice believed had led to the premature birth.

Seeking to understand Alice's experience when trying to feed Hope, the clinician asked, *"How do you know she is hungry?"* Alice responded, *"Because of the way she cries. Did you hear that loud cry? She only cries like that when she is hungry."* The clinician had only heard a brief cry, but she did not disconfirm Alice's misperception directly. She talked instead to the baby, saying, *"Your mom is trying to figure out what you need. Your mom was crying and maybe that made you sad too. You seem so happy now cuddled in your mom's arms. Maybe you just wanted your mommy to hold you."* Alice relaxed visibly. The clinician held a toy in the baby's line of vision, and Hope looked at it but did not reach for it. The clinician gave the toy to Alice, who put it next to the baby's hand, and Hope grabbed it and smiled. The clinician commented, *"Hope, you really prefer to be with your mother and to interact with her. You like it best when she gives you the toy."* The rationale behind this intervention was to foster a therapeutic connection in which Alice felt acknowledged as special to her baby. Alice felt inadequate as a mother. She also knew that the medical team was closely monitoring her competence through her baby's developmental progress. The clinician believed that the baby's weight gain and overall health could be promoted best by helping Alice feel special to her baby as the means of increasing her sense of agency as a mother.

When Alice and Hope returned for their second session, the clinician observed a repeat of the worrisome feeding interaction that had occurred in the first session. Hope cried, and Alice picked her up from the stroller and offered her the breast, which the baby avoided by turning her head away. As in the earlier session, Alice forced the breast into Hope's mouth as she said, *"If you don't eat, you will go to the hospital, they will put a tube inside you, and you will not have any other option, so just eat!"* Alice sounded frustrated and irritable, and the baby was making sounds of distress while continuing to avert her head away from the breast. Mother and baby were at an impasse that did not bode well for the establishment of a mutually satisfying experience around feeding and eating.

The clinician aligned herself with Alice's emotional experience as a way of promoting self-reflection. She said, *"You look very upset that she is not taking the breast. I am wondering, how do you feel when she turns her head in the opposite direction?"* Alice responded, *"I feel she is rejecting me. I just remembered when I was a child, I was hungry and my mother just ignored me when I asked to eat. I think that for many years I suffered from chronic hunger . . ."* The clinician reminded her that when she found out that she was pregnant her appetite decreased so much that she was not gaining weight. Alice responded, *"When my husband left, I wanted to die. He did not want us to have this baby . . ."* The clinician said, *"I see how hard you are trying to make Hope eat so she does not die. When you were pregnant, you wanted to die and you were not eating . . ."* Alice spontaneously linked what was happening between her and Hope with what she wished her mother had done for her. She said, *"I wish my mother had fed me when I was little and I was hungry. I wish she wanted to be with me during this pregnancy. I wish she could have been more available during the first part of my pregnancy, mainly after my husband left. She was very matter-of-fact about the whole thing."* The clinician acknowledged the pain Alice was experiencing and her fear about losing Hope. She then put Alice's feelings in the context of the emotional meaning of feeding and eating, saying, *"Even when you were little you knew that eating is a very special part of the relationship with one's mother. It is an intimate way of showing love and communicating with each other. For Hope, the pleasure of eating increases because she likes to be close to you. She likes you to hold her, because you are the most important person in her life. You now have a chance to feed Hope the way you wish your other had fed you.*"

The next time Hope cried and rooted toward the breast, she looked at her mother's face intently and reached out to Alice's mouth as her mother offered her the breast. Alice nibbled playfully on Hope's fingers, saying, "*This is yummy, I like it!*" Mother and baby continued this playful exchange while Hope fed. There was mutual pleasurable mirroring as Alice sucked her baby's fingers and her baby sucked at her mother's breast. The clinician thought to herself, "*Alice is repairing in her body the negative experience of feeding as a baby.*"

As the playfulness waned, Alice and Hope looked into each other's eyes as the baby continued to feed. Alice soon seemed a little bored, and the clinician suggested that Alice tell Hope a story while the baby was feeding. Alice remembered a story her grandmother used to tell her about three little pigs, each of whom wanted their milk prepared in a different way. She told the story to the clinician, saying that the mother pig prepared her piglets' cups of milk just the way each of them liked it. Alice said that her grandmother used to tell her this story while she was making food for Alice, and the clinician could sense Alice's longing to be fed both physically and metaphorically at this time of abandonment by her husband and her family.

The clinician used this "angel memory" to link Alice's benevolent childhood experience to her baby, turning to Hope and repeating the first words of the story Alice had told, "*Once upon a time there were three little pigs . . .*" Alice then took over in telling Hope the story. The clinician observed the typical elongated smiles, exaggerated facial nuances, and the rise and fall in the tone of voice that Daniel Stern called "normal baby voice." As Alice told Hope the story, the baby again put her hand in her mother's mouth as they smiled at each other.

When the clinician asked Alice how she felt this feeding had gone, Alice said with relief, "*So much better!*" She then revealed with a guilty expression that she had made it a habit to force-feed Hope in order to get her to gain weight, and she dreaded feeding times. The clinician commented sympathetically, "*I think food has a lot of meaning for you, both negative, because of your mom not listening to your hunger, and positive, because of your grandma's loving cooking for you. I think that now you can channel your grandma instead of your mom when you get ready to feed Hope.*" Alice responded that until this session she had not remembered the "Three Little Pigs" story, and it was amazing to realize how clear the details remained in her mind once she told the story aloud. The clinician commented that many childhood memories are like that—out of conscious awareness but exceedingly powerful once they emerge.

This vignette represents one significant moment in a 12-month course of treatment that ended when baby Hope turned 1 year old and was doing well both physically and developmentally. Developmental guidance, psychoeducation, and emotional support were integrated with targeted insight-oriented interpretation to elucidate the specific emotional obstacles that interfered with the establishment of mutuality in feeding between mother and baby. This intervention took place in the larger context of enabling Alice to differentiate between her enduring anger and grief at her husband's abandonment and her loving commitment to her baby. In this process, she became a "good enough mother" (Winnicott, 1971). Importantly, she also grew as a human being. While reflecting on the communication gulf that led to the end of her marriage, she said, *"I took for granted that he wanted what I wanted, and I never thought I needed to check with him before stopping birth control. I think he is a jerk for leaving me, but I also think I was readier to be a mother than he was to be a father. He wanted a long honeymoon, but I thought I knew better what was good for us because I wanted to settle down."* This empathic capacity to understand her husband's perspective while retaining her own point of view was a promising sign that Alice was moving from a wish-fulfillment stance toward adult relationships to a mature acknowledgment of the importance of communication to make these relationships work.

# Vignette 3. When Older Children Stay Behind: Helping Prepare Absent Siblings for a New Baby's Arrival

Preparing older children for the joys of a new sibling and the challenges of sharing parental love and attention is a normative stress of parenting, just as having a new sibling is a normative stress of childhood. This developmentally expectable life event becomes more stressful when there is a family separation. Many immigrant parents leave older children in the care of relatives in their home country in order to come to the United States in search of better opportunities to support them. They most often retain strong bonds of love and commitment to the children they left behind, along with a deep longing to be with them and an ongoing worry about their welfare. Distress for the separation is often compounded by guilt when they find new partners and create a new family. For the children left behind, the arrival of a new sibling they will not meet inevitably adds urgency to the questions all children have, with varying intensity, when they must accommodate to a new sibling: *"Does my parent still love me?"* *"Will the new baby replace me?"* These questions, whether spoken or unspoken, haunt parents who are separated from their older children, and must decide whether and how to tell these children about the new baby.

Involuntary migration to escape poverty and violence adds one more adversity to lives scarred by traumatic experiences that often begin in childhood and include traumatic events during the journey of migration. Avoidance and isolation of affect are two defense mechanisms that migrants often use to minimize the pain of family loss, particularly separation from their children. Other migrants report being preoccupied by thoughts about their absent children and by worries about their well-being. Phone calls can function either as a supportive mechanism to maintain family unity or as traumatic triggers for the pain of being apart and/or worries that the children are maltreated, neglected, or abused in the parents' absence. The effort to avoid these trauma triggers may result in a gradual loss of connection, as parents reduce the frequency of phone contact and children avoid meaningful exchanges with their parents during these calls.

Parental efforts at self-protection from the pain of separation from their older children can interfere with emotional investment in the new baby when avoidance and isolation of affect generalize across intimate relationships. The present vignette describes P-CPP interventions to help expectant parents integrate the new baby into an emotional framework that acknowledges their new circumstances and helps them grapple constructively with unresolved feelings about the sequelae of their migration decision.

## Including the Older Siblings to Make Space for the New Baby

Samantha was a 30-year-old Mexican immigrant who was 18 weeks pregnant with her third child when she came to treatment due to severe depression and PTSD symptoms that were first identified during her prenatal visits. During the first session, Samantha described the strain between her partner, Armando, and herself, because he was very happy anticipating the birth of his first child, while she was overwhelmed by guilt about her separation from her two older sons, ages 3 and 7. Armando was upset and disappointed that Samantha could not share in his joy for the new baby, but Samantha felt that celebrating this pregnancy entailed a betrayal of the older children by making the pain of separation less acute.

Samantha had come to the United States to escape from her violent and drug-abusing husband, leaving her children in her parents' care. Her husband saw the children occasionally and told them during these visits that he would "*hit her*" for leaving him. Her 7-year-old son described these threats during phone calls with Samantha, and said that he told his father that he would defend his mother but that his father laughed in response.

Samantha spoke more about her older children than about the baby she was expecting during the initial three sessions. She said she missed them immensely and wanted to do whatever was possible to reunify with them. She also talked about her husband's violence and the many losses that she had experienced throughout her life, including her beloved grandmother's death; losing part of her eyesight as the result of her husband's physical violence; and missing her country, parents, siblings, and most important, her two older children.

The content of these initial sessions made the clinician (G. O. B.) realize that Samantha's preoccupation with absences precluded her from enjoying the presence of a new life growing within her and the supportive presence of her relationship with Armando, a hardworking man who was lovingly committed to creating a family with her. This understanding framed the first goal of the therapy, which became helping her talk with her children about the topics that worried her about them. The clinician hoped that a meaningful dialogue with her children about the salient emotional topics that remained unspoken between them would free Samantha to make emotional space for Ramón—the name she and Armando had chosen for their unborn son.

Following this plan, the clinician asked Samantha during the fifth session how she told the children about her reasons for coming to the United States. Samantha responded that she had not told them because they were too small to understand. The clinician then asked whether the children knew about Ramón, and again Samantha said that they did not know. The clinician asked what she talks about with them during their weekly phone calls, and Samantha answered that she asks them about school and tells them to be good and obey their grandparents. She then added as an afterthought to her not telling the children about Ramón, *"How can I tell them that I'm pregnant? They know about Armando and they like him. Sometimes he talks to them when I call them, but I don't want them to feel that I stopped loving them, or that I'm replacing them with a new baby."*

The clinician commented that Samantha's feelings were understandable, but she wanted to offer a different point of view. She said that in her experience children do best when their parents talk with them about the important things that are happening in the family life, because that helps children not misunderstand or blame themselves for what is happening. In a long and emotional conversation over the following two sessions, the clinician and Samantha co-created an integrated trauma narrative and protective narrative that Samantha then used as a template to explain to her children her reasons for coming to the United States and for why she could not bring them with her and to tell them about her new pregnancy.

### Planning for a Courageous Long-Distance Conversation about Danger and Love

Highlights of this co-creation of a joint trauma/protective narrative involved the following dialogue. The clinician asked Samantha, *"How do you want them to understand what happened to all of you?"* Samantha was pensive, and after a silence responded, *"I want them to know that I love them with all my heart. That mommy didn't want them to keep seeing their father hitting and yelling at me. That is not good for anybody."* Samantha started crying. The clinician commented, *"It is hard to talk about feelings, especially when those feelings include difficult feelings, such as being hurt, scared, and abused."* Samantha kept crying. The clinician asked, *"Are you remembering those moments?"* Samantha nodded in assent. The clinician said, *"Now you are safe, and you are trying to keep your children safe.*" Samantha nodded. The clinician continued, "*You were brave to leave an abusive relationship, and you are being brave again in wanting to talk to your children about this. I think that telling them what you just said is very powerful. Maybe you can also talk with them about the feelings you think they have, so they know you understand them.*" Samantha responded, while crying, "*I didn't want to leave them behind, I wish I had them with me.*" The clinician responded, "*It was hard then, and I see how hard it continues to be.*"

Samantha then described the day she left her family. Her son was at school, and she was breastfeeding her 20-month-old son. She needed to begin her journey to the United States that day. After she finished breastfeeding, she passed her baby to her mother, hugged her mother and father, and left. She took the bus and did not look back, because it was very painful for her not knowing when she was going to see her baby again. She remembered her son crying and calling out, "*Mama, mama.*"

Samantha cried hard while describing these scenes, as if releasing tears for all the times that she had not cried before. Crying in a safe environment seemed to help her feel supported. From her posture and affect, the clinician was able to see that Samantha did not seem to be overwhelmed by her feelings. As the crying decreased, the clinician said, "*You allowed yourself to cry. How does it feel?*" "*It feels good,*" Samantha answered, and she and the clinician smiled together.

### Family Narrative and Family Album

Samantha came to the following session looking energized and holding a bag. "*I talked with them,*" she announced excitedly when she came into the office. "*Tell me about it,*" the clinician responded, matching her excitement. Samantha then described the conversation in minute detail, as follows.

"*Before talking with them, I called my mother to tell her that I wanted to tell them our story. She was worried that they would be upset, but I told her that is why I called, to ask her and my father to be more available to help them if they were sad and to confirm that what I told them was true. My mother was then open to my idea, and said that she would be with them in case they needed her. I called them by video. The two of them were together. I said, 'I want to tell you something. First of all, I want to tell you that I love you with all my heart.' Then I asked, 'Do you know why I came to the United States?' Emilio answered, 'I don't know, Mom, to send us money?' My little boy Tony shook his head. I said, 'Emilio, you are right. I came here to look for a better life for you. I didn't want to leave you behind, but I didn't have a choice. It was not safe to bring you with me, and I asked grandma and grandpa to take* good care of you. I sent them money so you can go to school, have food, and a place to live.' 'But we want you here, Mommy,' Tony said. I felt that my heart was breaking. I remember what you said, and I told them, 'I know that you miss me a lot, and you want me there with you. I miss you too. Sometimes you are scared or sad for not having me with you.' Tony started crying. I told him that our good-bye was hard, and I can't imagine how it was for him to not see mommy anymore. I reminded them of my promise to bring them here and to do whatever it takes to do it. Emilio said, 'I know Mommy that you always do what you promise.' I tried to be strong, even though I had a knot in my throat. I said, 'I also came here because when we were with your father you saw how he hit me and treated me badly. I don't want you to live like that anymore. That is not good for anybody.' Emilio told me, 'I won't allow him to hurt you anymore mom, I am a big boy now,' Emilio said. I told him that he is a little boy, and I'm trying to protect him from that by getting out of that situation. Then Emilio said, 'Now you live with Armando; does he hit you?' I was so sad he asked that, but I told him, 'Armando is nice to me. He is a good man, and we are going to have a baby.' Emilio smiled, and turned to Tony, and said, 'See I told you.' I asked him, 'What did you tell him, Emilio?' He said, 'I told him that you were pregnant.' 'How did you know?' I asked. 'I heard when grandma was telling grandpa, but they didn't see me,' Emilio said. 'What do you think?' I asked. 'I think that is OK that I have a little sibling, Mommy,' he said. Tony cried and hugged my mother. I said, 'Tony, Mommy still loves you very much, even though you are going to have a little brother.' 'A little brother!' Emilio said. 'Yes, a little brother,' I confirmed."

Samantha seemed to be back in the conversation while retelling it, as if in a reverie. When she stopped, she took out a handmade album from the bag that she was carrying. The front page had the title, "Our family." Samantha explained that she remembered that in one of the sessions the clinician had mentioned the idea of making an album for her children to help them feel included. She took the idea seriously, and went to the most popular tourist places in the city, taking a picture in each place of herself touching her belly and placing each photo next to a photo of Emilio and Tony. Armando was also included in some of the pictures. The clinician was happy and impressed with Samantha's creativity in making the album. Every page seemed to contain a lot of loving care. On each page, she explained where they were, and included their names, pictures, stickers, and tags. The clinician asked how the children responded when their mother showed them the album by video. "*They loved it,*" Samantha replied proudly. "*I promised that I was going to send it back home, so they could look at it every time that they missed me.*" "*What a great idea!*" the clinician said enthusiastically.

During this session, Samantha touched her belly more often, and the clinician took this opportunity to make an intervention, asking her if she could talk to Ramón. The mother agreed. Speaking to Ramón, the clinician said, *"Ramón, your mommy is so happy. She now knows how to talk to your siblings about you."* Samantha looked at her belly while touching it, and said, *"We are all a family, and soon we will be all together."* The clinician felt a pang in her heart thinking that this might not be a realistic plan in light of the enormous obstacles to immigrant family reunification in the current national climate, but she decided to echo the hope behind this understandable wish.

As Samantha became increasingly more comfortable talking with her children, she reported feeling better. Her mood improved, her energy level and interest in her bodily changes increased, and she actively prepared for the baby's arrival. These changes underscored the growing bond that she was feeling with her unborn child.

## Moments of Connection

Samantha had by now fully integrated Ramón into her inner life. She spoke much less about trauma, fear, and loss and much more about the details of everyday life with Ramón and Armando. During one session when Ramón was 4 months old, Samantha was talking about applications for day care, and the baby started taking his sock off. The mother absentmindedly put the sock back on the baby's foot. The clinician noticed that the same sequence happened at least three times, and asked, *"Can we pay attention to what is happening?"* Samantha seemed puzzled but agreed, and both women watched Ramón in silence. Ramón was lying on his back, moving his arms while kicking very fast in an effort to take the sock off again, while looking at his mother and making little effortful, but happy, noises. The clinician asked, *"Does it seem like he wants to play with you? Could this be a game?"* Samantha answered, *"Really?"* The clinician said, *"Let's see."* Samantha smiled, while putting the sock back on Ramón's foot, and asked, *"Do you want to play with mommy?"* Ramón smiled, while making some babbling noises, and moved his body very fast in an effort to take the sock off again, which he did. Samantha started laughing, while getting close to him, and gave him a kiss. They played the sock game for a little longer. The pleasurable reciprocity between them was palpable. Ramón had arrived home.

At the end of treatment, Ramón's development was on target, and Samantha's depressive and PTSD symptoms decreased considerably. Several years after the completion of treatment, Samantha called the clinician to let her know that her family was reunified and together.

Three distinct but intertwined processes were involved in this effort to integrate the unborn baby into Samantha's internal family constellation. First, the co-construction between Samantha and the clinician of a joint trauma/protective narrative enabled the mother to give expression and bring greater resolution to the many traumatic events she endured. Second, describing for her children the key components of the trauma/protective narrative in developmentally appropriate ways and responding to the emotions they expressed opened a more authentic emotional connection with them and helped Samantha relate to them as full participants in her daily life and not only as victims of her abandonment. Third, creating a physical object in the form of a family album that portrayed her children as present in the city where she now lived helped her give concrete expression to her hope for family reunification. Through these endeavors, Samantha was actively creating her new family configuration. In order to make space for baby Ramón, she needed to both grieve the separation from her older children and validate the space that they took up in her heart.

# Vignette 4. Sequelae of Childhood Parental Separation during Pregnancy

Childhood separation from one or both parents is a lifelong source of fear, anger, and pain, even in situations when the child's quality of attachment was marred by exposure to maltreatment (Bowlby, 1973). Attachment to absent and/or maltreating parents often has a toxic quality, because the expectation of love and suffering are deeply intertwined in the child's experience, creating internal models of intimate relationships that predispose the child to reexperience and reenact in adult relationships the early emotional experiences of childhood. The risks to mental health increase when the now-adult encounters adverse external circumstances, with pregnancy emerging as a particularly vulnerable period for the reemergence of unresolved traumatic responses that are enacted in the parent's relationship first with the fetus and then with the baby. The following clinical case illustrates how long-forgotten feelings associated with childhood separation from a parent reemerged during pregnancy in the context of the realistic fear of deportation for the woman's undocumented immigrant husband.

## Repairing Early Grief to Create Space for the Baby

*Prenatal Period: "I Want My Child to Grow Up with a Father"*

Sonia was a 28-year-old bicultural, bilingual Mexican American pregnant woman, who came to treatment at the end of her second trimester owing to high levels of anxiety that affected her health and her everyday functioning. She experienced two or three panic attacks a week that made her afraid of dying of a heart attack and left her shaken for hours afterward. The panic attacks began soon after she found out that she was pregnant, although both Sonia and her husband planned and wanted this pregnancy, and their families were excitedly awaiting the birth of the grandparents' first grandchild. The attacks were so frequent and intense that Sonia stopped working and was unable to leave home unless her husband was with her.

During the foundational phase of treatment Sonia reported that she had emigrated to the United States at age 14 with her mother and siblings to join her father, who had been living in California for many years and worked tirelessly to reunite his family with him. The family came with a permanent residency card and became American citizens years later. Sonia's husband Matias, on the other hand, arrived from Mexico alone at age 15 and had not been able to obtain permanent residency. Sonia described her fear that her husband might be deported at any moment, explaining that she felt overwhelmed by anxiety when she heard about raids targeting undocumented immigrants in workplaces. She described herself as always alert to Matias's whereabouts and panicking when he did not answer his cell phone. Her fears of being separated from him were so pervasive that she often forgot whether she was having a boy or a girl. She had to ask Matias to remind her, and he patiently repeated that they were having a baby boy every time she asked. She said that no matter how hard she tried she could not imagine what her baby would be like.

This description made the clinician (G. C.) understand the severity of Sonia's impaired functioning and the importance of an immediate clinical intervention to decrease her crippling anxiety level and redirect her emotional energies toward an affective bond with the fetus. After listening empathically to Sonia's story, the clinician made a supportive trial interpretation, saying, *"It makes sense that given the current situation with immigrants you are fearful that your husband will be deported and you will be separated from him. It reminds me of your growing up separated from your father. Do you think there is a connection between how you grew up, and how frightened you are now?"*

Sonia responded positively to this connection, enlarging on the clinician's opening interpretation. She said that as a child she saw her father very infrequently, at most twice a year. She added that she never had a chance to say good-bye to her father, because he always left the house when she was still sleeping. She said, *"Children need to be with both of their parents. I cannot imagine my son growing up without his father."*

Sonia's readiness to understand emotionally the parallels between growing up without her father and her fear that her son would grow up without his father created a solid template for the therapeutic alliance. The clinician used this foundation to guide Sonia in learning to identify triggers to her anxiety and to engage in breathing exercises and visualizations of comforting scenes to forestall panic attacks, to diminish their intensity, or to recover more readily from them. Sonia was encouraged to identify internal events (bodily sensations, thoughts, and emotions), and environmental signals (sights and sounds) when she noticed her anxiety level increasing.

As an example, Sonia reported, *"When I hear Matias closing the front door every morning on his way to work, my fear comes up, my heart pounds, and I have difficulty breathing."*

In response to this description, the clinician invited Sonia to use this memory to practice a deep abdominal breathing exercise. She asked Sonia to sit in a comfortable position, monitor the sensations in her body, and bring her attention to her breathing. She asked her to focus on the parts of her body where she felt the breathing sensations most vividly—perhaps in her belly, as it rose on the inhalation and fell on the exhalation; or in her nostrils, as the air passed in and then out; or in her chest, as the lungs and rib cage expanded and released.

The clinician also helped Sonia practice visualizations of a place where she felt safe. Sonia described her maternal grandmother's house as a beautiful place where she always felt safe and happy, and went on to remember in vivid detail the sounds and smells of her grandmother's kitchen. She discovered with joy that she had an impressive ability to place herself mentally in this comforting setting.

After learning these exercises, Sonia told the clinician that she practiced them daily and found them very helpful, especially in response to intrusive thoughts of her husband's imagined arrest and deportation. The panic attacks disappeared almost completely in the last trimester, and Sonia's unmodulated stress responses and painful muscular tension significantly decreased. Sonia began to enjoy her pregnancy. She no longer forgot that she was having a baby boy. She reported with deep emotion that she and Matias decided to name the baby Sebastian in honor of her beloved paternal grandfather, who had died just before she and her mother and siblings joined her father in California.

Baby Sebastian was born at 39 weeks of gestation after an uneventful delivery. Although Sonia's panic attacks had ceased during the last trimester, the baby's birth triggered a new manifestation of a "ghost in the nursery" that took up residence in Sonia's internal life during the immediate postnatal period.

### The Immediate Postnatal Period: "If I Sleep, People Disappear"

Sonia attended her weekly P-CPP sessions and made good use of the therapeutic space to continue processing her fears that Sebastian would grow up without a father, putting these fears in perspective, and deriving joy from her relationship with Sebastian.

When Sebastian was approximately 4 months old, Sonia started to report feeling increasingly frustrated because of the persistent lack of sleep that began after the baby's birth. Although Sebastian was now sleeping through the night, Sonia reported that she could not allow herself to sleep deeply. She got up several times during the night to go to the baby's room and check on him "*just to make sure he is in his crib,*" and she sometimes woke the baby up just to make sure of his presence. She described an increase in anxious feelings aggravated by exhaustion.

The clinician was alerted to the emotional weight of Sonia's need to make sure that the baby was in his crib, and she asked what made her think that Sebastian would not be there. Sonia responded: "*If I do not see him, I think that he is not here with me, that he disappeared. I have the urge to go to his bedroom and wake him up. I love the way he looks at me when I wake him up. But sometimes it is very difficult for him to go back to sleep. I am noticing that now Sebastian is the one who wakes up even before I go to his crib. It is getting very difficult to help him to go back to sleep.*"

The clinician understood that Sonia's actions were shaping Sebastian's sleep–wake rhythms, with the potential consequence of creating disrupted sleeping in the baby. Instead of providing developmental guidance about sleep hygiene, however, the clinician focused on Sonia's motivation for waking the baby as the most promising strategy for changing her behavior. She said, "*It seems that going to his bedroom and waking him up helps you to be certain that he is in his crib. Tell me what happens when he wakes up?*" Sonia thought for a moment, and said, "*Oh, I just remembered the feeling I had as a child of waking up in the morning and not seeing my Dad, and nobody explained to me what happened to him. He would come back when I was not expecting him, but he would disappear again without saying anything.*" Sonia remembered her anguish about not knowing where her father had gone but being scared to ask, for fear that asking where he was would get her in trouble. She added tearfully that it was not until she was about 8 years old that she realized that when her father "disappeared" he was returning to California after a family visit. Knowing that he actually was somewhere came as a big relief to her. Until then she had the idea that her father could simply disappear and reappear for no clear reasons. Nobody in the family thought that it would be helpful for a small child to give meaning to the father's absence and to say good-bye to the father she loved.

Sonia sounded very sad, and the clinician reflected, "*What a difficult experience for you, to have your father disappear without notice when you were so small. You probably thought that he disappeared during the night because you were still learning that people and things continue to exist even when we don't see them. You know, small children believe that things disappear when they don't see them. Of course you wished that your father would wake you up and reassure you that he would come back. I am thinking that maybe sleep became a threat for you, because bad things could happen while you were sleeping. Maybe you thought that separation from your dad meant that he abandoned you.*" Sonia looked thoughtful, and said, "*Separation . . . that is what I experienced when Sebastian was born. I remember feeling then what I feel now. Giving birth was a way of separating from the baby I held for 9 months . . .*"

This poignant statement illustrated Sonia's unconscious association of giving birth with being abandoned, as the baby that she felt as a visceral part of herself became a separate person with his own individuality who abandoned her just like her father had done. She equated the baby's absence from her body with her father's earlier absence from her life. Perhaps she was checking and confirming her own physical integrity in checking to confirm that Sebastian was where he belonged.

The clinician responded, "*Are you saying that you miss the feeling of Sebastian inside your body in the same way that you missed your father when you woke up in the morning?*" Sonia laughed briefly, and said, "*I think I really do! Do you think that is crazy?*" The clinician smiled back as she answered, "*It is not crazy at all! You are teaching me that separation can take many forms, but the feeling of missing the person remains the same.*"

This insight had a beneficial effect. Sonia looked more relaxed and well-groomed in the following session, and she reported that during the previous week she had told herself that her baby was where he belonged, she stopped waking up to check on him, and Sebastian was sleeping better. She continued talking about her fears as a child that people disappeared, adding that she wished her mother could have explained to her the reasons for her father's intermittent presence and repeated departures. She also disclosed that she had summoned her courage to ask her mother why she never told Sonia about her father's departures, and her mother responded that she wanted to protect Sonia from saying good-bye and feeling sad.

This conversation with her mother redefined Sonia's relationship with her. She made a shift in her identification with the "mother who did not protect her children from being raised without a father" to a more positive identification with the mother who wanted to spare her child pain. Her mother's benevolent motivation was sufficient to elicit Sonia's forgiveness for her misguided attempt to spare her daughter pain.

This vignette illustrates the long-term effects of early parental separation. In the words of Fraiberg et al. (1975), "The 'ghosts' that hover in the nursery are the painful remnants of the parents' past—the unresolved feelings associated with early relational disturbances and trauma in their childhood" (p. 388). The attainment of object constancy as a cognitive achievement had been derailed for Sonia by the emotionally charged, sudden, and unexplained disappearances of her father, giving rise to a lifelong fear that she could not rely on the stable presence of loved ones. The panic about her husband's deportation that had haunted Sonia earlier in her pregnancy derived its force from an unstable sense of object constancy at both the cognitive and emotional levels. Sonia released her baby from the grip of her ghostly fears of separation when she realized that she was equating her baby with her absent father and worrying that Sebastian would disappear in the night the way she once imagined her father had disappeared. Although the ever-present possibility of her husband's deportation remained an urgent concern, Sonia used her new self-understanding to better compartmentalize this fear so that it did not interfere as much with her daily functioning. Her newly found self-confidence showed that even painful realities can be manageable when not compounded by the projection of unresolved early affective experiences.

# Vignette 5.  Growing Up in Foster Care: Impact on Pregnancy and Motherhood

The inadequacies of foster care as a respite placement for maltreated children are well known, and it is beyond the scope of this vignette to describe its failures to fulfill its stabilizing and protective goals as a social institution in spite of the commitment and professionalism of many individuals involved with it in a variety of roles. Children who enter foster care are burdened by experiences of abuse and/or neglect and may show emotional and behavioral disturbances that pose caregiving challenges for foster parents and their families. Multiple changes in foster care placement, failed adoption efforts, maltreatment in the foster home, repeated failed family reunification, and differential treatment for children of color are frequent pathogenic institutional features of life for children in foster care (Smyke & Breidenstine, 2019). When these conditions occur, the chronic absence of supportive and dependable substitute caregiving relationships that help the child cope with the traumatic sequelae, sense of abandonment, and self-blame inherent in early maltreatment places the child at risk of marked disturbances in attachment that can arrest development and take a cumulative toll on the child's health and well-being over the lifespan. The present vignette describes how treatment addressed the impact of such experiences in a pregnant young woman who became overwhelmed by the physical changes in her body and the emotional challenges of caring for someone other than herself. The treatment helped her to address the urgent question she posed to the clinician (M. A. D.) as well as herself, namely, *"Nobody cared for me ever; how can I care for somebody else, including my own child?"*

## "Nobody's Child"

Shavon was a 25-year-old biracial African American/European American woman, who was 11 weeks pregnant with her first child when she came for treatment because of moderate depression and anxiety. The prenatal clinic social worker who made the referral told the clinician that Shavon's European American teenage mother abandoned her at a neighborhood church when she was 1 day old, and Shavon was placed in foster care, where she moved through several homes and failed adoptions until she gained emancipation at the age of 16. The social worker also reported that there were two substantiated instances of physical abuse when Shavon was in foster care, and that she had been in three different therapeutic group homes as an adolescent due to behavioral problems.

During the foundational phase of treatment, Shavon did not answer directly when the clinician asked about the circumstances of her pregnancy. Instead, she readily disclosed in a flood of words mixed with curses and street slang that she became sexually active at age 11, engaged in risky sexual behavior that included unprotected sex with multiple partners and a history of recurrent STDs, and she felt fortunate that she had not gotten pregnant as a teenager as her mother had. When the clinician asked Shavon how she explained her multiple relationships, she replied, "*I guess you ask 'cause I've been with a lot guys, right? I own that! You know, I'm looking for the love of my life; that person that gets me for who I am!*" She then said that she became pregnant following two sexual encounters in one night involving two different African American men she had met at a nightclub. She said she had seen the men at the club before but did not know them well, and decided to keep the pregnancy without telling them about it, because she refused to do what her mother did to her—namely, "*abandon the baby.*" She also explained that currently she was in a "*long-term relationship of 5 months with a white older man* [38 years old]," whom she met online and accepted to help take care of the baby. Shavon added that although she identified as black, she thought that because she was biracial it would be good for the baby to grow up with biracial parents and to get the message early on that biracial relationships were fine.

The initial phase of treatment involved a process of adaptation for the clinician, because Shavon used colloquial African American expressions that the clinician had to learn as well as language laced with profanities that required some personal adjustment. To begin addressing the goals of treatment, the clinician first helped Shavon address her depression and anxiety symptoms using body-based and mindfulness-based interventions that Shavon liked very much. The clinician also made some exploratory suggestions about possible links between Shavon's depression and anxiety symptoms and her growing-up experiences, but Shavon dismissed the possibility of these links and denied any impact of her life adversities on her mood or sense of self.

As treatment progressed, Shavon's distress about her growing body became a recurrent theme. She blamed the fetus for these unwelcome body changes and experienced pregnancy as an incessant series of aggravations. Her frankly expressed anger at these changes provided an opening for clinical progress.

At the 15th P-CPP session, Shavon greeted the clinician with a forced smile, sat down in her regular chair, looked at her belly with an annoyed facial expression, slapped it sharply, and said in a loud and angry voice, *"Hey, you are getting too big! My clothes are so tight."* Looking at the clinician, she added, *"Look at me! Soon I'll burst out of my clothes!"* The clinician was startled by the potential risk for future child abuse entailed by Shavon's act of slapping her belly. However, she chose not to focus on the slapping, because she thought that Shavon was testing whether the clinician could be trusted. Shavon was implicitly asking through her actions *"Will you report me to CPS* [child protective services]*? Will you tell me that I am bad? Will you abandon me? Will you kick me out like everybody else, because you think I am no good?"* The clinician saw Shavon's stance as an opportunity to model an empathic resonance with her intense affect that might lead to greater self-understanding and a shift in her negative attributions to the fetus. Following this line of thought, she said, *"You are right that Baby Sofia is growing so fast!"* Looking at Shavon's protuberant belly with an accepting demeanor, she added, *"I can see it too. That means your body is going through sooo many changes to make room for your growing baby. And yes, you are right. Your clothes do look a bit tight, and I bet you are feeling uncomfortable . . ."* Shavon nodded in agreement, and replied in a mortified tone of voice, *"It's sooo uncomfortable! I'm so annoyed by so many fucking changes! It's rough! I had no idea that being pregnant would be this brutal! I wasn't expecting this . . . first, the fucking nausea and puking up the first 3 months and now look at me. I didn't sign up for all this shit!"*

With the clinician's encouragement and support, Shavon went on to reflect on what her fantasies of *"carrying a baby"* had been prior to becoming pregnant, and how different the reality was from her fantasy. The clinician validated Shavon's difficulties adjusting to the normal body changes of pregnancy, saying, *"I can image how difficult it must be for you—you are experiencing these body changes for the first time—everything is so new and unexpected."* Shavon again nodded in agreement, but this time there was a slight shift in her affect, which now revealed a tint of sadness, similar to previous sessions when she recounted her upbringing in different foster homes. She simply responded, *"Yes, it's fucking tough . . ."*

Remembering that Shavon had shown motivation and interest in a somatic experiencing exercise during a previous session, the clinician suggested doing such an exercise now, so they could understand together how Shavon was experiencing the changes in her body. She said, *"Let's do something a little different . . . let's try an exercise where you get to close your eyes, take deep full breaths through your nose, and begin scanning your body, like that time when we did the body scanning exercise to let go of tension in your body, the stress you were carrying in your body. Do you remember that exercise?"* Shavon agreed with some curiosity and excitement. The clinician proceeded to say, *"Great! Let's take deep full breaths and start scanning your body. If you feel comfortable, please say out loud each physical change that you notice in the moment, as you are scanning different parts of your body. You can begin the exercise with any part of your body. It's completely up to you."* Shavon, smiling, with her eyes closed, took deep breaths and embarked on the exercise. She first expressed discontentment with the size of her belly, which she described as *"a big watermelon."* Chuckling, she next described her breasts getting fuller, and added, *"that is the one change I don't mind about being pregnant!"* She then described the overall changes in her body shape and size, saying that now her body was *"round like a balloon, with no sexy curves whatsoever,"* and went on to notice that even her feet were getting *"big as canoes!"* Shavon had indeed begun retaining water, which caused her to have swollen feet, and her doctor was monitoring her for preeclampsia. The similes Shavon used were notable, showing her rich imagination and preoccupation with herself as a sexual being.

After the conclusion of the exercise, the clinician normalized Shavon's observations and provided psychoeducation on the many changes that a pregnant woman's body goes through, both externally, as described by Shavon, but also internally. She explained that hormonal changes not only affect the woman's physical appearance, but can also affect mood and basic biological rhythms, such as sleep and appetite. Shavon had been listening attentively, and now exclaimed, *"You know, this is the first time I stop and think about each of the things that has changed in my body. Hmmm . . .* [She became pensive for a moment.] *No wonder I now have a hard time fitting into my clothes! Come to think about it even my shoes are uncomfortable!"*

Looking at Shavon's belly, the clinician said, *"Sofia, your mother and I have been talking about how fast you are growing. As you grow, we are trying to figure out ways to make your mommy feel a little more comfortable while you are inside her. You still have a few months left inside your mommy. It's tricky for mama right now, but we're trying to figure out how to make her feel a little better, more comfortable because these changes will continue to happen in your mama's body as you grow."* The clinician then asked Shavon, *"Are you having a hard time giving up your favorite clothes to wear maternity clothes?"* Shavon replied in a heartfelt manner, *"Aw yeah! I ain't want to look fat! Though I think I already do . . ."* The clinician sympathized with the feeling, and asked if Shavon's boyfriend thought she looked fat. Shavon replied, *"No, I don't think so but other guys do!"*

It became apparent again that Shavon was still quite interested in her sexual attractiveness outside of her relationship with her boyfriend, but the clinician chose to pursue a more reassuringly reality-oriented course of intervention, and said lightly that pregnancy was a time-limited state and that Shavon would soon regain the appearance she had before the pregnancy. Shavon expressed relief that this would be the case, and the clinician proceeded to ask, *"Do you have other clothes that are more comfortable for you and that also have a little more room for your baby?"* Shavon disclosed that earlier that day she had realized that it was time to switch to her maternity clothes but was having trouble getting used to the idea. The clinician reflected on her feelings, saying, *"Thank you for sharing your struggles with me. I'm glad you feel comfortable telling me how you feel."*

The clinician then looked at Shavon's high-heeled shoes, and asked, *"You mentioned your shoes also feel uncomfortable. How are those shoes?"* Shavon answered with disappointment that those were her favorite stiletto shoes, but that they were not safe for her now that she was so big. She went on to describe an *"embarrassing"* incident in which she almost fell on the street while getting off the bus, and acknowledged that *"sadly it is time to wear lower-heeled shoes."* Looking at Shavon's belly, the clinician said, *"Sofia, your mother is already thinking about ways of keeping both of you safe and protected."* She then acknowledged that many women have a hard time making the transition from being young, sexy, and fashionable to wearing clothes that made them feel older and bigger. She reiterated that this change was for a short time only, saying, *"Your favorite clothes and shoes will be waiting for you after Sofia is born."* Shavon shrugged her shoulders, as if unsure, and said, *"I will give it a try and let you know how it goes. I guess I can wear a couple of cute maternity tops I just got this week, but I'm not promising anything, OK? I will change my shoes though. It was embarrassing that I almost fell down on the street . . . my shoes are da bomb* [nice] *but I guess they ain't for me right now."* The clinician said in an accepting tone, *"Let's see how it goes. I look forward to hearing all about it next week. Changing your shoes to something more comfortable sounds like a good plan as well as considering the other changes. I can see how difficult these changes are for you . . . but you are still willing to try. Sofia, your mama is trying really, really hard to wear different clothes and be more comfortable so there is a little more room for you to grow comfortably too."*

Shavon arrived at the following session wearing lower-heeled shoes and a much looser top with low-cut cleavage, and then revealed proudly that she still had some weeks left wearing her favorite jeans because *"a hair band did the trick for now!"* She had cleverly expanded the waistband using an elastic hair band as a new buttonhole. She had learned *"this trick"* online and reported with delight that her jeans were much more comfortable now. Here again Shavon showed intelligence and creativity in pursuing what was important to her.

The clinician acknowledged the important changes Shavon had

made this past week so she could feel more comfortable, praising her creativity in finding a solution for her tight-waist jeans to allow for some more weeks of wear. Shavon was beaming with satisfaction and pride as she listened to the clinician say that she was impressed by her creativity. The clinician also used this opportunity to continue reflecting with Shavon on her struggles adapting to her pregnancy-related physical changes. Shavon, revealing slight sadness, agreed how difficult it had been for her to be pregnant and stated that she did not understand why she was struggling so much, when in fact she was the one who had decided to keep her pregnancy. A state of confusion was evident during this part of the session.

Shavon revealed drastic mood changes in a later session, particularly increased irritation and outbursts of anger directed toward her boyfriend. She described herself as cursing and insulting him for not answering the telephone when she called, even if he had a valid reason, such as being at work. The clinician helped Shavon recognize how her boyfriend's behavior triggered her feelings of abandonment and rejection, which were in turn connected with the maltreatment she experienced while growing up.

This conversation led to Shavon speaking about her defiant and aggressive behavior. She revealed that she had had *"a short fuse"* since she was a child, and said that everybody (social workers, foster parents, potentially adoptive parents, and teachers) criticized her for losing her temper quickly. She stated, *"I always jump salty fast!* [I always get very angry quickly.]" She added that her anger got worse as a teenager, and this was the reason *"for my landing in three therapeutic group homes where I was physically assaulted by a staff person after a fight."*

The clinician took this opportunity to ask, *"Is that short fuse the reason you slapped your belly when you were upset that Sofia was getting too big?"* Shavon responded, *"You bet! She really got on my nerves!"* The clinician asked, *"Did you know that at about this time in pregnancy babies in the womb can actually feel what happens to them?"* Shavon responded with surprise, saying she had no idea. The clinician commented that the people she depended on hit her as a way of punishing her, so it was only natural that she would learn to hit when she wanted to punish someone, including her unborn baby. Shavon looked very sad. The clinician said, *"Can we think together of ways that you can be angry without hitting so you don't hurt the people you love?"* Shavon nodded wordlessly.

It was soon after this exchange that Shavon disclosed that she had attempted suicide twice during her adolescence by cutting her wrists with a box cutter. This was a new and very worrisome revelation that led to several sessions in which the clinician helped Shavon explore the details of the connections between her outbursts of anger at her

boyfriend and at times at her unborn baby, and her despair while growing up at the many episodes of abandonment, abuse, and neglect that
she had endured.

Telling her story enabled Shavon to grieve for the many losses in
her life. She spoke tearfully sometimes, and angrily at other times,
about not knowing her biological parents, having nobody who claimed
her as their child, never experiencing a stable family environment, and
the emotional instability of so many unknowns in her life, such as who
her own parents and the father of her baby were and how she could
find them. Through this process, Shavon was able to explore, recognize, and understand that her outbursts of anger, sexual risk-taking
behaviors, alcohol abuse, experimentation with drugs, delinquent
behavior, and even suicide attempts to end her pain were efforts to
cope with an unbearable external and internal reality. The clinician
helped bring coherence and forgiveness to her trauma narrative by
helping her link her behaviors to the events that happened to her and
the feelings aroused by those events. The clinician also brought Shavon's attention to the small kindnesses that she remembered in her
experiences with others and to her own fortitude in standing up for
herself and seeking emancipation at 16 years of age. In this process of
self-understanding, Shavon's affect and body language began to shift
markedly from anger and defiance to soul-baring sadness and sorrow.

### "Let's Make Room for Two"

During one of these sessions, Shavon talked about her resentment
that being pregnant had completely changed her lifestyle. She could
no longer go out to bars with friends nor have an active sex life; she
had to keep a stable job to cover her new needs; and she needed to
wear "*old women's rags.*" She also elaborated on her wish to have the
freedom to choose what she wanted to do with her life instead of feeling trapped by pregnancy-related obligations. She said she wanted to
"*not depend on others or be tied to anyone.*" For Shavon, being a mother
meant renouncing her self-protective image as a sexy, young, desirable
woman. Throughout this time, the clinician was empathically present,
holding both Shavon and baby Sofia in mind. The clinician understood
that there was deep suffering beneath Shavon's anger and resentment
toward her unborn baby and her boyfriend. Shavon experienced her
pregnancy as a reminder that no one had created the physical and
emotional space for her, and she resented feeling pressured to do this
for somebody else—namely, her baby.

During this time in the treatment, Shavon grieved over the tragedy of being abandoned as an innocent newborn baby by her teenage

mother, and painfully remembered being "*bounced from one foster home to another as a young child*" because "*no one wanted*" her. With a mixture of sadness and anger, Shavon professed, "*No one gave me a home; no one loved me or cared about me. Many times I went hungry, and no one gave a damn about me! Why do I need to do this for someone else? I just don't know . . . no one ever did this for me.*" The clinician validated Shavon's reality by saying, "*It is so unfair that you had such a hard life as a young child. I now understand how hard it must be for you to make room in your heart and your life for somebody else . . . and also in your body for your baby girl . . . No one did that for you . . . You know it's so difficult to do something one has never experienced . . . no wonder it's so hard for you to do all these things.*"

The clinician's unfailingly empathic stance allowed Shavon to reveal in one of the sessions what she called her "*real fear*" that she would also abandon her baby once she was born, just as her mother did. She said very sadly, "*I was a burden for my mother. This may be too much for me to handle as well.*" It took a number of sessions of consistent emotional support to help Shavon entertain the possibility of relinquishing her baby for adoption without crippling guilt or fear of condemnation by the clinician. She became increasingly at ease as the clinician normalized both her wish and her fear of repeating her mother's story of relinquishing the baby for adoption. She accepted as realistic her worry that she did not have the support of a parent or relatives to raise her child. These sessions were very emotionally charged, with Shavon cursing loudly in anger or crying convulsively with much grief as she described her feeling devastated when prospective adoptive parents would "*give up on her*" owing to her continuous behavioral problems and she transitioned back to foster care.

During these sessions, the clinician normalized Shavon's feelings of anger for not having experienced the consistent care and support of caregivers to help her cope with so many traumatic changes and experiences in her early life. The clinician also provided psychoeducation about the effects of developmental trauma on child development, including placing children at risk of having behavioral problems and mood disorders, such as depression and anxiety. Shavon responded well to the developmental guidance, because it both validated her early experiences and gave her a deeper understanding of how much these adverse life experiences had affected her psychologically, physiologically, and relationally.

The benefit of this approach was clearly shown in Shavon's self-care. She kept all her prenatal care appointments in the latter stages of her pregnancy, and proactively obtained additional resources to improve her financial situation and increase her social support network. She enrolled in the Special Supplemental Nutrition Program for

Women, Infants, and Children (WIC), obtained a free car seat, and attended weekly prenatal support groups. To address her persistent fears of abandoning her baby after birth, the clinician helped her take note of how different her situation was from her teenage mother's situation, because she had supports her mother probably did not have. She also said that, should Shavon decide that she wanted Sofia to be adopted, the clinician could help her think through how she could do it safely in a way that was good both for Sofia and for herself, without having to leave the baby on the steps of a church as her own mother had done. It was noteworthy that Shavon never again slapped her belly even when she was very upset.

As her due date approached, Shavon spoke about her fears of going through labor and delivery, but was able to hold her baby's experience in mind, making comments such as, "*My little bae. You must be sooo squished in there.*" She also used wording that she heard the clinician use. While smiling and caressing her belly, she once said, "*Soon you'll come out and stretch out your little legs and arms. Mama has gotten you a tiny but cute crib, and you'll sleep next to me. You'll see. You'll like it. It's hot pink!*"

Sofia, a healthy 8-pound baby, was born without complications on Shavon's due date. Shavon responded to caregiving with a mixture of intense positive and negative feelings for her baby, struggling with impatience and anger but also experiencing "*more love than I ever felt in my life,*" and taking great pride and joy in the baby's responsiveness to her. She continued to contemplate what it would feel like for her to give her daughter up for adoption, but her love for the baby always prevailed. To support Shavon during this time of high stress and adjustment, the clinician and the pediatric social worker arranged for additional visits by the home-visiting nurse and made provisions to provide respite care for Shavon during the week.

During this time, Shavon also began contemplating looking for the two men she had slept with the night she got pregnant to try to figure out "*who the baby's daddy was*" and see whether he wanted to meet baby Sofia. These were very emotional sessions for Shavon, who expressed both her fears that these men would reject Sofia and her wish to protect her baby from this response because she knew firsthand how it felt to be rejected.

Treatment continued as needed for 5 years, to stabilize Shavon's complex psychopathology and to ensure her child's safety and well-being. Memories of physical abuse emerged forcefully during this period in response to Shavon's developmentally expected behaviors, including crying as a baby, temper tantrums as a toddler, and negativism and defiance as a preschooler. The treatment format was a combination of dyadic sessions using CPP and individual sessions with Shavon to consolidate her capacity for affect regulation and her integration of love and hate for Sofia and others who were close to her.

The termination phase lasted 6 months to enable Shavon to process safely her anger and despair at abandonment triggers. Sofia was a happy and healthy child with her mother's quick temper, but developing an age-appropriate capacity for self-regulation, good enough relationships with teachers and peers, and an exuberant interest in learning. Shavon had a stable job at a restaurant. She changed boyfriends several more times during these years. This part of her life remained edgy, but she protected Sofia by never bringing new lovers to the house. When she planned to stay out overnight, she left Sofia with the former foster parent who had supported her emancipation and had become a surrogate grandmother for her daughter. She was also conscientious with birth control after a series of conversations with the clinician in which she explored how many children she wanted, and decided that she would not get pregnant again until she was sure she met the love of her life.

This case illustrates the value of a flexible approach to treatment whereby the decision to end treatment is dictated by clinical stability and not by external considerations, such as agency policies, funding constraints, and the dictates of an intervention model. Society had failed Shavon in major ways by not providing her with a safe caregiving environment. It was only fair that she be allowed to find a place to heal from her lifelong maltreatment in her own time and at her own pace.

# Vignette 6.  Rage in Pregnancy:
# Reenacting Childhood Exposure to Domestic Violence

Witnessing domestic violence, also referred to previously as intimate partner violence or IPV, places children at risk for developmental and psychosocial problems that can adversely affect later development, with emotion dysregulation and problems in impulse control as salient features that play a major role in adjustment difficulties (see Section I, and Schechter, Willheim, Suardi, & Serpa, 2019, for a review). It is important to note that IPV frequency and lethality is highest when it involves male violence against their female partners, but in a study we conducted with 101 women seeking prenatal care at our county hospital we found that the women self-reported high rates of perpetrating as well as being the targets of IPV (Narayan et al., 2017). Although the IPV rates decreased during pregnancy, a significant portion of the women reported that the violence continued during the pregnancy. Specifically, 56% of the women reported that their partners perpetrated IPV against them before the pregnancy, and 14% said that the violence was ongoing during the present pregnancy. In close comparison, 54% of the women reported that they were physically aggressive with their partners before their pregnancy, and 20% acknowledged that they continued to perpetrate IPV during the current pregnancy. These figures, reported by women attending prenatal care who were neither receiving nor seeking mental health services, highlight the importance of asking pregnant women about both being victimized by and perpetrating IPV.

The present vignette describes how specific components of P-CPP were implemented with a pregnant woman who was distraught about her physical aggression against her partner and the father of her baby, but felt unable to control her outbursts of violence. The mostly egodystonic nature of her aggression was an important prognostic feature of her readiness for change. Treatment involved a combination of psychoeducation about the etiology of aggressive behavior and the impact of IPV on adult and infant health; insight-oriented exploration linking memories of her parents' violence as manifested against each other, her, and her siblings; and body-based and mindfulness interventions.

## When Maternal Aggression Endangers the Infant's Safety

Alessia, a 24-year-old European American woman, was referred for treatment when she was 16 weeks pregnant owing to current moderately severe depression and a history of episodic major depressive episodes starting in adolescence. She also described several incidents of perpetrating IPV in the course of her 4-year relationship with Johnny, the baby's father, ranging from mutual verbal abuse to Alessia's hitting and throwing objects at Johnny. She denied that Johnny was ever physically aggressive with her.

### "I Can't Stop My Rage!"

During the foundational phase of treatment, Alessia downplayed the severity of her depression, and focused instead on wanting treatment to control her aggressive outbursts, because she was afraid that Johnny would leave her and that she could hurt her baby. When the clinician (M. A. D.) asked her about her memories of anger while growing up, Alessia responded that when she was 7 years old she saw her mother hit her father on the head with a broom. Remembering her feelings at the time, she said, "*I was proud that my mom fought back. She later told me that my father never hit her again, because she taught him a lesson.*"

The clinician thought to herself that Alessia had likely suppressed her fear and horror in witnessing what must have been a loud and frightening scene. She preserved instead what her mother wanted her to learn: to overcome victimization by aggressively fighting back. Indeed, Alessia went on to report with pride, "*My mother told me I should never let a man hit me, and I should always defend myself if a man ever tried to hurt me.*" The clinician took note of the contrast between Alessia's earlier statement that she wanted treatment to help control her aggression and her present identification with her mother's admonishment that she should fight back in order to protect herself. Here again the suppression of vulnerable feelings in response to witnessing her parents' violence was likely at work.

After a tumultuous marriage, Alessia's parents divorced when she was 9 years old. Her father later remarried, moved to a distant city, and had three more children with his new wife. Alessia reported that she had a close relationship with her mother, but that she lost contact with her father except for greetings over the Christmas holidays and birthdays. Her father's abandonment following his wife's "*standing up for herself*" might have echoes in the present in Alessia's fear that Johnny would leave her if she continued to be physically aggressive with him.

When Alessia arrived to her sixth therapy appointment, she seemed distracted and almost tripped over a chair on her way into the office. The clinician expressed concern and asked Alessia if she was all right. Alessia minimized the incident, responding, "*It wasn't as bad as it looked. I was close to falling down but I didn't.*" The clinician expressed relief she did not fall and said, "*Many people get frightened even if they don't actually fall.*" Alessia listened attentively, and then said, "*Come to think of it, my heart is still beating fast . . . It was scary that I almost fell down, especially because I'm pregnant. But like I said, I'm glad that it didn't happen. I just need to be more careful when I am walking and pay attention to where I am going.*"

Something in Alessia's heavy tone of voice made the clinician think not all was well, and she asked Alessia how things were for her. Looking sad and remorseful, Alessia said that she was feeling absent-minded because "*something*" had happened the night before. The clinician replied, "*So there is something that seems to be worrying you.*" Alessia then told the clinician that she had "*once again lost her temper*" and hit Johnny in the face and chest several times with a closed fist following an argument. The clinician commented that this outburst was indeed worrisome, and asked Alessia to describe what prompted her aggression. Alessia looked down at her belly, and remained quiet for a few seconds as she wiped off the tears that had begun rolling down her face. As she began speaking, however, her sadness quickly turned to anger. She said that she became "*enraged*" when she discovered that Johnny had lied to her "*again.*" She explained that Johnny had told her that he would be at work all day, but instead he spent the afternoon with his 6-year-old son and ex-wife. She followed this brief description with a torrent of curses about Johnny's untrustworthiness, spoken in loud voice and with a contorted facial expression.

The clinician commented that she could see how angry Alessia was that Johnny lied to her, and then said, "*I noticed something that I want to check with you. Just before you started describing how Johnny lied to you and became so angry, you looked very sad and quiet for a moment, and started crying. Then you changed suddenly from sadness to anger. Did I see it right? Is that how you also felt?*" Alessia responded that the clinician was right, she was sad at first, because she hated it when she hit Johnny, but then she remembered how "*sneaky*" Johnny had been, and the sadness turned into anger.

The clinician commented, "*You know, something I notice a lot is that it is easier for many people to be angry than to be sad, because anger makes us feel strong.*" Alessia agreed with interest. The clinician went on, "*What do you think about slowing down a little so you can tell me step-by-step the events that led up to your hitting Johnny and the feelings in your body when that was happening?*" Alessia agreed. She first described feeling tense and angry with Johnny when she could not reach him on his cellular phone. When he finally answered the phone, he told her that he was still at work. However, Alessia could hear his son in the background calling him. When Alessia realized that Johnny was not at work but with his son, she threw the phone against the wall, began pacing the room, and felt overwhelming anger *"taking over"* her. The clinician asked Alessia to describe how it felt in her body to be taken over by this anger. Alessia thought for a while, and spoke slowly and reflectively as she replied, *"My blood began to boil, and I felt how it rushed to my face. I felt hot all over my body. I felt like I was going to explode in anger, like a ticking bomb, ready to explode. I felt like I was blazing in anger. It felt awful!"*

When Johnny finally arrived home, Alessia said that she began yelling and hitting him on the face and chest with her fists as hard as she could. In response, Johnny simply covered himself to avoid being hit in the face. The clinician then asked Alessia whether she remembered how she felt as she was hitting Johnny. She stated, *"Everything happened so fast, and the only thing I remembered was feeling furious at Johnny. I was shaking in rage for his having lied to me."* When she no longer could hit Johnny, she described being inundated by a feeling of relief, but also guilt at the realization of what she had done to Johnny. Alessia then began sobbing as she told the clinician, *"I know what I did was wrong, but I couldn't control myself. My anger once again took over me. I cannot reason when I get angry."*

The clinician helped Alessia process these conflicting feelings, and explored with her other situations when she had felt like this in the past. She recalled several incidents when she *"lost control of herself"* involving her ex-boyfriends starting during adolescence. Every one of these episodes had involved perceived betrayals: the boy flirting with someone else, or not showing up for a date, or breaking up with her. The clinician asked, *"Do you think there could be a connection with your father in what all these episodes have in common?"* Alessia denied it, saying that she never liked her father and was glad when her mother left him. Over time, however, the clinician kept bringing up Alessia's father, his remarriage, his three new children, and his walking out of Alessia's life. In one particular session, the clinician asked Alessia how she felt about Johnny having another son. She said, *"I hate that kid! He never has enough of his father; he is always calling Johnny for one thing or another."* Over time, she came to realize that she was feeling protective of her own baby, worried that Johnny would leave her and the baby to return to his older son and make her and their baby feel abandoned as her own father did.

Along with making connections between past and present, the clinician also provided psychoeducation about the impact of violence on the fetus and on the baby and explained that young children learn to express anger safely when they learn how from their parents. Alessia said sadly, *"I could never learn that because my parents never taught me."* The clinician responded, *"You are right. It is very sad that you did not have that chance when you were little, but you are learning now just in time to share your new learning with your baby."* Alessia replied, *"I want to give my child everything that my parents didn't give me. I want to give my baby a home where there are no fights or yelling, because I know how much that affected me. I remember feeling helpless when my father hit my mother. I want my child to grow up with parents who love her and who love each other, not hate or hurt each other."*

The clinician acknowledged and validated Alessia's wishes, and helped her recognize that by coming to therapy she had taken the first step in achieving her goals. She then spoke about anger and sadness as a normal part of the spectrum of human feelings everybody experiences, giving her permission to feel intensely without enacting those feelings in ways that hurt. The clinician concluded the session by teaching Alessia body-based self-regulation techniques (e.g., breathing, visualization, and grounding exercises) to practice during the week. She also did a verbal no-violence contract with Alessia, in which she agreed not to be physically aggressive with Johnny during the week and committed herself to practice one of the exercises she had learned whenever she felt that her anger was taking over her.

# Vignette 7. Father–Daughter Incest: Its Long Shadow on Pregnancy and Motherhood

Incest violates the basic need of children to be protected from developmentally inappropriate experiences. Usually coerced to keep it secret, children subjected to incest tend to experience confusion, shame, and self-blame. In their book *The Relational Trauma of Incest,* Marcia Sheinberg and Peter Fraenkel (2001) describe the maelstrom of conflicted emotions experienced by children in this situation. They write:

> When a child is sexually abused, she struggles with a number of relational binds, contradictions, confusions, and dilemmas. Some of these are about what to do: for instance, whether to attempt to resist the person who offended, or when this is impossible because of his threats, how to participate physically without participating emotionally. If he tells her that disclosing the abuse will break apart the family and hurt her mother and other family members, she may struggle between the desperate need to protect herself and her wish not to threaten the unity of the family. If she does decide to disclose, she may wonder if it is best to tell the nonoffending parent—who the child may fear will blame and be angry with her, or will side with the person who offended, or just not believe her—or to tell someone else and risk having the parent be angry that she wasn't told directly.
>
> Other confusions revolve around identity and meaning; how to reconcile her experience of the offending family member as a person who in some ways seems to love her, and even takes care of her, with her experience of him as someone who violates her trust, her personhood, her body; how to view the nonoffending parent as someone who can protect her in the future, when she hasn't in the past; how to view herself as a girl her own age, after participating in activities she may know are meant for adults; how to feel about her body once she has been violated; how to think that she is worth loving and protecting, and is a good person, when she has been abused; how to think of her whole family—as a good, safe family, or a bad, dangerous family. (pp. 3–4)

The psychological picture becomes even more complicated when the young girl is terrified and alienated from her abusive mother, perceives the father as the one reliably loving and protective attachment figure, and thinks of herself as the father's sexual partner and his source of comfort. The association of precocious sexual pleasure with the father as the person who inflicts both pleasure and pain creates confusion about the boundaries between sexual and nonsexual forms of intimacy. Women whose fathers sexually abused them have more negative scores than controls on measures of depression, sexual satisfaction, and communication with their partners about sex (Stroebel et al., 2012).

The psychological sequelae of childhood incest can have a powerful influence on the woman's response to pregnancy and becoming a mother. The present vignette illustrates some aspects of the treatment of a pregnant woman with a history of incest, whose love and loyalty for her father created conflicts in her relationship with her boyfriend and with her baby boy. Treatment addressed the couple's conflicts as well as the mother's conscious and unconscious attributions to the baby and ambivalence about physical contact with him.

## Anxiety, Emotional Numbness, and Rage in the Couple Relationship

Kezia was a 27-year-old European American woman in her 29th week of pregnancy when the medical social worker referred her for treatment owing to intense anxiety, self-reports of feeling disconnected from the unborn baby in spite of her approaching due date, and bouts of explosive anger toward her boyfriend Esben.

As the clinician (G. O. B.) explored with Kezia during the initial meeting how she understood her emotional difficulties, Kezia revealed that her father regularly had sex with her between the ages of 7 and 12 years, and added, "*I was never scared, I got used to it.*" She seemed unaware of the contrast between her conscious conviction that she "*got used to it*" and the anxiety, numbness, and outbursts of rage that brought her to treatment. When the clinician asked whether she had told anybody what her father was doing to her, Kezia responded, "*No. I think I didn't want to get him in trouble, and maybe I was afraid they would blame me because I allowed it to happen.*" She added, "*Things stopped when one day, my mother and my little sister arrived to the house unexpectedly and almost found us in bed. I guess he thought he was going to get caught. I felt relieved that I didn't have intercourse with him anymore, because I knew that it was not OK even though he told me that it was OK.*" Kezia's body language and tone of voice conveyed an affect of sad resignation while she spoke.

It is noteworthy in understanding the dynamics of Kezia's relationship with her father that he was the one protective figure that she mentioned when the clinician asked her about childhood moments when she felt loved, safe, and understood (evoking "angels in the nursery") during the foundational phase assessment. She narrated specific episodes when he protected her from her mother's harsh punishments, played with her, and taught her to bicycle, swim, and go on long hikes in the beautiful nature preserve surrounding her hometown. It was clear from her wistfulness as she described these memories that her conscious mental representations of her father identified him as her primary attachment figure, with the incest as an emotionally compartmentalized experience.

Kezia's boyfriend emerged as the primary target of her anger during the initial sessions. She had told him about the incest early in their relationship and, after his initial shock, he seemed to make his peace with this aspect of his girlfriend's early life. After they became unexpectedly pregnant, however, he became increasingly incensed in response to Kezia's ongoing contact with her father and insisted that she stopped seeing him, except during family reunions. Kezia refused to do so on the grounds that her father loved her, posed no threat to her, and needed her help with everyday chores that were easy for her to do as both of her parents became older and less independent. Kezia's pregnancy exacerbated the couple's conflict, because Esben demanded that Kezia's father have no contact with their son after the birth, and Kezia felt that such an estrangement would destroy her ties with her family members, who ostensibly were unaware of the sexual abuse.

The clinician offered to see the parents together as the first focus of treatment, because of the increasing frequency and intensity of their fights, which always remained verbal but were taking a toll on Kezia's well-being and did not bode well for the baby. The parents agreed with relief, saying that they had run out of options in how to talk with each other because their disagreement about the role of Kezia's father in their lives was coloring all aspects of their relationship, and they were feeling increasingly estranged from one another.

The following scene is emblematic of how the clinician addressed this relationship impasse. Kezia and Esben arrived to the sixth session on time, looking glum. Esben started the session saying, *"Her parents called her again"* in a defiant tone of voice, while glancing sideways at Kezia as if he expected her to scold him. Kezia looked back at him with a reproving expression, as if he was betraying her by bringing the topic up yet again. After a tense silence, the clinician asked, *"What happened?"* Looking annoyed, Kezia explained that her parents called to ask how she was doing, and Esben disapproved of her speaking cordially to her father. Kezia said that she felt in a conundrum about how to speak with her mother but not with her father when they called. Esben said to the clinician, *"I don't understand how she can talk to him again. I think that she is better off not talking to him at all. Both of her parents have hurt her a lot. I can tolerate her mother being around, but not him."*

The clinician responded, "*It sounds like you are very clear that you want to protect Kezia and your baby. You want to make sure that they are safe.*" Esben nodded. The clinician then turned to Kezia and said, "*I hear you saying that you see things differently, that you want to continue contact with your mother and also with your father and feel that it is safe to continue talking to him.*" Kezia nodded and said, "*I decreased my contacts with them. I know that Esben is right, I should cut contact with him, but how can I do it if my parents live together, and my mother does not know what happened. I'm trying to cut off ties but at the same time . . .*" She stopped. "*It seems that you want some kind of relationship with your mother but also with your father,*" the clinician added. Kezia smiled and said, "*Yes.*" There was a silence, as Kezia and Esben looked at each other. The clinician commented, "*Each of you has very strong feelings that are legitimate from your own different perspectives. What we can do together is to look for a solution that each of you can live with, even if it is not exactly what you want.*" This seemed like a novel idea for the parents, who looked at the clinician expectantly. The clinician continued, "*It will take some time to get there, but I think that as you try to explain your point of view to each other, maybe you can find points of agreement. For example, Kezia just said that you are right, Esben, and that she is decreasing contact with her father, even though she wants to continue some kind of relationship with him. Maybe you can think about what kind of relationship would be manageable for you. While you work on that, it is worthwhile thinking that your lives include much more than Kezia's father. You are a young couple, and you can do many enjoyable things together. And you are about to have a baby, and that is a lot to prepare for.*"

The tenor of the exchanges between Kezia and Esben changed in the course of preparing for the baby's birth following this session, because both of them became more aware that their conflict about Kezia's relationship with her father was only one aspect of the much larger commitment that they felt for each other. However, there continued to be many moments of great tension. The clinician helped the couple manage these moments by using breathing techniques and affect regulation exercises as ways of creating a respite in their mutual recriminations and of restoring a willingness to resume a respectful dialogue. The most frequent theme in these difficult encounters was Esben's worry about Kezia's and the baby's safety, invariably countered by Kezia's heated contention that she was safe with her mother and father and that she could ensure the baby's safety.

A transformational moment occurred when Kezia tearfully told Esben about the many ways that her father had protected her from her mother. She said, "*I had nobody else. He was the one who taught me to swim, to ride a bike; he was the one who stopped my mother from hitting me many times.*" The clinician commented, "*When you were little you needed your father even though he did things to you that a father should not do. If you gave up on him, you would have been all alone, with nobody to protect you."* Kezia burst into tears, and Esben looked at her silently. The clinician added, *"Do you think that maybe there is a part of you that is grateful to him, and now you feel you need to be there for him because he is older and more infirm?"* Kezia nodded, continuing to cry. For Esben, this moment revealed the ways in which Kezia had depended on her father while she was growing up. He said in a choked voice, *"I don't want you to ever be alone with him, but if you want to be with him when other people are around I will learn to live with that."*

Esben's statement became the basis for an agreement that brought a measure of resolution to both Kezia and Esben, because it accommodated both his safety concerns and her continued need for a relationship with her father. The clinician understood that Kezia's wish for a continued relationship with her father had unconscious layers of motivation that were more complex than her gratitude for the moments of goodness she perceived him as providing. However, the exploration of these unconscious motives was outside the agreed-upon goals of treatment, which consisted of removing the emotional obstacles to Kezia's loving relationship with her baby and her boyfriend. A recurrent task of P-CPP clinicians is to delineate the boundaries between the more circumscribed goal of creating a safe psychological space for the baby in the parent's psyche and the terminable and interminable process of deepening parental insight about internal conflicts once the infant-focused goals are achieved.

### Whose Baby Is This?: Little DeAndre as a Trigger for Maternal and Paternal Attributions

The birth of baby DeAndre opened up new manifestations of the conflict between the parents. When he was 2 months old, the parents started a conversation about who he resembled in the family. Esben believed that he looked like Esben's mother and older brother—placing DeAndre squarely within the paternal genealogical line. Kezia immediately disagreed by saying, *"He looks just like my father; every time I look at him is like I'm seeing my father."* There was an awkward silence, and the clinician asked her, *"How is that like for you?"* Kezia responded with a smile, *"It's strange that DeAndre looks just like my father after everything that we have been talking about."* Esben answered sharply that DeAndre did not look like Kezia's father. In this exchange, it seemed as if Esben was striving to assert his own paternity to counter Kezia's implicit unconscious fantasy that her father was DeAndre's "real" father.

There was again an awkward silence, interrupted by Esben

pointing out that DeAndre had started smiling and that his smile was particularly quick and broad when directed at Kezia. This was a loving attempt at repairing the conflict between them, and the clinician chose to reinforce this conciliatory gesture by asking Kezia whether she had noticed that DeAndre smiled more readily at her. Kezia responded that she had not noticed it, but she now recognized in hindsight that what Esben observed was probably true. The clinician took this opportunity to affirm Esben's special role as a father by saying to the baby, *"DeAndre, your daddy is getting to really know you. He is noticing the new things that you do and how much you like it when your mom comes close to you."* Both parents smiled with pleasure, but the clinician knew that Kezia's statement that she saw her father every time she looked at her baby was a clear demonstration of the emotional force that the incest continued to have in her inner life and in her perceptions of the baby. Decreasing the power of Kezia's fantasy of an incestuous baby would require tactful but sustained insight-oriented therapeutic work.

### The Baby as Erotic Trigger: Moving to a Dyadic Treatment Format

In a subsequent session, Kezia said that she was having difficulty sleeping, because DeAndre moved a lot during the night, and this was causing problems for her because she needed to wake up early to go to work. The ensuing conversation revealed that Kezia and DeAndre slept in the same bed since the baby's birth and Esben slept in the guest room—ostensibly because DeAndre fussed when he was put in his crib, and his nighttime wakings prevented Esben from feeling rested for work in the mornings.

This theme brought up the family's sleeping arrangements, an important topic for new parents. Cultural norms are changing from earlier recommendations that babies should learn to sleep on their own to a greater acceptability of infants sleeping with their parents into their toddler years and sometimes later. Parents make choices about family sleeping arrangements based on multiple factors, including cultural traditions, pragmatic considerations, and psychodynamic needs. In the specific case of Kezia and Esben, the clinician believed that the choice of Esben sleeping in a separate room from his wife and son might be consciously based on practical considerations, but it also meant that at an emotional level the son was replacing the father as a partner in the mother's bed.

The concept of an "oedipal baby"—the fantasized product of Kezia's sexual relationship with her father—was very much in the clinician's mind as she pondered the meaning of the family sleeping arrangements, which did not conform to the parents' cultural traditions. A spontaneous statement from Kezia provided support for this clinical hypothesis when she said, "*I can't sleep well also because I try to stay away from DeAndre. I don't understand it, but I feel like there is a barrier between us. I don't feel comfortable sleeping close to him.*" The clinician asked, "*What does the barrier feel like?*" Hesitating, Kezia responded, "*Sometimes I get pictures of my father and me when I am lying down with DeAndre.*" Esben looked very uncomfortable as she spoke. The clinician commented, "*That must make it difficult to sleep, and I am thinking maybe DeAndre feels your tension, and that makes him move so much at night—what do you think?*" Kezia seemed pensive and nodded in agreement. The clinician turned to DeAndre and said, "*Your mom is telling me that things at night are difficult for the three of you, your mommy has difficult memories coming to her mind, and you move a lot, and Daddy has to sleep in another room.*" By speaking to the baby, the clinician was making him an integral participant in the treatment, addressing his restlessness at night as worthy of attention as a possible response to his mother's unease over physical closeness with him.

The emergence of the baby as a trigger for Kezia's incestuous memories and sensations called for a change in the treatment format. The clinician felt the need to create the kind of emotional boundaries that Kezia had not experienced as a young child by creating a private space where she could free-associate about her incestuous experience without imposing those experiences on Esben, thus protecting him from becoming a symbolic witness to the incest. Striving for a tactful way of proposing a changed treatment format, the clinician addressed both Kezia and Esben by saying, "*Lots of parents take a while to find the right sleeping arrangement for themselves and their babies. I am thinking that maybe for you both finding the right arrangement is more complicated than usual because Kezia learned as a little girl to accept that her father came into her bed and did not let her sleep as a young child should. How would you feel if we change the way we meet for a while, and Kezia comes to see me alone with DeAndre to talk more freely about the barrier that she feels about sleeping with him?*" Esben agreed immediately, saying that he was becoming increasingly angry and uncomfortable listening to Kezia speak about her father when they were coming to treatment to talk about themselves as parents. The clinician said supportively, "*I can understand that. It can get difficult when one's private life spills into one's life as a parent and as a couple. Kezia, I can see how honest you are in trying to understand yourself. Do you think that coming alone with DeAndre will help you speak more freely?*" Kezia said that she felt supported by Esben's presence, but was willing to accept the new format.

The changed format facilitated the emergence of Kezia's sexual feelings toward DeAndre. While opening herself to exploring the sexual meaning that the baby had for her, she also demonstrated the sturdy defenses she had developed to protect both the baby and herself from reenacting the incest she had experienced by moving from victim to perpetrator. These defenses kept the impulses at bay but filled her with anxiety. She spoke, for example, about distressing intrusive memories of her father kissing her when she moved toward DeAndre to kiss him, her fear of touching him sexually when changing his diaper, her profound shame at finding herself looking at his genitals, and remembering her father's genitals. She also said that she felt an urgent need to be present whenever Esben changed DeAndre's diaper to make sure "*nothing inappropriate*" was happening to the baby.

The clinician spoke to the powerful protective impulses Kezia was describing. She said, "*I'm wondering if you feel the need to put a barrier between you and DeAndre to protect him. Do you think that the barrier that you feel about getting close to him tells us that part of you is making sure that you have the strength and the will to not do to him what your father did to you?*" Kezia seemed sad as she nodded. At the end of session, Kezia expressed relief that she could tell the clinician about her feelings and her fears, because they had been making her very anxious since the baby was born.

In subsequent sessions, the clinician helped Kezia process in the moment her bodily sensations as she held DeAndre, diapered him, and expressed affection for him. It is noteworthy that Kezia only bottle-fed the baby. She had decided since before giving birth that she would not nurse DeAndre—another expression of the protective barrier she needed to create between them and one that the clinician did not attempt to modify. Both the clinician and Kezia felt reassured by the mother's increased capacity in the course of treatment to differentiate between her fear of sexually abusing him and her confidence that the pleasure she felt in touching and holding her baby were normal expressions of her affection for him.

The clinician's comfort in speaking openly about sexuality was a key factor in the success of treatment. Although the clinician did not address the sexual relationship between the parents directly, she spoke in a matter-of-fact manner about both the pleasures and the challenges inherent in a long-term sexual relationship, including the inevitable changes brought about by the birth of a baby and the need for patient and open communication about the partners' different needs and preferences. This comfort with body sensations enabled the clinician to help the parents accept DeAndre's exploration of his own body and the discovery of his genitals as he entered toddlerhood.

Treatment continued until DeAndre was 17 months old, using both dyadic and triadic formats depending on the salient clinical issues. Kezia became increasingly more conscious of the fear and pain her father had inflicted on her, and grieved the loss of the idealized image she had created that minimized her father's sexual abuse for so many years. DeAndre and Kezia were both fortunate that Esben was a solid, loving, reliable man who provided a secure emotional base for both of them. There were recurrent episodes of relational conflict about the role of Kezia's father in their life, but Esben grew as a partner, a father, and a man as he learned to assert his demand that Kezia and DeAndre only see her father in the presence of her mother or other people. DeAndre started sleeping in his crib in a room adjoining the parents' bedroom when he was 14 months old, and Esben returned to the couple's bed—a graphic statement that everyone was now where they belonged.

# Vignette 8.
# When the Mother's Mother Died in Childbirth: Pregnancy after a History of Maternal Loss

Learning to define oneself as a mother by identifying with one's own mother carries enormous psychological peril when the woman's mother died giving birth to her. Women who lost their mothers at birth inevitably carry the burden of causing the mother's death. The pregnant woman faces an existential conundrum: identifying with her dead mother entails the danger of death, whereas a safe childbirth may create guilt for surviving while being the agent of her mother's death. Women in these circumstances often experience clinical levels of anticipatory anxiety, sadness, and guilt. The psychological reorganization that occurs during pregnancy can promote emotional growth when the woman can forge a life-affirming identification with her dead mother that allows her to honor her memory and redeem her death by making a new life possible. The present vignette describes the use of P-CPP to promote this process. Therapeutic interventions included a clear acknowledgment of the social determinants of maternal mortality and the health disparities represented by the exponentially higher maternal mortality rate of African American women when compared with European American women in the United States (Review to Action, 2018).

## Resolution of Unconscious Traumatic Grief as a Prelude to Healthy Bonding

Aisha was a 38-year-old married African American woman who was 16 weeks pregnant with her second child when she sought treatment for severe depression. There was a 9-year gap between her first child, a boy, and her current planned pregnancy. During the first session of the foundational phase, Aisha spontaneously revealed that her own mother had died while giving birth to her as the result of a hemorrhage caused by uterine rupture, but said that this loss did not affect her, because her grandmother raised her and was a loving mother to her. She reported that she had experienced intermittent bouts of depression throughout her life, and attributed this to a genetic propensity inherited from her father. She also said she felt mildly anxious and always concerned about safety because, although she lived in a safe neighborhood, she was always alert to the dangers that her husband and her son faced as African American males, who often encountered experiences of racism in everyday life. The initial assessment revealed no childhood trauma in addition to her mother's death. Aisha also grew up with a maternal aunt whom she described as a supportive and caring figure in her life, and she stated feeling blessed to have a closely knit extended family. Her father had remarried and had two daughters significantly younger than Aisha. She spent weekends with her father and his new family, and reported feeling jealous of her sisters because her father was more spontaneously affectionate with them, and the girls treated her as if she were their fun older playmate but not an integral part of the family. She felt loved by her grandmother and her aunt, who provided her with a sense of unconditional support. They often told her that she looked just like her mother and that her mother would be proud of her.

Aisha's symptoms worsened significantly in the second trimester, when fetal movement started and her ultrasound revealed that the baby was a girl. Aisha disclosed the sex of the baby during a telephone conversation with the clinician (M. A. D.), who noticed that Aisha seemed surprised by the news as she described in an overly bright tone of voice that her husband and son were happy that the baby was a girl. She pointedly left herself out of this statement. When Aisha came in for her weekly therapy session, the clinician greeted her in the waiting area and immediately noticed dark circles under her eyes and a sullen expression on her face. As Aisha was entering the therapy room, she yawned and commented, "*I feel very tired today.*" The clinician responded sympathetically, "*You do look tired today. Did you get enough rest last night?*" As Aisha's red, puffy eyes met the clinician's eyes, she answered with a tone of uncertainty, "*I don't know why, but these past days I've been sleeping badly.*" The clinician took the opportunity to reinforce Aisha's commitment to the therapy by saying appreciatively, "*You are very tired, but you still came to see me.*" Aisha whispered with a forced smile, "*I wanted to come see you. I really don't know what's going on with me . . . what's happening to me. I can't sleep, I can't eat, I am really sad and irritable. Everything gets on my nerves.*"

The clinician explored a possible connection between the increase in Aisha's symptoms and the results of the ultrasound by asking when she began feeling this way. Aisha, now sitting with her arms crossed and looking physically exhausted, replied, "*It has only been a few days ago that I started waking up at 2:00 or 3:00 A.M. and am unable to fall back asleep. Hmmm . . . I think it started on Monday night, and it has gotten worse as the days went by.*" The clinician asked Aisha to describe what usually happened after she woke up in the middle of the night. Sighing in frustration, she replied, "*I toss and turn and begin thinking about different things that I cannot get out of my head. My mind gets so loud that I cannot shut it down! So I get out of bed, and walk around the house to clear my mind.*" The clinician responded, "*It sounds like there is something that is worrying you . . . that is keeping you awake, weighing on your mind . . . that even made you lose your appetite and feel edgy and irritable.*" Aisha fidgeted nervously, and said with a preoccupied frown on her face, "*I've been having dreams about something bad happening to me. It is so hard to go back to sleep after such dreams . . .*" The clinician asked Aisha whether she could remember the details of her dreams. Aisha replied, as tears welled up in her eyes, "*I dreamed of dying three times this week . . . the dreams were so intense that I woke up screaming. My husband tried to calm me, but I had to get out of bed and started walking around the house and turning on lights because I was so upset.*" As she was speaking, tears began rolling down her face and her speech turned into loud, anguished sobbing. She sunk into her chair, burying her face in her hands as she continued crying.

The clinician remained quiet for a few minutes, sensing the importance of this moment and giving Aisha a supportive space to experience these intense feelings. She then handed Aisha a tissue and tried to help her bring meaning to her experience, saying, "*These dreams must have been very scary for you . . . for so many reasons. I can only imagine how you must have felt then and how you are feeling right now as you are remembering these dreams.*" Aisha continued crying loudly, now anxiously gripping her hands together, and replied in a broken voice, "*I'm scared. I wish I were having a baby boy. I don't want to have a girl . . . Why is this happening to me?*" She let out a louder cry, as she touched her forehead and said, "*I don't feel well . . . my head is hurting . . . I feel sick.*"

The knowledge that she was having a baby girl had created intense fear in Aisha, eliciting psychophysiological reactions connected to losing her mother in childbirth. Before exploring this connection, the clinician opted to first use body-based techniques to decrease Aisha's physiological arousal. She offered Aisha a glass of water, saying in a calm voice, "*It sounds like your body is reacting to what you are telling me. I think taking small sips of cold water can help.*" Aisha quickly accepted the glass and, as she took the first sip of water, the clinician said, "*Now, feel the cold water in your mouth . . . as you swallow, feel that water go down your throat slowly. That's it . . . just concentrate on drinking the water.*" The clinician repeated the exercise until Aisha finished the water. She then suggested that Aisha join her in a short breathing exercise, reminding her that this exercise had calmed her nervous system down in previous sessions when she was upset. Aisha seemed more grounded and engaged with the clinician at the end of the breathing exercise, although her deep distress was still manifest in a distraught facial expression and shaky voice.

The next step was to help Aisha understand what the dreams were telling her about herself. The clinician told Aisha, *"Now that you feel a little calmer, let's go back to the frightening recurrent dream you've been having."* Aisha took a deep breath and nodded her head in agreement. The clinician continued, *"You mentioned that you dreamed three times about dying . . . that you are scared . . . that you wish you were having a baby boy, not a baby girl. Could it be that you are scared that something bad will happen to you because you are having a baby girl?"*

As she wiped off her tears, Aisha said, *"Yes . . . I'm sooo scared. I'm scared of dying like my mother did when she had me . . . I always felt that I caused her death. I worry that this baby girl can cause my own death too."* A few seconds of intense silence invaded the room.

The clinician acknowledged Aisha's heavy burden of guilt over her mother's death and fear about her own dying by saying, *"That must be so hard for you. No wonder you cannot sleep, you cannot eat, you are so upset and frightened."* With her eyes still swollen from crying and in a choked voice, Aisha responded, *"Yes, it is scary and difficult to even talk about this. I always felt guilty about my mother's death . . . I always felt that I killed her. That's why I didn't want to have a family of my own until I met my husband. So when I got pregnant the first time with a boy, my prayers were answered. The Lord gave me a beautiful boy. I felt safe carrying him in my belly. I was hoping this time would be the same way to, so I was shocked at first when I was told I was having a baby girl. Good thing my husband was there with me, and you called me afterward."*

The clinician spoke to the trauma of Aisha's mother's death. *"It was such a tragedy what happened to your mother. You were an innocent newborn baby girl that was coming into the world to be with her mother, to be cared for, to be loved, to be protected and raised by her mother. How difficult it must have been for you as a fragile newborn baby girl not to have the much-needed love and warmth of your mother. I can only imagine how much you missed not having your mother there with you."*

Aisha listened attentively with tears in her eyes. She replied, *"I don't remember anything from when I was a baby though . . . How can I miss what I don't remember?"* The clinician validated Aisha's experience as a newborn, saying, *"You are right. Newborn babies do not have words to describe what happened to them, but they do experience the world with each sense in their bodies. A baby feels her mother's touch, smells her mother's scent, gazes into her mother's eyes, hears her mother's voice, and feeds from her mother's breasts. A newborn baby can experience through her senses the many losses of not having her mother with her, not being in her mother's arms. Babies do feel the loss of their mothers, because they cannot experience their mothers through their senses.*" Aisha, still tearful, said, "*I guess I did need and miss my mother when I was a newborn baby . . . also later on in my life. I always felt a void in my life, so alone without her . . . even though I grew up in a big family. As a child, I remember daydreaming about having a mother. I remember that my aunt Lakisha would tell me stories about my mother as a child; she said my mother was a very playful and sweet girl who became a very strong woman. When I was an adolescent, I struggled with the feeling I didn't deserve to be here, that I would be better off dead. And now as a grown woman I still wish my mother could be here with me . . . I missed having my mother. Life is so unfair and cruel . . ."*

The clinician validated Aisha's experience, saying, "*You missed your mother as a baby and throughout your life, and you wish she was here as you are becoming a mother for the second time. And you are right: life situations can be very unfair and cruel at times.*" Aisha nodded silently. There was a quiet sense of attunement between the two of them.

The clinician then addressed Aisha's fear of dying in the context of the higher maternal mortality rate among African American women. She articulated the appropriate reality appraisal of Aisha's fear by saying, "*I can also understand why you are so worried about dying. Maternal death in childbirth happens very unfairly to women in your community; it did happen to your own mother. But it is also important to recognize how you are preparing yourself to make it less likely that something like this will happen to you. Your prenatal checkups show that this is a healthy pregnancy. You are following the recommendations of your prenatal care team, although this week has been hard, but you are trying really hard to follow your diet plan. I can attest to that. Your doctor knows that your mother had a hemorrhage from a uterine rupture and died when she gave birth to you, and she is extra alert to respond quickly in an emergency. All those things make it more likely that things go well during delivery.*" Aisha replied, "*You are right. I am doing a lot. I hadn't thought about that. Sometimes I forget how much time and effort I am dedicating to this pregnancy. Thanks for reminding me of this.*"

During the following sessions, Aisha continued processing the immense guilt she had felt all her life for her mother's death. Aisha also shared details of her close relationship with her maternal aunt Lakisha. She commented, "*Aunt Lakisha helped my grandma raise me in a loving, large, close-knit family in spite of not having much money.*" In one session, Aisha described her aunt's recollections of her mother's pregnancy with her. She said, "*My aunt told me that my mother was very happy to be expecting a baby girl and made many plans for my arrival. She fixed my crib, bought baby clothes, and even kept ultrasound photos.*" She also disclosed that her aunt had given her pictures of her mother, including one when she was pregnant with Aisha, which "*she had kept in a shoebox, tucked away somewhere in her garage.*"

As treatment progressed, Aisha understood and accepted that she was not responsible for her mother's death and was able to integrate this event as an external tragedy in her life rather than an event she had caused. She also began to anticipate becoming the mother of a baby girl as an opportunity for healing by offering her daughter experiences that her mother could not give her. A week before the healthy delivery of a baby girl, Aisha framed one of her mother's pictures and hung it in the baby's room so that "grandma could watch over baby Janae." She named the baby Janae after her own mother.

# Section V

# Monitoring Fidelity

*The "What" and "How" of P-CPP*

Practicing a treatment model with fidelity means implementing the intervention in the way it was intended, with clinicians trained and supervised to the extent necessary to enable them to show clinical competence and adherence to the theoretical principles and therapeutic strategies of the model as outlined in the treatment manual or protocol (Sharpless & Barber, 2009). The fidelity measures presented in this section serve as guidelines for monitoring clinician competence and adherence to the principles and modalities that comprise P-CPP.

The introduction to this book describes our conceptualization of P-CPP as a manualized application of CPP for the treatment and prevention of trauma in pregnancy and the perinatal period. As with CPP (Lieberman et al., 2015), we do not prescribe adherence to a standardized, step-by-step approach to treatment, because we believe that treatment at its best involves a co-creation between the clinician and the recipient(s) of the treatment, with the clinician responding to the themes and emotional tone of the clinical moment. This manual provides clinicians with a toolkit that consists of a clear theoretical approach, a range of intervention modalities, comprehensive clinical illustrations, and research support for the effectiveness of the treatment. Reflective and didactic training and supervision are necessary to translate the written text to the clinical situation with fidelity to the goals and intervention modalities of the model. Once clinicians have gained competence in understanding the conceptual principles, in developing a clear clinical formulation and treatment plan, and in applying the P-CPP intervention modalities, they are encouraged to rely on their clinical judgment to appraise the domain of intervention and choose the specific therapeutic strategy that might be the most promising to promote positive change at any given moment.

# Pillars of a Therapeutic Attitude

Section II of this book includes a subsection titled "Pillars of a Therapeutic Attitude." These pillars, already described in Section II (pp. 51–53), provide the overarching attitudinal frame that guides clinical judgment and serves as the basis for the fidelity measures.

- *Notice feelings in the moment.* This pillar involves attunement to present emotional experience as a port of entry to understanding. It also involves tracking body movement and posture as other ports of entry to identifying the manifestations of traumatic reminders and other strong emotions in the body.
- *Speak the unspeakable: Dare to use concrete words to describe the trauma.* Guilt and shame can silence a person's voice. Hearing the clinician model how to articulate unspeakable experiences, overwhelming feelings, and bodily reactions using a calm and supportive stance can normalize the experience and restore a sense of belonging rather than alienation from self and others.
- *Find connections between experiences.* Following the person's free associative flow of thoughts and feelings can guide the clinician to an understanding of unconscious motives, fears, and wishes and make them amenable to reflection and the creation of new meaning.
- *Remember the suffering under the rage.* Anger is often a form of self-protection against unmanageable fear. Offering protection, safety, and understanding helps to modulate rage, promotes self-understanding, and relieves shame and guilt.
- *Seek out the benevolence in the conflict.* Bitter disagreements often stem from a clash between competing but equally legitimate values and priorities. Bowlby (1969) described security of attachment after infancy as a "goal-corrected partnership" in which both partners endeavor to negotiate mutually acceptable solutions when conflicts arise. Building reciprocal emotional relationships involves a conscious effort to understand and legitimize the other's perspective even when it is not feasible to agree with it.
- *Offer kindness.* This component of the therapeutic attitude involves remaining empathically curious and nonjudgmental. Kindness and compassion generate healing by relieving the self-recrimination, shame, and guilt that are universal components of traumatic stress.
- *Encourage hope.* Trusting that things can get better provides the emotional energy and commitment to action to make it happen. The effectiveness of treatment relies on trust in the possibility of improving the present and the future. Clinicians need to foster this trust by noticing and highlighting examples of the treatment participants' strengths and harnessing these examples to the goals of treatment.

# Six Fidelity Strands

CPP developed a multidimensional fidelity framework consisting of six interconnected fidelity strands informed by the pillars of a therapeutic attitude (Ghosh Ippen & Lieberman, 2019; Ghosh Ippen, Lieberman, & Van Horn, 2012). This framework and the accompanying measures have proven very effective in CPP training and clinical practice. For this reason, P-CPP has adopted it as its fidelity framework, with some adaptations to account for the different but overlapping developmental stages and clinical problems addressed by each model. Specifically, CPP treats traumatized children under age 6 and their (often traumatized) caregivers, whereas P-CPP treats expectant parents with histories of trauma that endanger their healthy bond with their unborn baby and continues into at least the first 6 months of the baby's life, with treatment extended as clinically necessary for the safety and healthy development of the infant.

The fidelity strands are described next. An extensive description of the CPP fidelity model is available in Lieberman et al. (2015).

## Strand 1: Reflective Practice Fidelity

All psychodynamically informed interventions highlight the importance of the clinician's self-awareness as critical to effective intervention. Countertransference reactions can promote a strong therapeutic alliance that supports positive change or create obstacles to clinical improvement by generating negative feelings, a judgmental stance, overidentification, or other departures from sound clinical judgment. P-CPP clinicians' capacity for self-reflection about these issues needs to be cultivated at different levels—that is, in the present clinical moment, in retrospect in thinking back about what transpired during each session, and in continually monitoring clinical improvement in the course of treatment.

## Strand 2: Emotional Process Fidelity

The capacity to feel, understand, tolerate, and modulate the experience and the expression of emotions in developmentally appropriate and culturally accepted ways is at the core of mental health across the lifespan. The first pillar of the therapeutic attitude is the clinician's readiness to notice feelings in the moment. The second pillar is the clinician's ability to identify and articulate affective connections between successive emotional expressions in order to create meaning and promote greater self-understanding. The P-CPP clinician's attunement to the client's emotional experience needs to guide all interventions, regardless of the specific therapeutic modality that the clinician may choose at any given moment.

## Strand 3: Dyadic Relational Fidelity

The quality of emotional attunement between two partners in an intimate relationship—such as between the parent and the fetus, the parent and the child, two spouses, or the two parents of a child—is a major contributor to the harmony or dissension in a relationship. Affective mismatches are inevitable, but the motivation to seek repair and restore reciprocity of positive affect are hallmarks of a healthy and resilient affective bond. Bowlby (1969) defined security of attachment after infancy as a goal-corrected partnership whereby both members of the dyad find ways of reconciling competing agendas for the sake of the relationship. The P-CPP clinician may start treatment meeting with the pregnant woman either individually or with her and her partner. Before birth, the unborn infant is a silent interlocutor actively present in the form of parental attributions, often triggered by maternal physical sensations and health conditions associated with the period of gestation. After childbirth, the physical baby becomes an integral participant in the treatment.

The P-CPP clinician endeavors to be attuned simultaneously to the individual emotional experience of each partner, to the quality of the emotional connection between them, and to the match or mismatch between their respective psychological perspectives. Parental mental representations of the fetus/baby are explicitly evoked and addressed both before and after the baby's birth.

Keeping different perspectives simultaneously in mind means that the clinician extends the second emotional process fidelity strand to this third strand. The clinician must attend at the same time to the individual participant and to the relationship between each of the treatment participants without losing sight of their varied experiences. Interventions are geared toward building bridges of connection, empathy, understanding, and repair whenever the participants' divergent perspectives signal misunderstanding, anger, or alienation that if left unaddressed, could have a negative impact on the functioning of the dyadic or triatic unit.

## Strand 4: Trauma Framework Fidelity

This strand distinguishes both CPP and P-CPP from other infant/early childhood mental health treatments, because screening for trauma exposure and addressing traumatic reminders are defining component of both treatment models. The Israeli poet Yehuda Amichai (2004) wrote, "I fear/What the past will do to me/In the future." Clinicians providing treatment to traumatized people of all ages share the poet's fear on behalf of those they treat, because they witness what the past is doing to them in the present and anticipate how present suffering may unfold in the person's future and the generations to come. By definition, the traumatic moment occurs unpredictably and overwhelms the capacity to think and to reflect: the person is assaulted by terrifying stimuli (sights, sounds, smells, and tactile and kinetic sensations) that overwhelm the senses and trigger automatic body responses involving fight, flight, and freezing that are enacted outside conscious volition and are cut off from logical thinking and rational planning. One cannot "unsee" or "unhear" what was once seen and heard. The experiences continue to exist, often outside consciousness, but also in the form of intrusive images and intense unpleasant physical sensations that offer no respite. The sense of predictable safety is the first casualty of trauma, because traumatized people lose the subjective expectation of reliable protection.

Systematic screening for trauma exposure is an integral component of the P-CPP foundational phase. The P-CPP clinician starts treatment with the assumption that trauma exposure is such a prevalent social phenomenon that it may explain the etiology of the presenting problems in expectant mothers and fathers that come for treatment, even when they themselves do not know the impact of their past and current stressors on the emotional difficulties they report. P-CPP shares with CPP the assumption that "speaking the unspeakable" holds the key to healing, because it provides reason and meaning to explain seemingly inexplicable fear, rage, despair, overreaction, inability to feel love, physical discomfort, and absence of joy. When the parent has experienced trauma, the clinician explores the possible connections between the experience of trauma and the presenting clinical problems, creating a clinical formulation triangle that links adverse and traumatic circumstances with presenting symptoms, and presents a treatment plan that includes the hope of healing.

The trauma framework fidelity strand consistently emerges as the most demanding aspect of both CPP and P-CPP. Clinicians whose professional training involved a "wait until the client is ready" approach to treatment express concern that asking about trauma exposure at the beginning of treatment risks "scaring people away" or retraumatizing them. This trepidation is particularly notable for clinicians who provide treatment to pregnant women. Many clinicians, regardless of their level of professional experience, express concern that opening up the topic of trauma can induce psychological disorganization at a vulnerable developmental stage and that this emotional disorganization can negatively affect the outcome of the pregnancy.

We hold that the opposite is more likely to be true. Tactful, supportive inquiry about the difficult circumstances of a person's life can offer relief from the shameful burden of "knowing what you are not supposed to know and feeling what you are not supposed to feel" (Bowlby, 1988). Pregnant women often report the resurfacing of intrusive images and physical sensations from their traumatic experiences that raise their anxiety levels and make them feel overwhelmed, helpless, and drained of motivation and energy. The clinician's supportive stance in normalizing traumatic responses and helping to differentiate between remembering the past and reliving it can transform the meaning of the intrusive images and physical sensations from threats to psychological and physical integrity into tools for self-understanding and self-compassion for what the person went through. One woman in her 38th week of pregnancy said to her clinician at the end of the foundational phase, "*I feel as if you sat me down in your living room and showed me a movie picture of my life, frame by frame. Everything came together in a way I never understood before.*" She gave birth the following day to a healthy baby, as if signaling that she had completed an internal process of labor and delivery that could now have concrete expression in the birth of her child.

There is great release from learning that terrible truths can finally be shared with someone who can offer empathy and understanding rather than shame, blame, punishment, threats, and the overt or covert demand that "you shall not know and you shall not tell, or else. . . ." Unless the clinician leads by example, showing the possibility of articulating what until now could not be said, the traumatized person may remain for a long time in frozen suffering with her daunting secret, assuming that if the "expert" does not ask, then surely one must not tell, surely it is not important.

Chandra Ghosh Ippen developed a metaphor that compares trauma therapists to firefighters, who engage in the counterintuitive move of walking toward a fire when everyone else moves away from it. She describes trauma clinicians as performing the counterintuitive move of speaking directly about the trauma. For this move to be affirming rather than threatening, the clinician (like the firefighter) needs to be well trained, well equipped, and able to rely on team support (Ghosh Ippen & Lieberman, 2019). This book is part of the "first-response equipment" that provides effective treatment to pregnant women and their partners exposed to traumatic experiences. Extensive training, clinical supervision, and access to consistent mentoring and peer support are also indispensable to prevent vicarious trauma. Many clinicians are "wounded healers" (Jung, 1951/1982), and having access to consistent clinical support can help them remember the power of hope to find purpose and transcend pain.

### Strand 5: Procedural Fidelity

All the treatment phases of P-CPP share the common theme of the clinician's active emotional support and therapeutic engagement with the themes that emerge in order to co-create the goals of treatment and monitor progress. The initial foundational phase provides the forum in which to demonstrate this clinical attitude as the basis for effective therapeutic engagement and the co-creation of a therapeutic working relationship. During the core phase of treatment, the clinician needs to remain aware of the concrete demands of preparing for labor, delivery, and the postpartum period, while also maintaining a focus on the clinical themes that emerge. The termination phase involves attention to the possible reemergence of earlier conflicts, while also affirming the gains made and preparing for life after treatment. The procedural fidelity strand directs the clinician's attention to the fulfillment of the procedures that guide and organize the work across the three phases of treatment.

The procedural strand also includes a consideration of the most appropriate format for the sessions if both parents participate in the treatment. In general, individual sessions are conducted with each parent separately when both of them are involved in order to offer opportunities to disclose sensitive personal information that the parents may not have disclosed to each other. The clinician speaks openly with the parents about their expectations for confidentiality regarding the sharing of information with the other parent, and creates a consensus that joint sessions will be the forum for sharing of information about each other.

Effective engagement during the foundational phase calls for four interconnected activities:

***1. Gathering relevant clinical and demographic information in an emotionally attuned manner that generates trust in the clinician's empathy and support.*** The foundational phase involves combining information gathering and initial interventions to explore the range of treatment modalities that promote positive change. The use of structured measures in clinical practice to screen for trauma exposure is highly recommended, because their use conveys the message that traumatic events are a regular feature of human experience and offers the clinician and the respondent a shared frame to talk about these difficult events.

Structured interviews to assess for depression and PTSD are also recommended. These measures are administered after the trauma screening to enable the clinician to start finding connections between the adverse and traumatic events in the parents' life and their current psychological functioning and affective picture. Structured clinical interviews also provide a baseline measure of symptomatology that allows the clinician to track progress in treatment. Clinicians need to remember that structured measures probe for disclosure of intimate experiences that may be associated with intense negative feelings, including sadness, anger, guilt, and shame. The clinician's genuine interest and support must pervade all information-gathering procedures, including the administration of structured measures.

As described in discussing Strand 4, the trauma framework, many clinicians find that screening for exposure to adversity and trauma is the most challenging element of learning to implement P-CPP. They report a fear of being perceived as intrusive or retraumatizing the parent(s) by asking directly about difficult events in their lives. The procedural fidelity strand guides the clinician in explaining to the parents the rationale for asking about their personal history as an indispensable first step in creating a shared dialogue about the goals of treatment. The rationale involves an emotionally supportive explanation that what happened to the parents while growing up has an effect on how they feel about themselves and about other people, including how the parents respond to the present pregnancy and to the prospect of becoming parents. The clinician also states that many parents find that they understand themselves better when they recount in a supportive environment the conditions of their growing-up years and the feelings that they had in response to important events, both difficult and positive. In the course of listening to a parent's description of specific traumatic events, the clinician is actively engaged in therapeutic interventions that may involve empathic listening, normalizing the traumatic response, intervening if emotional dysregulation occurs, providing psychoeducation about the negative impact of trauma, and guiding the identification of trauma reminders.

Screening for adversity and trauma is always paired with assessing for protective and supportive memories (the "angels in the nursery" concept). People are influenced not only by the painful events in their lives. Encouraging parents to recall and articulate experiences of feeling loved, supported, and protected helps promote affect modulation in the aftermath of sharing difficult experiences and fosters psychological integration of positive and negative experiences. The clinician's knowledge of positive experiences also promotes nuance in the clinical formulation by incorporating protective factors as well as risk factors in the clinician's perception of the parents. It is optimal to assess for positive events and memories in the session devoted to screening for trauma and symptoms in order to help the parent remember self-affirming as well as difficult experiences and to create an integration of the trauma narrative and the protective narrative from the beginning of treatment. Ending the session with a hope-affirming theme is also emotionally sustaining, as parent and clinician part ways until the next session.

2. *Organizing the emerging information to give it clinical meaning.* Information gathering is not an end in itself. The clinician must be alert to the clinical implications of the information and to the emotional tone with which the parent provides the information, both through verbal communication and through unspoken messages conveyed in different forms of body language. The foundational phase provides the first opportunity to assess the parent's psychological strengths and vulnerabilities, including a capacity for self-reflection, insightfulness, and affect regulation, and the interplay between her defense structure and adaptive coping strategies.

Trial interventions are an important strategy for assessing the clinical meaning of the emerging information. The clinician engages in an internal process whereby she or he observes the parent's affect in the moment, develops clinical hypotheses about possible connections between different experiences, and decides on an intervention strategy to assess the clinical usefulness of the hypothesis. Trial interventions test out how the parent responds to the clinician's emerging clinical formulations. For example, some parents may welcome interventions that help them understand the connections between their childhood experiences and their current adult circumstances, whereas other parents may initially dismiss their past experiences and may prefer to focus on their current challenges with concrete problem-solving strategies. The foundational phase equips the clinician with a preliminary set of intervention modalities that hold the greatest promise for successful therapeutic engagement as the basis for treatment.

3. *Offering feedback, and presenting the clinical formulation triangle.* The feedback session marks the culmination of the foundational phase. The goal of this session is to engage the parents in co-creating an integrated trauma narrative and protective narrative that will provide the organizing themes of treatment. In preparing for this session, clinicians review what they learned during the previous sessions and develop a clinical formulation triangle that includes how the parents' life events and current circumstances affect their sense of themselves, their relationship with the baby's other parent, attitudes toward the pregnancy, and positive and negative attributions to the unborn baby,

and also outlines how treatment can help attain their goals for themselves and their baby.

This clinical understanding is shared with the parent(s) using the format of the clinical formulation triangle. In the context of presenting the formulation, the clinician makes use of specific moments during the previous sessions when therapeutic meaning was co-created between the parent and the clinician about the links between their past and present experiences, and how these links have shaped their sense of self and their emotional responses to the pregnancy and the unborn baby. When both parents participate in the treatment, the feedback session is conducted jointly in order to create a shared understanding of what each parent brings to the clinical situation.

**4. Offering treatment.** The offer of treatment emerges organically from the presentation of the clinical formulation triangle. The clinician engages the parents in the co-creation of a treatment plan, which includes the goals of treatment and agreements about the treatment participants, the expected length of the treatment, the location of the treatment, and the frequency and length of each treatment session. The clinician may refer back to helpful trial interventions as examples of possible ways of fostering the treatment goals.

The foundational phase does not always result in an invitation to engage in P-CPP. Alternative services or forms of treatment may take priority in certain clinical situations, including ongoing IPV, active and severe substance use, cognitive disabilities, and psychiatric conditions that prevent the formation of a therapeutic alliance on behalf of the baby. In those situations, the clinician endeavors to make appropriate referrals and to engage the parent in successful follow-up to make use of those referrals. When appropriate, the clinician may leave open the possibility of returning for P-CPP treatment once the obstacles to its successful implementation have been addressed.

### Strand 6: Content Fidelity

This component of the P-CPP treatment fidelity framework guides clinicians in monitoring the responsiveness of their interventions to the clinical themes and the needs of the treatment participants, which may change in the course of treatment. The goals and objectives of treatment tend to remain the same in the course of treatment, but fluctuations in the psychological state of the parents, the baby's developmental course, changes in real-life circumstances, and the deepening of the clinical work may call for recalibrating how these goals are pursued and what intervention modalities are used. The components of Content Fidelity are an elaboration of the pillars of a therapeutic attitude that integrates the previous five strands of self-reflection (Strand 1, Reflective Practice); attunement to the emotional experience of each participant (Strand 2, Emotional Process); simultaneous attunement to the different perspectives of the treatment participants (Strand 3, Dyadic Relational); trauma lens (Strand 4, Trauma Framework); and attention to implementation (Strand 5, Procedural). Clinicians strive to internalize a therapeutic road map that keeps the following treatment goals, objectives, and mechanisms in mind throughout the different phases of treatment:

- Offering kindness and conveying hope as the key ingredients of a therapeutic stance.
- Maintaining a reflective empathic stance toward the self and the treatment participants.
- Promoting environmental and interpersonal safety.
- Fostering affect regulation.
- Encouraging mutual understanding and positive emotional reciprocity.
- Including themes of trauma and protection in giving meaning to behavior.

## Fidelity Items

The items provided in the following checklists help clinicians monitor the "goodness of fit" between P-CPP as a treatment model and the clinician's therapeutic interventions. Although the items are presented as statements, there is no expectation that the clinician will respond with a binary "yes" or "no" answer. As an aid to promoting best clinical practice, each item is intended as a prompt that guides the clinician's attention to the key components of P-CPP, whether she or he implemented one or more of these components during the session, and the obstacles that prevented their implementation.

The checklists may be used for reflection following each session or at regular intervals in the course of treatment, and are particularly helpful when there is a lack of progress in meeting the treatment goals. The checklists may be used individually by the clinician or as a tool to promote greater understanding during supervision or consultation.

### Strand 1: Reflective Practice Fidelity

1. The clinician felt emotionally present and regulated as the prevailing internal stance during the session.

2. The clinician experienced internal confusion about the goals, purpose, and/or course of the session.
3. The clinician had a prevalence of negative feelings toward the parent(s), parent–baby dyad, or family triad. These feelings may have involved helplessness, worry, disapproval, anger, fear, and/or other responses that interfered with the ability to act kindly and promote hope.
4. The clinician experienced distress about the mismatch between her or his cultural values and expectations and the cultural values and expectations of the parent(s), the parent–baby dyad, or family triad.
5. Competing goals with other systems of care (e.g., medical team, child protective services, or legal system) interfered with the clarity of the clinician's role in the course of the sessions.
6. The clinician used external supports (e.g., peer consultation, supervision, other) to aid in self-reflection and gain greater self-understanding.

### Strand 2: Emotional Process Fidelity

1. The clinician endeavored to understand the emotional processes underlying the statements and behavior of the treatment participant(s).
2. The clinician prioritized safety in monitoring the emotional processes and behaviors of the participant(s) and intervened decisively when needed to preserve or restore safety.
3. The clinician retained a clarity of clinical formulation in response to the expression of intense emotion in the participant(s).
4. The clinician conveyed an understanding of and support for the emotional experience of the participant(s) through verbal and/or nonverbal responses.
5. The clinician created a therapeutic context that supported the reflective functioning of the participant(s) vis-à-vis the self and/or other (baby or partner).
6. The clinician made use of P-CPP treatment modalities that deepened self-understanding in the treatment participant(s).
7. The clinician made use of P-CPP treatment modalities that promoted emotional regulation in the treatment participant(s).

### Strand 3: Dyadic Relational Fidelity

1. The clinician enabled each treatment participant to make use of the clinical space during the session.
2. The clinician maintained simultaneous clinical awareness of the competing or divergent individual emotional experiences of each participant.

3. The clinician conveyed empathic understanding for each participant's individual perspective without alienating the other participant(s).
4. The clinician acted as an effective translator to promote greater understanding among the treatment participants of each other's emotional experience and point of view.
5. The clinician used P-CPP treatment strategies that promoted the participants' capacities for conflict resolution and problem solving.

## Strand 4: Trauma Framework Fidelity

1. The clinician listened to the treatment participant, keeping in mind possible connections between the themes unfolding during the session and adverse/traumatic events in the parent's past.
2. The clinician listened for the potential trauma-based etiology of parental attributions to the fetus/infant.
3. The clinician listened for the potential trauma-based etiology of parental attributions to each other and their couple relationship, with particular focus on their parenting collaboration.
4. The clinician used P-CPP treatment modalities to explore and address possible links between parental attributions to the baby and the parent's trauma experiences.
5. The clinician explored the potential impact of historical trauma and current circumstances on the parent's perceptions of the baby and behaviors toward the baby, and toward each other, if working with both parents.
6. The clinician used P-CPP treatment modalities to address affect dysregulation.
7. The clinician used P-CPP treatment modalities to correct parental misperceptions of the baby.
8. The clinician used P-CPP treatment modalities to raise parental awareness of safe and risky childrearing practices and promote protective caregiving.

## Strand 5: Procedural Fidelity

1. During the foundational phase, the clinician addressed the topics relevant to this phase of treatment:
   • Presentation of P-CPP as an opportunity to prepare for the baby's arrival by reflecting on how the woman is feeling about herself and the people important to her, including the baby and the baby's father.
   • Informed consent for treatment and a discussion of legal constraints on confidentiality.

- Duration of treatment, estimated date for the end of treatment, and an explanation that they can be revised as treatment progresses in response to parental needs and other considerations, which may involve, for example, agency regulations regarding treatment length and funding sources.
- Circumstances of the pregnancy and whether the woman and her partner have similar or different views about the pregnancy, including whether or not it was planned and wanted by either the woman, her partner, or both; how the woman and her partner each responded to learning about the pregnancy; and what each of their respective feelings are now.
- Relationship with the intimate partner/father of the baby, his personal characteristics as perceived by the mother, and consideration of his possible involvement in treatment.
- Safety issues involving the intimate partner/father of the baby.
- Specific information about the woman's life history and current circumstances, including her relationship with attachment figures, positive experiences, adversities and traumatic events (including violence in intimate relationships), and a description of current support networks. Structured assessment instruments are clinically useful to elicit systematic information about trauma exposure and life circumstances as a way of creating acceptance for "speaking the unspeakable" and normalizing traumatic events that routinely engender shame and guilt as a painful but frequent aspect of human experience.
- Specific information about the mother's symptoms, with a particular focus on symptoms of depression and posttraumatic stress.
- Perception, attitudes, and feelings about the fetus and hopes and fears for the baby, including positive and negative attributions that reflect the woman's internal world in relation to the fetus and baby-to-be.
- Psychological strengths and vulnerabilities, including the woman's capacity for self-reflection, insightfulness, and affect regulation; her defense structure; her coping strategies; and her openness to trial clinical interpretations.
- The meaning that the woman gives to her real-life circumstances and psychological experiences, including her sense of self as an individual and as a mother; the role of the baby's father; and pathogenic beliefs about herself, the baby, and others that may interfere with psychological growth and the capacity to love.
- Cultural background, including historical trauma and culturally rooted values and attitudes about pregnancy and childrearing practices.

2. The clinician conducted a feedback session and presented the clinical formulation triangle to the parent(s).

3. The clinician extended an invitation to treatment when clinically appropriate that included the co-creation of a treatment plan, containing clear agreements about the format of treatment, about the frequency and length of sessions, and about who would participate in treatment.

4. During the core phase of treatment, the clinician employed P-CPP treatment modalities to attend to the relevant issues involving labor and delivery and the postpartum period, including the co-creation of a birth plan, coordination with the medical team and other service providers as appropriate, and plans about contact during the postpartum period.

5. During the core phase of treatment, the baby was physically present as an integral participant in treatment.

6. During the termination phase, the clinician engaged the parent in a recapitulation of the clinical themes that emerged during treatment to affirm therapeutic progress and provide anticipatory guidance about future challenges.

## Strand 6: Content Fidelity

1. Offering kindness and conveying hope as the key ingredients of a therapeutic stance:
   - The clinician underscored areas of strength, achievement, and resilience in the treatment participant's functioning to emphasize that positive change is possible.
   - The clinician provided realistic examples of potential pathways to healing.
   - The clinician reframed the parent's self-defeating perceptions by describing the adaptive and benevolent aspects of conflictual situations.
   - The clinician maintained a positive and supportive stance to promote the participant's sense of being valued.

2. Maintaining a reflective empathic stance toward the self and the treatment participants:
   - The clinician monitored her or his emotional responses and behaviors to uphold a supportive therapeutic stance.
   - The clinician encouraged each participant's self-reflection by consistently showing interest in the possible origins and the motives underlying distressing feelings and maladaptive behaviors.

3. Promoting environmental and interpersonal safety:
   - The clinician helped the participant reflect on her or his history of physical and emotional endangerment and how the

experiences affect current expectations and behaviors involving danger and safety.

- The clinician addressed supportively but firmly lapses in safe behavior and used P-CPP therapeutic modalities to promote actions that increased physical and interpersonal safety.
- The clinician used P-CPP therapeutic modalities to correct distorted perceptions of danger and safety.
- The clinician engaged with the participant in concrete strategies to safeguard or restore safety.

4. Fostering affect regulation:
   - The clinician helped the participant identify and reflect on moments of emotional dysregulation.
   - The clinician used P-CPP therapeutic modalities to promote affect regulation in caregivers and/or the infant.
   - The clinician helped the participant explore trauma triggers for emotional dysregulation.

5. Encouraging mutual understanding and positive emotional reciprocity:
   - The clinician helped the parents identify and explore negative perceptions and feelings toward intimate others and the baby.
   - The clinician helped the parents respond contingently to the baby's signals of physical and social needs.
   - The clinician used P-CPP therapeutic modalities to promote each participant's increased understanding of the other's point of view.

6. Including themes of trauma and protection in giving meaning to behavior:
   - The clinician used P-CPP therapeutic strategies to normalize the traumatic stress response by contextualizing it and describing its adaptive function.
   - The clinician promoted a deep emotional acknowledgment of the impact of trauma, while helping the participant differentiate between remembering and reliving the traumatic experience.
   - The clinician helped the parents identify the unconscious reenactment of past traumatic experiences in their perceptions of and behaviors toward the baby.
   - The clinician helped the participant create a trauma narrative that integrated the pain of the past with proactive engagement with developmental goals for the present and the future.

## Training Guidelines

Training in P-CPP is organized by the UCSF Child Trauma Research Program. The training is designed to promote adherence to the model using the fidelity guidelines just described. We know that many clinicians implement excellent therapeutic interventions with pregnant women and with expectant fathers individually, as couples, or in a group format, and Section I provides an overview of several models of intervention that show successful outcomes in achieving their goals. However, therapeutic competence in working with expectant mothers and fathers does not by itself equip clinicians to implement P-CPP with adherence to this specific model. Similarly, although P-CPP is an application of CPP to pregnancy and the perinatal period, CPP clinicians do not necessarily have the specialized knowledge about normative and pathological processes during pregnancy and the perinatal period to enable them to translate their CPP expertise to P-CPP without additional training. For these reasons, we strongly recommend seeking P-CPP training before implementing the model. Information about this training will be posted on the Child Trauma Research Program website, and it can be obtained from the first author (A. F. L.) of the book.

# References

Abajobir, A. A., Maravilla, J. C., Alati, R., & Najman, J. M. (2016). A systematic review and meta-analysis of the association between unintended pregnancy and perinatal depression. *Journal of Affective Disorders, 192,* 56–63.

Abraído-Lanza, A. F., Echeverría, S. E., & Flórez, K. R. (2016). Latino immigrants, acculturation, and health: Promising new directions in research. *Annual Review of Public Health, 37,* 219–236.

Ainsworth, M. D. S., Blehar, M. C., Waters, E., & Wall, S. N. (1978). *Patterns of attachment: A psychological study of the Strange Situation.* Hillsdale, NJ: Erlbaum.

Alvarez-Segura, M., Garcia-Esteve, L., Torres, A., Plaza, A., Imaz, M. L., Hermida-Barros, L., . . . Burtchen, N. (2014). Are women with a history of abuse more vulnerable to perinatal depressive symptoms?: A systematic review. *Archives of Women's Mental Health, 17*(5), 343–357.

American Psychiatric Association. (2013). *Diagnostic and statistical manual of mental disorders* (5th ed.). Arlington, VA: Author.

Amichai, Y. (2004). Concrete poem. *The New Republic, 231*(24), 32–33.

Armstrong, D., & Hutti, M. (1998). Pregnancy after perinatal loss: The relationship between anxiety and prenatal attachment. *Journal of Obstetric, Gynecologic, and Neonatal Nursing, 27*(2), 183–189.

Asling-Monemi, K., Peña, R., Ellsberg, M. C., & Persson, L. A. (2003). Violence against women increases the risk of infant and child mortality: A case-referent study in Nicaragua. *Bulletin of the World Health Organization, 81*(1), 10–16.

Atzl, V. M., Narayan, A. J., Rivera, L. M., & Lieberman, A. F. (2019). Adverse childhood experiences and prenatal mental health: Type of ACEs and age of maltreatment onset. *Journal of Family Psychology, 33*(3), 304–314.

Bader, A. P. (1995). Engrossment revisited: Fathers are still falling in love with their newborn babies. In J. L. Shapiro, M. J. Diamond, & M. Greenberg (Eds.), *Becoming a father* (pp. 224–233). New York: Springer.

Baer, R. A. (2003). Mindfulness training as a clinical intervention: A conceptual and empirical review. *Clinical Psychology: Science and Practice, 10,* 125–143.

Barnett, K. (1972). A theoretical construct of the concepts of touch as they relate to nursing. *Nursing Research, 21,* 102–110.

Becker, K. D., Stuewig, J., & McCloskey, L. A. (2010). Traumatic stress symptoms of women exposed to different forms of childhood victimization and intimate partner violence. *Journal of Interpersonal Violence, 25*(9), 1699–1715.

Beebe, B., Lachmann, F., & Jaffe, J. (1997). Mother–infant interaction structures and presymbolic self- and object representations. *Psychoanalytic Dialogues, 7*(2), 133–182.

Behnke, M., Smith, V. C., & Committee on Substance Abuse. (2013). Prenatal substance abuse: Short- and long-term effects on the exposed fetus. *Pediatrics, 131*(3), 1009–1024.

Benedek, T. (1970). The psychobiology of pregnancy. In E. J. Anthony & T. Benedek (Eds.), *Parenthood: Its psychology and psychopathology* (pp. 137–151). New York: Little, Brown.

Bennett, C., Underdown, A., & Barlow, J. (2013). Massage for promoting mental and physical health in typically developing infants under the age of six months. *Cochrane Database of Systematic Reviews, 4*.

Benoit, D., Parker, K. C., & Zeanah, C. H. (1997). Mothers' representations of their infants assessed prenatally: Stability and association with infants' attachment classifications. *Journal of Child Psychology and Psychiatry, 38*, 307–313.

Bernet, W., & Freeman, B. W. (2000). Child maltreatment. In B. J. Sadock & V. A. Sadock (Eds.), *Kaplan and Sadock's comprehensive textbook of psychiatry* (7th ed., pp. 2878–2889). Baltimore: Lippincott Williams & Wilkins.

Beydoun, H. A., Al-Sahab, B., Beydoun, M. A., & Tamim, H. (2010). Intimate partner violence as a risk factor for postpartum depression among Canadian women in the Maternity Experience Survey. *Annals of Epidemiology, 20*(8), 575–583.

Bibring, G. L. (1959). Some considerations of the psychological processes in pregnancy. *Psychoanalytic Study of the Child, 14*, 77–121.

Bibring, G., Dwyer, T., Huntington, D., & Valenstein, F. (1961). A study of the psychological processes in pregnancy and of the earliest mother–child relationship: I. Some propositions and comments. *Psychoanalytic Study of the Child, 16*, 9–24.

Bion, W. R. (1959). *Splitting and projective identification.* Northvale, NJ: Jason Aronson.

Birksted-Breen, D. (2000). The experience of having a baby: A developmental view. In J. Raphael-Leff (Ed.), *'Spilt milk': Perinatal loss and breakdown* (pp. 17–27). London: Institute of Psychoanalysis.

Bogat, G. A., DeJonghe, E., Levendosky, A., Davidson, W., & von Eye, A. (2006). Trauma symptoms among infants exposed to intimate partner violence. *Child Abuse and Neglect, 30*(2), 109–125.

Bollas, C. (1987). *The shadow of the object: Psychoanalysis of the unthought known.* London: Free Association Books.

Boris, N. W., Renk, K., Lowell, A., & Kolomeyer, E. (2019). Parental substance abuse. In C. H. Zeanah, Jr. (Ed.), *Handbook of infant mental health* (4th ed., pp. 187–202). New York: Guilford Press.

Bowlby, J. (1969). *Attachment and loss: Vol. 1. Attachment.* New York: Basic Books.

Bowlby, J. (1973). *Attachment and loss: Vol. 2. Separation: Anxiety and anger.* New York: Basic Books.

Bowlby, J. (1980). *Attachment and loss: Vol. 3. Loss, sadness, and depression.* New York: Basic Books.

Bowlby, J. (1988). *A secure base: Parent–child attachment and healthy human development.* New York: Basic Books.

Bradley, E. (2000). Pregnancy and the internal world. In J. Raphael-Leff (Ed.), *'Spilt milk': Perinatal loss and breakdown* (pp. 28–38). London: Institute of Psychoanalysis.

Brazelton, B. (2006). *Touchpoints birth to 3: Your child's emotional and behavioral development* (2nd ed.). Cambridge, MA: Da Capo Lifelong Books.

Brennan, A., Ayers, S., Ahmed, H., & Marshall-Lucette, S. (2007). A critical review of the Couvade syndrome: The pregnant male. *Journal of Reproductive and Infant Psychology, 25*(3), 173–189.

Brennan, A., Marshall-Lucette, S., Ayers, S., & Ahmed, H. (2007). A qualitative exploration of the Couvade syndrome in expectant fathers. *Journal of Reproductive and Infant Psychology, 25*(1), 18–39.

Bronfenbrenner, U. (1979). *The ecology of human development: Experiments by nature and design.* Cambridge, MA: Harvard University Press.

Bruschweiler-Stern, N. (2009). The neonatal moment of meeting—Building the dialogue, strengthening the bond. *Child and Adolescent Psychiatric Clinics of North America, 18*(3), 533–544.

Buckwalter, J. G., Buckwalter, D. K., Bluestein, B. W., & Stanczyk, F. Z. (2001). Pregnancy and postpartum: Changes in cognition and mood. *Progress in Brain Research, 133,* 303–319.

Burke Harris, N. (2018). *The deepest well: Healing the long-term effects of childhood adversity.* New York: Houghton Mifflin Harcourt.

Carlson, M., & Earls, F. (1997). Psychological and neuroendocrinological sequelae of early social deprivation in institutionalized children in Romania. In C. S. Carter, I. I. Lederhendler, & B. Kirkpatrick (Eds.), *Annals of the New York Academy of Sciences, Vol. 807: The integrative neurobiology of affiliation* (pp. 419–428). New York: New York Academy of Sciences.

Carpenter, G. L., & Stacks, A. M. (2009). Developmental effects of exposure to intimate partner violence in early childhood: A review of the literature. *Children and Youth Services Review, 31*(8), 831–839.

Centers for Disease Control and Prevention. (2019). Pregnancy Mortality Surveillance System. Retrieved from *www.cdc.gov/reproductivehealth/maternalinfanthealth/pregnancy-mortality-surveillance-system.htm.*

Cha, S., Chapman, D. A., Wan, W., Burton, C. W., & Masho, S. W. (2016). Discordant pregnancy intentions in couples and rapid repeat pregnancy. *American Journal of Obstetrics and Gynecology, 214*(4), 494.e1–494.e12.

Charles, P., & Perreira, K. M. (2007). Intimate partner violence during pregnancy and 1-year postpartum. *Journal of Family Violence, 22,* 609–619.

Child Welfare Information Gateway. (2019). Child abuse and neglect fatalities 2017: Statistics and interventions. Retrieved from *www.childwelfare.gov/pubPDFs/fatality.pdf.*

Chugani, H. T., Behen, M. E., Muzik, O., Juhász, C., & Chugani, D. C. (2001).

Local brain functional activity following early deprivation: A study of postinstitutionalized Romanian orphans. *NeuroImage, 14,* 1290–1301.

Cicchetti, D., & Sroufe, L. A. (2000). The past as prologue to the future: The times, they've been a-changin'. *Development and Psychopathology, 12*(3), 255–264.

Coker, A. L., Sanderson, M., & Dong, B. (2004). Partner violence during pregnancy and risk of adverse pregnancy outcomes. *Paediatric and Perinatal Epidemiology, 18*(4), 260–269.

Commission for Historical Clarification. (1999). Guatemala: Memory of silence. Report of the Commission for Historical Clarification, Conclusions and Recommendations (CEH). Retrieved from *www.aaas.org/sites/default/files/s3fs-public/mos_en.pdf.*

Cowan, P. A., Cowan, C. P., Pruett, M. K., & Pruett, K. D. (2018). Supporting father involvement: A father-inclusive couples group approach to parenting interventions In H. Steele & M. Steele (Eds.), *Handbook of attachment-based interventions* (pp. 466–492). New York: Guilford Press.

Cowan, P. A., Cowan, C. P., Pruett, M. K., & Pruett, K. D. (2019). Fathers' and mothers' attachment styles, couple conflict, parenting quality, and children's behavior problems: An intervention test of mediation. *Attachment and Human Development, 21*(5) 532–550.

Darvill, R., Skirton, H., & Farrand, P. (2010). Psychological factors that impact on women's experiences of first-time motherhood: A qualitative study of the transition. *Midwifery, 26*(3), 357–366.

Davis, L., Edwards, H., Mohay, H., & Wollin, J. (2003). The impact of very premature birth on the psychological health of mothers. *Early Human Development, 73*(1-2), 61–70.

Dube, S. R., Anda, R. F., Felitti, V. J., Edwards, V. J., & Croft, J. B. (2002). Adverse childhood experiences and personal alcohol abuse as an adult. *Addictive Behaviors 27*(5), 713–725.

Eckenrode, J., Ganzel, B., Henderson, C. R., Smith, E., Olds, D., Powers, J., . . . Sidora, K. (2000). Preventing child abuse and neglect with a program of nurse home visitation: The limiting effects of domestic violence. *JAMA, 284*(11), 1385–1391.

Edelstein, R. S., Wardecker, B. M., Chopik, W. J., Moors, A. C., Shipman, E. L., & Lin, N. J. (2014). Prenatal hormones in first-time expectant parents: Longitudinal changes and within-couple correlations. *American Journal of Human Biology, 27*(3), 317–325.

Edleson, J. L., & Williams, O. J. (Eds.). (2006). *Parenting by men who batter: New directions for assessment and intervention.* London: Oxford University Press.

El Kady, D., Gilbert, W. M., Xing, G., & Smith, L. H. (2005). Maternal and neonatal outcomes of assaults during pregnancy. *Obstetrics and Gynecology, 105*(2), 357–363.

Emde, R. N. (1990). Mobilizing fundamental modes of development: Empathic availability and therapeutic action. *Journal of the American Psychoanalytic Association, 38*(4), 881–913.

Fadiman, A. (1997). *The spirit catches you and you fall down: A Hmong child, her*

*American doctors, and the collision of two cultures.* New York: Farrar, Straus & Giroux.

Feijo, L., Hernandez-Reif, M., Field, T., Burns, W., Valley-Gray, S., & Simco, E. (2006). Mothers' depressed mood and anxiety levels are reduced after massaging their preterm infants. *Infant Behavior and Development, 29*(3), 476–480.

Feldman, R., Gordon, I., & Zagoory-Sharon, O. (2011). Maternal and paternal plasma, salivary, and urinary oxytocin and parent–infant synchrony: Considering stress and affiliation components of human bonding. *Developmental Science, 14*(4), 752–761.

Felitti, V. J., Anda, R. F., Nordenberg, D., Williamson, D. F., Spitz, A. M., Edwards, V., . . . Marks, J. S. (1998). Relationship of childhood abuse and household dysfunction to many of the leading causes of death in adults: The Adverse Childhood Experiences (ACE) Study. *American Journal of Preventive Medicine, 14*(4), 245–258.

Field, T. (2014). Massage therapy research review. *Complementary Therapies in Clinical Practice, 20*(4), 224–229.

Field, T., Diego, M., & Hernandez-Reif, M. (2010). Preterm infant massage therapy research: A review. *Infant Behavior and Development, 33*(2), 115–124.

Field, T., Hernandez-Reif, M., Diego, M. A., Schanberg, S. M., & Kuhn, C. M. (2005). Cortisol decreases and serotonin and dopamine increase following massage therapy. *International Journal of Neuroscience, 115*(10), 1397–1413.

Finer, L. B., & Zolna, M. R. (2016). Declines in unintended pregnancy in the United States, 2008–2011. *New England Journal of Medicine, 374*(9), 843–852.

Finkelhor, D., Ormrod, R., Turner, H., & Hamby, S. L. (2005). The victimization of children and youth: A comprehensive, national survey. *Child Maltreatment, 10*(1), 5–25.

Finnbogadóttir, H., Dykes, A., & Wann-Hansson, C. (2014). Prevalence of domestic violence during pregnancy and related risk factors: A cross-sectional study in southern Sweden. *BMC Women's Health, 14*(63), 1–13.

Fivaz-Depeursinge, E., & Corboz-Warnery, A. (1999). *The primary triangle: A developmental systems view of mothers, fathers, and infants.* New York: Basic Books.

Fleming, A. S., Corter, C., Stallings, J., & Steiner, M. (2002). Testosterone and prolactin are associated with emotional responses to infant cries in new fathers. *Hormones and Behavior, 42*(4), 399–413.

Flores, Y. G. (2013). *Chicana and Chicano mental health: Alma, mente y corazón.* Tucson: University of Arizona Press.

Flores-Ortíz, Y., Valdez Curiel, E., & Andrade, P. (2002). Intimate partner violence and couple interaction among women from Mexico City and Jalisco. *Journal of Border Health, 7*(1) 33–42.

Fonagy, P. (1998). Moments of change in psychoanalytic theory: Discussion of a new theory of psychic change. *Infant Mental Health Journal, 19*(3), 346–353.

Fraiberg, S. (Ed.). (1980). *Clinical studies in infant mental health: The first year of life.* New York: Basic Books.

Fraiberg, S., Adelson, E., & Shapiro, V. (1975). Ghosts in the nursery: A psychoanalytic approach to the problems of impaired infant–mother relationships. *Journal of the American Academy of Child Psychiatry, 14*(3), 387–421.

Freud, S. (1959). Inhibitions, symptoms and anxiety. In J. Strachey (Ed. & Trans.), *Standard edition of the complete psychological works of Sigmund Freud* (Vol. 20, pp. 75–175). London: Hogarth Press. (Original work published 1926)

Gaudet, C., Séjourné, N., Camborieux, L., Rogers, R., & Chabrol, H. (2010). Pregnancy after perinatal loss: Association of grief, anxiety and attachment. *Journal of Reproductive and Infant Psychology, 28*(3), 240–251.

Ghosh Ippen, C., & Lieberman, A. F. (2019). *The Child–Parent Psychotherapy fidelity framework: A guide for conducting relationship-based trauma-informed interventions.* Unpublished manuscript.

Ghosh Ippen, C., Lieberman, A. F., & Van Horn, P. (2012). Child–Parent Psychotherapy fidelity instruments. Retrieved from *http://childparentpsychotherapy.com/providers/implementationtools/fidelity.*

Gipson, J. D., Koenig, M. A., & Hindin, M. J. (2008). The effects of unintended pregnancy on infant, child, and parental health: A review of the literature. *Studies in Family Planning, 39*(1), 18–38.

Gloria, A. M., & Castellanos, J. (2016). Latinas poderosas: Shaping mujerismo to manifest sacred spaces for healing and transformation. In T. Bryant-Davis & L. Comas-Díaz (Eds.), *Womanist and mujerista psychologies: Voices of fire, acts of courage* (pp. 93–119). Washington, DC: American Psychological Association.

Goodwin, M. M., Gazmararian, J. A., Johnson, C. H., Gilbert, B. C., & Saltzman, L. E. (2000). Pregnancy intendedness and physical abuse around the time of pregnancy: Findings from the Pregnancy Risk Assessment Monitoring System, 1996–1997. *Maternal and Child Health Journal, 4*(2), 85–92.

Gordon, I., Zagoory-Sharon, O., Leckman, J. F., & Feldman, R. (2010). Prolactin, oxytocin, and the development of paternal behavior across the first six months of fatherhood. *Hormones and Behavior, 58*(3), 513–518.

Gratz, K. L., & Gunderson, J. G. (2006). Preliminary data on an acceptance-based emotion regulation group intervention for deliberate self-harm among women with borderline personality disorder. *Behavior Therapy, 37*(1), 25–35.

Gratz, K. L., & Tull, M. T. (2010). Emotion regulation as a mechanism of change in acceptance- and mindfulness-based treatments. In R. A. Baer (Ed.), *Assessing mindfulness and acceptance processes in clients: Illuminating the theory and practice of change* (pp. 107–133). Oakland, CA: Context Press/New Harbinger.

Gray, P. B., & Anderson, K. G. (2010). *Fatherhood: Evolution and human paternal behavior.* Cambridge, MA: Harvard University Press.

Gray, S. A., Jones, C. W., Theall, K. P., Glackin, E., & Drury, S. S. (2017). Thinking across generations: Unique contributions of maternal early life and prenatal stress to infant physiology. *Journal of the American Academy of Child and Adolescent Psychiatry, 56*(11), 922–929.

Gross, J. J. (1998). The emerging field of emotion regulation: An integrative review. *Review of General Psychology, 2*(3), 271–299.

Grossman, P., Niemann, L., Schmidt, S., & Walach, H. (2004). Mindfulness-based stress reduction and health benefits: A meta-analysis. *Journal of Psychosomatic Research, 57*(1), 35–43.

Grossmann, K., Grossmann, K. E., Kindler, H., & Zimmerman, P. (2008). A wider view of attachment and exploration: The influence of mothers and fathers on the development of psychological security from infancy to young adulthood. In J. Cassidy & P. R. Shaver (Eds.), *Handbook of attachment: Theory, research, and clinical applications* (2nd ed., pp. 857–879). New York: Guilford Press.

Groves, B. M., Van Horn, P., & Lieberman, A. F. (2007). Deciding on fathers' involvement in their children's treatment after domestic violence. In J. L. Edleson & O. J. Williams (Eds.), *Parenting by men who batter: New directions for assessment and intervention* (pp. 65–84). New York: Oxford University Press.

Hall, J. A., Benton, L., Copas, A., & Stephenson, J. (2017). Pregnancy intention and pregnancy outcome: Systematic review and meta-analysis. *Maternal and Child Health Journal, 21*(3), 670–704.

Hamilton, B. E., Martin, J. A., Osterman, M. J. K., Curtin, S. C., & Mathews, T. J. (2015). Births: Final data for 2014. *National Vital Statistics Reports, 64*(12). Retrieved from *www.cdc.gov/nchs/data/nvsr/nvsr64/nvsr64_12.pdf.*

Herman, J. L. (1992). *Recovery: The aftermath of violence, from domestic abuse to political terror.* New York: Basic Books.

Hill, A., Pallitto, C., McCleary-Sills, J., & Garcia-Moreno, C. (2016). A systematic review and meta-analysis of intimate partner violence during pregnancy and selected birth outcomes. *International Journal of Gynecology and Obstetrics, 133*(3), 269–276.

Hinshaw, S. P. (2013). Child maltreatment. In T. P. Beauchaine & S. P. Hinshaw (Eds.), *Child and adolescent psychopathology* (2nd ed., pp. 3–28). Hoboken, NJ: Wiley.

Hofmann, S. G., Sawyer, A. T., Witt, A. A., & Oh, D. (2010). The effect of mindfulness-based therapy on anxiety and depression: A meta-analytic review. *Journal of Consulting and Clinical Psychology, 78*(2), 169–183.

Hohmann-Marriott, B. (2009). The couple context of pregnancy and its effects on prenatal care and birth outcomes. *Maternal and Child Health Journal, 13*(6), 745–754.

Hopping-Winn, A. (2012). Supporting children of parents with co-occurring mental illness and substance abuse. National Abandoned Infants Assistance Resource Center (AIA) Research to Practice Brief. Retrieved from *www.ct.gov/dmhas/lib/dmhas/cosig/BriefSupportingChildren.pdf.*

Hrdy, S. B. (1999). *Mother nature: A history of mothers, infants, and natural selection.* New York: Pantheon.

Hughes, K. E., Bellis, M. A., Hardcastle, K. A., Sethi, D., Butchart, A. R., Mikton, C., . . . Dunne, M. P. (2017). The effect of multiple adverse childhood experiences on health: A systematic review and meta-analysis. *The Lancet Public Health, 2*(8), e356–e366.

Hughes, P., Turton, P., Hopper, E., & Evans, C. D. H. (2002). Assessment of guidelines for good practice in psychosocial care of mothers after still-birth: A cohort study. *The Lancet, 360*(9327), 114–118.

Huth-Bocks, A. C., Levendosky, A. A., & Bogat, G. A. (2002). The effects of domestic violence during pregnancy on maternal and infant health. *Violence and Victims, 17*(2), 169–185.

Huth-Bocks, A. C., Levendosky, A. A., Theran, S. A., & Bogat, G. A. (2004). The impact of domestic violence on mothers' prenatal representations of their infants. *Infant Mental Health Journal, 25*(2), 79–98.

James L., Brody, D., & Hamilton, Z. (2013). Risk factors for domestic violence during pregnancy: A meta-analytic review. *Violence and Victims, 28*(3), 359–380.

Jasinski, J. L. (2004). Pregnancy and domestic violence: A review of the literature. *Trauma, Violence, and Abuse, 5*(1), 47–64.

Johnson, P. J., Hellerstedt, W. L., & Pirie, P. L. (2002). Abuse history and non-optimal prenatal weight gain. *Public Health Reports, 117*(2), 148–156.

Jones, D. J., Zalot, A., Foster, S., Sterrett, E., & Chester, C. (2007). A review of childrearing in African American single mother families: The relevance of a coparenting framework. *Journal of Child and Family Studies, 16*(5), 671–683.

Jones, L., Hughes, M., & Unterstaller, U. (2001). Post-traumatic stress disorder (PTSD) in victims of domestic violence: A review of the research. *Trauma, Violence, and Abuse, 2*(2), 99–119.

Jung, C. (1966). Fundamental questions of psychotherapy. In *Collected works* (Vol. 16, p. 121). London: Routledge. (Original work published 1951)

Jung, C. (1982). Fundamental questions of psychotherapy. In S. H. Read, M. Fordham, G. Adler, & W. McGuire (Eds.), *Collected works of C. G. Jung: Practice of psychotherapy* (Vol. 16, pp. 116–129). Princeton, NJ: Princeton University Press. (Original work published 1951)

Karst, P., & Stevenson, G. (2000). *The invisible string.* Camarillo, CA: DeVorss & Company.

Kelly, U. A. (2009). "I'm a mother first": The influence of mothering in the decision-making processes of battered immigrant Latino women. *Research in Nursing and Health, 32*(3), 286–297.

Kendler, K. S., Myers, J., & Prescott, C. A. (2007). Specificity of genetic and environmental risk factors for symptoms of cannabis, cocaine, alcohol, caffeine, and nicotine dependence. *Archives of General Psychiatry, 64*(11), 1313–1320.

Kersting, A., Kroker, K., Steinhard, J., Lüdorff, K., Wesselmann, U., Ohrmann, P., . . . Suslow, T. (2007). Complicated grief after traumatic loss. *European Archives of Psychiatry and Clinical Neuroscience, 257*(8), 437–443.

Kersting, A., & Wagner, B. (2012). Complicated grief after perinatal loss. *Dialogues in Clinical Neuroscience, 14*(2), 187–194.

Kim, P., Rigo, P., Mayes, L. C., Feldman, R., Leckman, J. F., & Swain, J. E. (2014). Neural plasticity in fathers of human infants. *Social Neuroscience, 9*(5), 522–535.

Kim, S., Iyengar, U., Mayes, L. C., Potenza, M. N., Rutherford, H. J., & Strathearn, L. (2017). Mothers with substance addictions show reduced reward responses when viewing their own infant's face. *Human Brain Mapping, 38*(11), 5421–5439.

Kimbrough, E., Magyari, T., Langenberg, P., Chesney, M., & Berman, B. (2010). Mindfulness intervention for child abuse survivors. *Journal of Clinical Psychology, 66*(1), 17–33.

Kitzman, H. J., Olds, D. L., Cole, R. E., Hanks, C. A., Anson, E. A., Arcoleo, K. J., . . . Holmberg, J. R. (2010). Enduring effects of prenatal and infancy home visiting by nurses on children: Follow-up of a randomized trial among children at age 12 years. *Archives of Pediatrics and Adolescent Medicine, 164*(5), 412–418.

Klein, H. (1991). Couvade syndrome: Male counterpart to pregnancy. *International Journal of Psychiatry in Medicine, 21*(1), 57–69.

Klein, M. (1980). *Envy and gratitude: And other works, 1946–1963*. London: Hogarth Press. (Original work published 1946)

Kofman, S., & Imber, R. (2005). Pregnancy. In S. F. Brown (Ed.), *What do mothers want?: Developmental perspectives, clinical challenges* (pp. 151–170). New York: Analytic Press.

Korenman, S., Kaestner, R., & Joyce, T. (2002). Consequences for infants of parental disagreement in pregnancy intention. *Perspectives on Sexual and Reproductive Health, 34*(4) 198–205.

Kost, K., & Lindberg, L. (2015). Pregnancy intentions, maternal behaviors, and infant health: Investigating relationships with new measures and propensity score analysis. *Demography, 52*(1), 83–111.

Kotelchuck, M., & Lu, M. (2017). Father's role in preconception health. *Maternal and Child Health Journal, 21*(11), 2025–2039.

Kubička, L., Matějček, Z., David, H., Dytrych, Z., Miller, W., & Roth, Z. (1995). Children from unwanted pregnancies in Prague, Czech Republic revisited at age thirty. *Acta Psychiatrica Scandinavica, 91,* 361–369.

Lahiri, J. (2004). *The namesake*. New York: First Mariner Books.

Lamb, M. E. (1976a). Effects of stress and cohort on mother– and father–infant interaction. *Developmental Psychology, 12*(5), 435.

Lamb, M. E. (1976b). Interactions between two-year-olds and their mothers and fathers. *Psychological Reports, 38*(2), 447–450.

Lamb, M. E. (1978). Qualitative aspects of mother– and father–infant attachments. *Infant Behavior and Development, 1,* 265–275.

Landi, N., Montoya, J., Kober, H., Rutherford, H. J., Mencl, W. E., Worhunsky, P. D., . . . Mayes, L. C. (2011). Maternal neural responses to infant cries and faces: Relationships with substance use. *Frontiers in Psychiatry, 2*(32), 1–13.

Lavi, I., Gard, A. M., Hagan, M., Van Horn, P., & Lieberman, A. F. (2015). Child–Parent Psychotherapy examined in a perinatal sample: Depression, posttraumatic stress symptoms and child-rearing attitudes. *Journal of Social and Clinical Psychology, 34*(1), 64–82.

Lefèber, Y., & Voorhoeve, H. W. (1998). *Indigenous customs in childbirth and child care*. Assen, the Netherlands: Van Gorcum.

Leifer, M. (1977). Psychological changes accompanying pregnancy and motherhood. *Genetic Psychology Monographs, 95*(1), 55–96.

Letourneau, N. L., Fedick, C. B., & Willms, J. D. (2007). Mothering and domestic violence: A longitudinal analysis. *Journal of Family Violence, 22,* 649–659.

Levendosky, A. A., Leahy, K. L., Bogat, G. A., Davidson, W. S., & von Eye, A. (2006). Domestic violence, maternal parenting, maternal mental health, and infant externalizing behavior. *Journal of Family Psychology, 20*(4), 544–552.

Lieberman, A. F. (1983). Infant–Parent Psychotherapy during pregnancy. In S. Provence (Ed.), *Infants and parents: Clinical case reports* (pp. 84–141). New York: International Universities Press.

Lieberman, A. F. (1999). Negative maternal attributions: Effects on toddlers' sense of self. *Psychoanalytic Inquiry, 19*(5), 737–756.

Lieberman, A. F., & Blos, P. (1980). Make way for baby. In S. Fraiberg & L. Fraiberg (Eds.), *Clinical studies in infant mental health: The first year of life* (pp. 242–259). New York: Basic Books.

Lieberman, A. F., Diaz, M. A., & Van Horn, P. (2009). Safer beginnings: Perinatal Child–Parent Psychotherapy for newborns and mothers exposed to domestic violence. *Zero to Three, 29,* 17–22.

Lieberman, A. F., Diaz, M. A., & Van Horn, P. (2011). Perinatal Child–Parent Psychotherapy: Adaptation of an evidence-based treatment for pregnant women and babies exposed to intimate partner violence. In S. A. Graham-Bermann & A. A. Levendosky (Eds.), *How intimate partner violence affects children* (pp. 47–66). Washington, DC: American Psychological Association.

Lieberman, A. F., Ghosh Ippen, C., & Van Horn, P. (2006). Child–Parent Psychotherapy: Six month follow-up of a randomized control trial. *Journal of the American Academy of Child and Adolescent Psychiatry, 45*(8), 913–918.

Lieberman, A. F., Ghosh Ippen, C., & Van Horn, P. (2015). *Don't hit my mommy: A manual for Child–Parent Psychotherapy with young witnesses of family violence* (2nd ed.). Washington, DC: Zero to Three.

Lieberman, A. F., Padron, E., Van Horn, P., & Harris, W. W. (2005). Angels in the nursery: The intergenerational transmission of benevolent parental influences. *Infant Mental Health Journal, 26,* 504–520.

Lieberman, A. F., & Van Horn, P. (2005). *"Don't hit my mommy!": A manual for Child–Parent Psychotherapy with young witnesses of family violence.* Washington, DC: Zero to Three.

Lieberman, A. F., & Van Horn, P. (2008). *Psychotherapy with infants and young children: Repairing the effects of stress and trauma on early attachment.* New York: Guilford Press.

Lieberman, A. F., Van Horn, P. J., & Ghosh Ippen, C. (2005). Toward evidence-based treatment: Child–Parent Psychotherapy with preschoolers exposed to marital violence. *Journal of the American Academy of Child and Adolescent Psychiatry, 44,* 1241–1248.

Lindberg, L. D., & Kost, K. (2014). Exploring U.S. men's birth intentions. *Maternal and Child Health Journal, 18*(3), 625–633.

Londono Tobon, A., Condon, E., Holland, M., Slade, A., Mayes, L. C., & Sadler, L. (2018). Lasting effects of Minding the Baby® Home Visiting Program for young families. *Journal of the American Academy of Child and Adolescent Psychiatry, 57*(10S), S159.

Luborsky, L. (1984). *Principles of psychoanalytic psychotherapy: A manual for supportive-expressive treatment.* New York: Basic Books.

Lutenbacher, M. (2002). Relationships between psychosocial factors and abusive parenting attitudes in low-income single mothers. *Nursing Research, 51*(3), 158–167.

Maeda, A., Bateman, B. T., Clancy, C. R., Creanga, A. A., & Leffert, L. R. (2014). Opioid abuse and dependence during pregnancy: Temporal trends and obstetrical outcomes. *Journal of the American Society of Anesthesiologists, 121*(6), 1158–1165.

Main, M., Hesse, E., & Kaplan, N. (2005). Predictability of attachment behavior and representational processes at 1, 6, and 19 years of age: The Berkeley Longitudinal Study. In K. E. Grossmann, K. Grossman, & E. Waters (Eds.), *Attachment from infancy to adulthood: The major longitudinal studies* (pp. 245–304). New York: Guilford Press.

Main, M., Kaplan, N., & Cassidy, J. (1985). Security in infancy, childhood, and adulthood: A move to the level of representation. *Monographs of the Society for Research in Child Development, 50*(1–2), 66–104.

Marmar, C. R., Foy, D., Kagan, B., & Pynoos, R. S. (1993). An integrated approach for treating posttraumatic stress disorder. In J. Oldham, J. M. Riba, & A. Tasman (Eds.), *Review of psychiatry* (pp. 239–272). Washington, DC: American Psychiatric Press.

Martin, S. L., Beaumont, J. L., & Kupper, L. L. (2003). Substance use before and during pregnancy: Links to intimate partner violence. *American Journal of Drug and Alcohol Abuse, 29*(3), 599–617.

Martin, S. L., Mackie, L., Kupper, L. L., Buescher, P. A., & Moracco K. E. (2001). Physical abuse of women before, during, and after pregnancy. *JAMA, 285*(12), 1581–1584.

Martin, S. L., Macy, R. J., Sullivan, K., & Magee, M. L. (2007). Pregnancy-associated violent deaths: The role of intimate partner violence. *Trauma, Violence, and Abuse, 8*(2), 135–148.

McHale, J. P., Salman-Engin, S., & Coovert, M. D. (2015). Improvements in unmarried African-American parents' rapport, communication, and problem-solving following a prenatal coparenting intervention. *Family Process, 54*(4), 619–629.

Menchú, R. (1984). *I, Rigoberta Menchú: An Indian woman in Guatemala.* Brooklyn, NY: Verso Books.

Monk, C., Feng, T., Lee, S., Krupska, I., Champagne, F. A., & Tycko, B. (2016). Distress during pregnancy: Epigenetic regulation of placenta glucocorticoid-related genes and fetal neurobehavior. *American Journal of Psychiatry, 173*(7), 705–713.

Moog, N. K., Buss, C., Entringer, S., Shahbaba, B., Gillen, D. L., Hobel, C. J., & Wadhwa, P. D. (2016). Maternal exposure to childhood trauma is associated during pregnancy with placental–fetal stress physiology. *Biological Psychiatry, 79*(10), 831–839.

Moog, N. K., Entringer, S., Heim, C., Wadhwa, P. D., Kathmann, N., & Buss, C.

(2017). Influence of maternal thyroid hormones during gestation on fetal brain development. *Neuroscience, 342,* 68–100.

Morland, L. A., Leskin, G. A., Block, C. R., Campbell, J. C., & Friedman, M. J. (2008). Intimate partner violence and miscarriage: Examination of the role of physical and psychological abuse and posttraumatic stress disorder. *Journal of Interpersonal Violence, 23*(5), 652–669.

Muzik, M., Cameron, H., Fezzey, A., & Rosenblum, K. (2009). Motherhood in the face of trauma: PTSD in the childbearing year. *Zero to Three, 29*(5), 28–34.

Nabokov, V. (1955). *Lolita.* London: Weidenfeld & Nicolson.

Narayan, A. J., Ghosh Ippen, C., Harris, W. W., & Lieberman, A. F. (2017). Assessing angels in the nursery: A pilot study of childhood memories of benevolent caregiving as protective influences. *Infant Mental Health Journal, 38*(4), 461–474.

Narayan, A. J., Ghosh Ippen, C., Harris, W. W., & Lieberman, A. F. (2019). Protective factors that buffer against the intergenerational transmission of trauma from mothers to young children: A replication study of angels in the nursery. *Development and Psychopathology, 31*(1), 173–187.

Narayan, A. J., Oliver Bucio, G., Rivera, L. M., & Lieberman, A. F. (2016). Making sense of the past creates space for the baby: Perinatal Child–Parent Psychotherapy for pregnant women with childhood trauma. *Zero to Three, 36,* 22–28.

Narayan, A. J., Rivera, L. M., Bernstein, R. E., Castro, G., Gantt, T., Thomas, M., . . . Lieberman, A. F. (2017). Between pregnancy and motherhood: Identifying unmet mental health needs in pregnant women with lifetime adversity. *Zero to Three, 37,* 4–13.

Narayan, A. J., Rivera, L. M., Bernstein, R. E., Harris, W. W., & Lieberman, A. F. (2018). Positive childhood experiences predict less psychopathology and stress in pregnant women with childhood adversity: A pilot study of the Benevolent Childhood Experiences (BCEs) scale. *Child Abuse and Neglect, 78,* 19–30.

Natalucci, G., Bucher, H. U., Von Rhein, M., Tolsa, C. B., Latal, B., & Adams, M. (2017). Population based report on health related quality of life in adolescents born very preterm. *Early Human Development, 104,* 7–12.

Nemeth, J. M., Mengo, C., Kulow, E., Brown, A., & Ramirez, R. (2019). Provider perceptions and domestic violence (DV) survivor experiences of traumatic and anoxic–hypoxic brain injury: Implications for DV advocacy service provision. *Journal of Aggression, Maltreatment and Trauma, 28*(6), 744–763.

Nugent, J. K., Keefer, C. H., Minear, S., Johnson, L. C, & Blanchard, Y. (2007). *Understanding newborn behaviour and early relationships: The Newborn Behavioral Observations (NBO) system handbook.* London: Brookes.

Office of the Surgeon General. (2005, March 30–31). *Implementing innovations of a public health approach.* Publication from the Surgeon General's Workshop on Making Prevention of Child Maltreatment a National Priority, National Institutes of Health, Bethesda, MD. Retrieved from *www.ncbi.nlm.nih.gov/books/NBK47486.*

Ogden, T. H. (1982). *Projective identification and psychotherapeutic technique.* New York: Jason Aronson.

Oh, D. L., Jerman, P., Silvério Marques, S., Koita, K., Purewal Boparai, S. K., Burke Harris, N., & Bucci, M. (2018). Systematic review of pediatric health outcomes associated with childhood adversity. *BMC Pediatrics, 18*(1), 83.

Olds, D. L., Kitzman, H., Hanks, C., Cole, R., Anson, E., Sidora-Arcoleo, K., . . . Bondy, J. (2007). Effects of nurse home visiting on maternal and child functioning: Age-9 follow-up of a randomized trial. *Pediatrics, 120*(4), e832–e845.

Olff, M., Langeland, W., & Gersons, B. P. (2005). The psychobiology of PTSD: Coping with trauma. *Psychoneuroendocrinology, 30*(10), 974–982.

Onozawa, K., Glover, V., Adams, D., Modi, N., & Kumar, R. C. (2001). Infant massage improves mother–infant interaction for mothers with postnatal depression. *Journal of Affective Disorders, 63*(1–3), 201–207.

Ordway, M. R., Sadler, L. S., Holland, M. L., Slade, A., Close, N., & Mayes, L. C. (2018). A home visiting parenting program and child obesity: A randomized trial. *Pediatrics, 141*(2). Retrieved from *https://pediatrics.aap-publications.org/content/pediatrics/141/2/e20171076.full.pdf.*

Ostler, T. (2009). Mental illness in the peripartum period. *Zero to Three, 29*(5), 4–9.

Pallitto, C. C., Campbell, J. C., & O'Campo, P. (2005). Is intimate partner violence associated with unintended pregnancy?: A review of the literature. *Trauma, Violence, and Abuse, 6*(3), 217–235.

Pally, R. (2001). A primary role for nonverbal communication in psychoanalysis. *Psychoanalytic Inquiry, 21*(1), 71–93.

Patrick, S. W., Schumacher, R. E., Benneyworth, B. D., Krans, E. E., McAllister, J. M., & Davis, M. M. (2012). Neonatal abstinence syndrome and associated health care expenditures: United States, 2000–2009. *JAMA, 307*(18), 1934–1940.

Petersen, E. E., Davis, N. L., Goodman, D., Cox, S., Mayes, N., Johnston, E., . . . Barfield, W. (2019). Vital signs: Pregnancy-related deaths, United States, 2011–2015, and strategies for prevention, 13 States, 2013–2017. *Morbidity and Mortality Weekly Report, 68,* 423–429.

Pollack, W. S. (1995). A delicate balance: Fatherhood and psychological transformation—A psychoanalytic perspective. In J. L. Shapiro, M. J. Diamond, & M. Greenberg (Eds.), *Becoming a father: Contemporary social, developmental, and clinical perspectives* (pp. 316–331). New York: Springer.

Powell, J. A., & Menendian, S. (2016). The problem of othering: Towards inclusiveness and belonging. *Othering and Belonging: Expanding the Circle of Human Concern, 1,* 14–39. Retrieved from *www.otheringandbelonging.org/the-problem-of-othering.*

Pruett, K. D. (2000). *Fatherneed: Why father care is as essential as mother care for your child.* New York: Free Press.

Pruett, K., & Pruett, M. P. (2009). *Partnership parenting: How men and women parent differently—Why it helps your kids and can strengthen your marriage.* Cambridge, MA: Da Capo Press.

Pynoos, R. S., Steinberg, A. M., & Piacentini, J. C. (1999). A developmental psychopathology model of childhood traumatic stress and intersection with anxiety disorders. *Biological Psychiatry, 46*(11), 1542–1554.

Review to Action. (2018). Building U.S. capacity to review and prevent maternal deaths: Report from nine maternal mortality review committees. Retrieved from *http://reviewtoaction.org/Report_from_Nine_MMRCs*.

Rosenblum, K. L., Muzik, M., Morelen, D. M., Alfafara, E. A., Miller, N. M., Waddell, R. M., . . . Ribaudo, J. (2017). A community-based randomized controlled trial of Mom Power parenting intervention for mothers with interpersonal trauma histories and their young children. *Archives of Women's Mental Health, 20*(5), 673–686.

Rutter, M. J. (1972). *Maternal deprivation reassessed.* Hammondsworth, UK: Penguin Books.

Sadler, L. S., Slade, A., Close, N., Webb, D. L., Simpson, T., Fennie, K., & Mayes, L. C. (2013). Minding the baby: Enhancing reflectiveness to improve early health and relationship outcomes in an interdisciplinary home visiting program. *Infant Mental Health Journal, 34*(5), 391–405.

Saleem, H. T., & Surkan, P. J. (2014). Parental pregnancy wantedness and child social–emotional development. *Maternal and Child Health Journal, 18*(4), 930–938.

Salisbury, A., Law, K., LaGasse, L., & Lester, B. (2003). Maternal–fetal attachment. *JAMA, 289*(13), 1701.

Saltzman, W., & Ziegler, T. E. (2014). Functional significance of hormonal changes in mammalian fathers. *Journal of Neuroendocrinology, 26*(10), 685–696.

Sanchez, S. E., Pineda, O., Chaves, D. Z., Zhong, Q., Gelaye, B., Simon, G. E., . . . Williams, M. A. (2017). Childhood physical and sexual abuse experiences associated with post-traumatic stress disorder among pregnant women. *Annals of Epidemiology, 27,* 716–723.

Saxbe, D., Corner, G. W., Khaled, M., Horton, K., Wu, B., & Khoddam, H. L. (2018). The weight of fatherhood: Identifying mechanisms to explain paternal perinatal weight gain. *Health Psychology Review, 12*(3), 294–311.

Scacciati, L. C. (2015). Ultrasound scan and internal process. In G. F. Mori (Ed.), *From pregnancy to motherhood: Psychoanalytic aspects of the beginning of the mother–child relationship* (pp. 65–81). New York: Routledge.

Schechter, D. S., & Willheim, E. (2009). Disturbances of attachment and parental psychopathology in early childhood. *Child and Adolescent Psychiatric Clinics of North America, 18*(3), 665–686.

Schechter, D. S., Willheim, E., Suardi, F., & Serpa, S. R. (2019). The effects of violent experiences on infants and young children. In C. H. Zeanah, Jr. (Ed.), *Handbook of infant mental health* (4th ed., pp. 219–238). New York: Guilford Press.

Schwerdtfeger, K. L., & Goff, B. S. (2007), Intergenerational transmission of trauma: Exploring mother–infant prenatal attachment. *Journal of Traumatic Stress, 20*(1), 39–51.

Scorza, P., Duarte, C. S., Hipwell, A. E., Posner, J., Ortin, A., Canino, G., & Monk, C. (2018). Research review: Intergenerational transmission of disadvantage: Epigenetics and parents' childhoods as the first exposure. *The Journal of Child Psychology and Psychiatry, 60*(2), 119–132.

Seligman, S. (1999). Integrating Kleinian theory and intersubjective infant research observing projective identification. *Psychoanalytic Dialogues, 9*(2), 129–159.

Seng, J. S., Low, L. K., Sperlich, M., Ronis, D. L., & Liberzon, I. (2009). Prevalence, trauma history, and risk for posttraumatic stress disorder among nulliparous women in maternity care. *Obstetrics and Gynecology, 114*(4), 839–847.

Shah, P. E., Browne, J., & Poehlmann-Tynan, J. (2019). Prematurity: Identifying risks and promoting resilience. In C. H. Zeanah, Jr. (Ed.), *Handbook of infant mental health* (4th ed., pp. 203–218). New York: Guilford Press.

Shapiro, J. L. (1987). *When men are pregnant: Needs and concerns of expectant fathers.* San Luis Obispo, CA: Impact.

Sharfstein, S. (2006). New task force will address early childhood violence. *Psychiatric News, 41*(3), 3.

Sharpless, B. A., & Barber, J. P. (2009). A conceptual and empirical review of the meaning, measurement, development, and teaching of intervention competence in clinical psychology. *Clinical Psychology Review, 29*(1), 47–56.

Sharps, P. W., Laughon, K., & Giangrande, S. K. (2007). Intimate partner violence and the childbearing year: Maternal and infant health consequences. *Trauma, Violence, and Abuse, 8*(2), 105–116.

Sheinberg, M., & Fraenkel, P. (2001). *The relational trauma of incest: A family-based approach to treatment.* New York: Guilford Press.

Silverman, J. G., Decker, M. R., Reed, E., & Raj, A. (2006). Intimate partner violence victimization prior to and during pregnancy among women residing in 26 U.S. states: Associations with maternal and neonatal health. *American Journal of Obstetrics and Gynecology, 195*(1), 140–148.

Silverman, R. C., & Lieberman, A. F. (1999). Negative maternal attribution, projective identification, and the intergenerational transmission of violent relational patterns. *Psychoanalytic Dialogues, 9*, 161–186.

Simmons, L. E., Rubens, C. E., Darmstadt, G. L., & Gravett, M. G. (2010). Preventing preterm birth and neonatal mortality: Exploring the epidemiology, causes, and interventions. *Seminars in Perinatology, 34*(6), 408–415.

Slade, A., & Cohen, L. J. (1996). Processes of parenting and the remembrance of things past. *Infant Mental Health Journal, 17*(3), 217–238.

Slade, A., Holland, M. L., Ordway, M. R., Carlson, E. A., Jeon, S., Close, N., . . . Sadler, L. S. (2019). Minding the Baby®: Enhancing parental reflective functioning and infant attachment in an attachment-based, interdisciplinary home visiting program. *Development and Psychopathology, 14*, 1–15.

Slade, A., & Sadler, L. S. (2019). Pregnancy and infant mental health. In C. H. Zeanah, Jr. (Ed.), *Handbook of infant mental health* (4th ed., pp. 25–40). New York: Guilford Press.

Slade, A., Simpson, T. E., Webb, D., Albertson, J. G., Close, N., & Sadler, L. S. (2018). Minding the baby: Complex trauma and attachment-based home intervention. In H. Steele & M. Steele (Eds.), *Handbook of attachment-based interventions* (pp. 151–173). New York: Guilford Press.

Smyke, A. T., & Breidenstine, A. S. (2019). Foster care in early childhood. In C. H. Zeanah, Jr. (Ed.), *Handbook of infant mental health* (4th ed., pp. 553–566). New York: Guilford Press.

Spielman, E., Herriott, A., Paris, R., & Sommer, A. R. (2015). Building a model program for substance-exposed newborns and their families: From needs assessment to intervention, evaluation, and consultation. *Zero to Three, 36*(1), 47–55.

Sroufe, L. A., Egeland, B., Carlson, E. A., & Collins, W. A. (2005). *The development of the person: The Minnesota Study of Risk and Adaptation from Birth to Adulthood.* New York: Guilford Press.

St-Pierre, J., Laurent, L., King, S., & Vaillancourt, C. (2016). Effects of prenatal maternal stress on serotonin and fetal development. *Placenta, 48*(1), S66–S71.

Steen, M., Downe, S., Bamfort N., & Edozien, L. (2012). Not-patient and not-visitor: A metasynthesis fathers' encounters with pregnancy, birth and maternity care. *Midwifery, 28*(4), 422–431.

Stern, D. N. (1985). *The interpersonal world of the infant: A view from psychoanalysis and developmental psychology.* London: Karnac Books.

Stern, D. N. (1995). *The motherhood constellation: A unified view of parent–infant psychotherapy.* New York: Basic Books.

Stern, D. N. (2005). The psychic landscape of mothers. In S. F. Brown (Ed.), *What do mothers want?: Developmental perspectives, clinical challenges* (pp. 3–18). New York: Analytic Press.

Stern, D., & Bruschweiler-Stern, N. (1998). *The birth of a mother: How motherhood experience changes you forever.* New York: Basic Books.

Stern, G., & Kruckman, L. (1983). Multi-disciplinary perspective on postpartum depression: An anthropological critique. *Social Science and Medicine, 17*(15), 1027–1041.

Stevens, J., Ammerman, R. T., Putnam, F. G., & Van Ginkel, J. B. (2002). Depression and trauma history in first-time mothers receiving home visitation. *Journal of Community Psychology, 30*(5), 551–564.

Storey, A. E., Walsh, C. J., Quinton, R. L., & Wynne-Edwards, K. E. (2000). Hormonal correlates of paternal responsiveness in new and expectant fathers. *Evolution and Human Behavior, 21*(2), 79–95.

Stover, C. S., & Carlson, M. (2017). Interventions for perpetration of intimate partner violence: Special populations. In P. Sturmay (Ed.), *The Wiley handbook of violence and aggression* (Vol. 2, pp. 1–15). New York: Wiley.

Stroebel, S. S., O'Keefe, S. L., Beard, K. W., Kuo, S. Y., Swindell, S. V., & Kommor, M. J. (2012). Father–daughter incest: Data from an anonymous computerized survey. *Journal of Child Sexual Abuse, 21*(2), 176–199.

Substance Abuse and Mental Health Services Administration. (2014). *Results from the 2013 National Survey on Drug Use and Health: Summary of national findings* (NSDUH Series H-48, HHS Publication No. [SMA] 14-4863). Rockville, MD: Author.

Suchman, N. E., DeCoste, C., Borelli, J. L., & McMahon, T. J. (2018). Does improvement in maternal attachment representations predict greater maternal sensitivity, child attachment security and lower rates of relapse to substance use?: A second test of mothering from the inside out treatment mechanisms. *Journal of Substance Abuse Treatment, 85*, 21–30.

Suchman, N. E., Pajulo, M., & Mayes, L. C. (Eds.). (2013). *Parenting and substance abuse: Developmental approaches to intervention.* London: Oxford University Press.

Taylor, F. M., Ko, R., & Pan, M. (1999). Prenatal and reproductive health care. In E. J. Kramer, S. L. Ivey, & Y. Ying (Eds.), *Immigrant women's health problems and solutions* (pp. 121–135). San Francisco: Jossey-Bass.

Telles, E. (2007). Discrimination against indigenous peoples: The Latin American context. *UN Chronicle, XLIV*(3). Retrieved from *www.un.org/en/chronicle/article/discrimination-against-indigenous-peoples-latin-american-context.*

Tilden, V. P. (1980). A developmental conceptual framework for the maturational crisis of pregnancy. *Western Journal of Nursing Research, 2*(4), 667–678.

Toth, S. L., Michl-Petzing, L. C., Guild, D., & Lieberman, A. F. (2018). Child–parent psychotherapy: Theoretical bases, clinical applications, and empirical support. In H. Steele & M. Steele (Eds.), *Handbook of attachment-based interventions* (pp. 296–317). New York: Guilford Press.

Tronick, E., Thomas, R., & Daltbuit, M. (1994). The manta pouch: A regulatory system for Peruvian infants at high altitude. *Children's Environments, 11*(2), 142–146.

U.S. Advisory Board on Child Abuse and Neglect. (1995). *A nation's shame: Fatal child abuse and neglect in the United States.* Washington, DC: Administration for Children, Youth, and Families (DHHS).

U.S. Department of Health and Human Services, Children's Bureau. (2019). Child maltreatment 2017. Retrieved from *www.acf.hhs.gov/cb/resource/child-maltreatment-2017.*

Valentine, D. P. (1982). The experience of pregnancy: A developmental process. *Family Relations, 31*(2), 243–248.

van der Kolk, B. A. (2014). *The body keeps the score: Brain, mind, and body in the healing of trauma.* New York: Penguin Books.

Whitfield, C. L., Anda, R. F., Dube, S. R., & Felitti, V. J. (2003). Violent childhood experiences and the risk of intimate partner violence in adults: Assessment in a large health maintenance organization. *Journal of Interpersonal Violence, 18*(2), 166–185.

Winnicott, D. W. (1956). Primary maternal preoccupation. In *Collected papers: Through paediatrics to psychoanalysis* (pp. 300–305). New York: Basic Books.

Winnicott, D. W. (1960). The theory of the parent–infant relationship. *International Journal of Psychoanalysis, 41*, 585–595.

Winnicott, D. W. (1965). *The maturational processes and the facilitating environment: Studies in the theory of emotional development.* New York: International Universities Press.

Winnicott, D. W. (1971). *Playing and reality.* Oxford, UK: Penguin.

Woods, S. J. (2005). Intimate partner violence and post-traumatic stress disorder symptoms in women: What we know and need to know. *Journal of Interpersonal Violence, 20*(4), 394–402.

World Bank. (2003). *A World Bank country study: Poverty in Guatemala.* Washington, DC: Author.

Wright, C. L., Dallas, R., Moldenhauer, R., & Carlson, E. A. (2018). Practice and policy considerations for parents with opioid use disorders. *Zero to Three, 38*(5), 10–16.

Yehuda, R., & Ledoux, J. D. (2007). Response variation following trauma: A translational neuroscience approach to understanding PTSD. *Neuron, 56*(1), 19–32.

Yost, N. J., Bloom, S. L., McIntire, D. D., & Leveno, K. J. (2005). A prospective observational study of domestic violence during pregnancy. *Obstetrics and Gynecology, 106*(1), 61–65.

Zero to Three. (2016). *Diagnostic classification of mental health and developmental disorders of infancy and early childhood: Revised edition (DC:0–5).* Washington, DC: Author.

# Index

Note. *f* following a page number indicates a figure.